Neuroimaging Tropical Disease

Guest Editor

RAKESH K. GUPTA, MD

NEUROIMAGING CLINICS OF NORTH AMERICA

www.neuroimaging.theclinics.com

Consulting Editor
SURESH K. MUKHERJI, MD

November 2011 • Volume 21 • Number 4

SAUNDERS an imprint of ELSEVIER, Inc.

W.B. SAUNDERS COMPANY
A Division of Elsevier Inc.

1600 John F. Kennedy Boulevard • Suite 1800 • Philadelphia, Pennsylvania 19103-2899

http://www.theclinics.com

NEUROIMAGING CLINICS OF NORTH AMERICA Volume 21, Number 4
November 2011 ISSN 1052-5149, ISBN 13: 978-1-4557-2371-3

Editor: Joanne Husovski
Developmental Editor: Donald Mumford

Neuroimaging Clinics of North America (ISSN 1052-5149) is published quarterly by Elsevier Inc., 360 Park Avenue South, New York, NY 10010-1710. Months of issue are February, May, August, and November. Business and editorial offices: 1600 John F. Kennedy Blvd., Suite 1800, Philadelphia, PA 19103-2899. Business and editorial offices: 6277 Sea Harbor Drive, Orlando, FL 32887-4800. Periodicals postage paid at New York, NY, and additional mailing offices. Subscription prices are USD 314 per year for US individuals, USD 436 per year for US institutions, USD 158 per year for US students and residents, USD 363 per year for Canadian individuals, USD 546 per year for Canadian institutions, USD 461 per year for international individuals, USD 546 per year for international institutions and USD 226 per year for Canadian and foreign students and residents. To receive student/resident rate, orders must be accompanied by name of affiliated institution, date of term, and the *signature* of program/residency coordinator on institution letterhead. Orders will be billed at individual rate until proof of status is received. Foreign air speed delivery is included in all *Clinics* subscription prices. All prices are subject to change without notice. POSTMASTER: Send address changes to *Neuroimaging Clinics of North America*, Elsevier Health Sciences Division, Subscription Customer Service, 3251 Riverport Lane, Maryland Heights, MO 63043. Telephone: 1-800-654-2452 (U.S. and Canada); 314-447-8871 (outside U.S. and Canada). Fax: 314-447-8029. E-mail: journalscustomerservice-usa@elsevier.com (for print support); journalsonlinesupport-usa@elsevier.com (for online support).

Reprints. For copies of 100 or more of articles in this publication, please contact the Commercial Reprints Department, Elsevier Inc., 360 Park Avenue South, New York, NY 10010-1710. Tel.: 212-633-3812; Fax: 212-462-1935; E-mail: reprints@elsevier.com.

Neuroimaging Clinics of North America is covered by *Excerpta Medical/EMBASE*, the RSNA Index of Imaging Literature, *MEDLINE/PubMed (Index Medicus)*, MEDLINE/MEDLARS, SciSearch, Research Alert, and Neuroscience Citation Index.

Printed and bound by CPI Group (UK) Ltd, Croydon, CR0 4YY

Transferred to Digital Print 2011

GOAL STATEMENT

The goal of *Neuroimaging Clinics of North America* is to keep practicing radiologists and radiology residents up to date with current clinical practice in radiology by providing timely articles reviewing the state of the art in patient care.

ACCREDITATION

The *Neuroimaging Clinics of North America* is planned and implemented in accordance with the Essential Areas and Policies of the Accreditation Council for Continuing Medical Education (ACCME) through the joint sponsorship of the University of Virginia School of Medicine and Elsevier. The University of Virginia School of Medicine is accredited by the ACCME to provide continuing medical education for physicians.

The University of Virginia School of Medicine designates this enduring material activity for a maximum of 15 *AMA PRA Category 1 Credit*(s)™ for each issue, 60 credits per year. Physicians should claim only the credit commensurate with the extent of their participation in the activity.

The American Medical Association has determined that physicians not licensed in the US who participate in this CME enduring material activity are eligible for a maximum of 15 *AMA PRA Category 1 Credit*(s)™ for each issue, 60 credits per year.

Credit can be earned by reading the text material, taking the CME examination online at http://www.theclinics.com/home/cme, and completing the evaluation. After taking the test, you will be required to review any and all incorrect answers. Following completion of the test and evaluation, your credit will be awarded and you may print your certificate.

FACULTY DISCLOSURE/CONFLICT OF INTEREST

The University of Virginia School of Medicine, as an ACCME accredited provider, endorses and strives to comply with the Accreditation Council for Continuing Medical Education (ACCME) Standards of Commercial Support, Commonwealth of Virginia statutes, University of Virginia policies and procedures, and associated federal and private regulations and guidelines on the need for disclosure and monitoring of proprietary and financial interests that may affect the scientific integrity and balance of content delivered in continuing medical education activities under our auspices.

The University of Virginia School of Medicine requires that all CME activities accredited through this institution be developed independently and be scientifically rigorous, balanced and objective in the presentation/discussion of its content, theories and practices.

All authors/editors participating in an accredited CME activity are expected to disclose to the readers relevant financial relationships with commercial entities occurring within the past 12 months (such as grants or research support, employee, consultant, stock holder, member of speakers bureau, etc.). The University of Virginia School of Medicine will employ appropriate mechanisms to resolve potential conflicts of interest to maintain the standards of fair and balanced education to the reader. Questions about specific strategies can be directed to the Office of Continuing Medical Education, University of Virginia School of Medicine, Charlottesville, Virginia.

The faculty and staff of the University of Virginia Office of Continuing Medical Education have no financial affiliations to disclose.

The authors/editors listed below have identified no professional/financial affiliations for themselves or their spouse/partner:
Ahmed Abdel Khalek Abdel Razek, MD; Vikas Agarwal, MD, DM; Cem Calli, MD; Mauricio Castillo, MD; Sandeep Chauhan, MD, FICP; Chi-Jen Chen, MD; Swati Chinchure, MD; Patricia M. Desmond, MSc, MD, FRANZCR; Ajay Garg, MD; Christine Goh, MBBS, FRANZCR; Rakesh K. Gupta, MD (Guest Editor); Vivek Gupta, MD; Sanjeev Kumar Handique, MD; Yen-Lin Huang, MD; Nuzhat Husain, MD; Joanne Husovski, (Acquisitions Editor); Chandrasekharan Kesavadas, MD; N. Khandelwal, MD, Dip NBE, FICR; Osman Kızılkılıc, MD; Praveen Kumar, MSc; Sunil Kumar, MD; S.K. Susheel Kumar, MD; Pramit M. Phal, MBBS, FRANZCR; Shilpa S. Sankhe, MD; P. Satishchandra, DM (Neuro), FAMS, FIAN; Lubdha M. Shah, MD (Test Author); Paramjeet Singh, MD; Sanjib Sinha, MD, DM; and Arvemas Watcharakorn, MD.

The authors listed below have identified the following professional/financial affiliations for themselves or their spouse/partner:
Suresh K. Mukherji, MD (Consulting Editor) is a consultant for Philips.
C.C. Tchoyoson Lim, MBBS, FRCR, MMed (DiagRadiol) is a patent holder for A*Star, is an Editorial Board Member and Reviewer for Singapore Medical Journal, is a reviewer for Biomed Central, Neuroradiology, Cerebrovascular Diseases, Parkinsonism and Related Disorders, Yonsei Medical Journal, Neurology India, Acta Paediatrica, Journal of Pharmaceutical and Biomedical Analysis, Journal of Neuroimaging, Parasite Immunology, Journal of Signal Processing Systems, Magnetic Resonance Imaging, European Journal of Neurology, Journal of Neurology, Neurosurgery, and Psychiatry, Annals, Academy of Medicine, Singapore Medical Journal, Singapore General Hospital Proceedings, Neurological Journal of South East Asia, and is a grant reviewer for SingHealth Research Grants, Biomedical Research Council, National Health Group, and National Medical Research Council.

Disclosure of Discussion of Non-FDA Approved Uses for Pharmaceutical Products and/or Medical Devices
The University of Virginia School of Medicine, as an ACCME provider, requires that all faculty presenters identify and disclose any off-label uses for pharmaceutical and medical device products. The University of Virginia School of Medicine recommends that each physician fully review all the available data on new products or procedures prior to clinical use.

TO ENROLL

To enroll in the Neuroimaging Clinics of North America Continuing Medical Education program, call customer service at 1-800-654-2452 or sign up online at http://www.theclinics.com/home/cme. The CME program is available to subscribers for an additional annual fee of USD 196.

Neuroimaging Clinics of North America

THE CLINICS ARE NOW AVAILABLE ONLINE!

Access your subscription at:
www.theclinics.com

Contributors

CONSULTING EDITOR

SURESH K. MUKHERJI, MD, FACR
Professor and Chief of Neuroradiology, and
Head and Neck Radiology; Professor of
Radiology, Otolaryngology Head and Neck
Surgery, Radiation Oncology, Periodontics and
Oral Medicine, University of Michigan Health
System, Ann Arbor, Michigan

GUEST EDITOR

RAKESH K. GUPTA, MD
Professor, MR Section, Department of
Radiodiagnosis, Sanjay Gandhi Postgraduate
Institute of Medical Sciences, Lucknow,
Uttar Pradesh, India

AUTHORS

AHMED ABDEL KHALEK ABDEL RAZEK, MD
Diagnostic Radiology Department, Mansoura
Faculty of Medicine, Mansoura, Egypt

VIKAS AGARWAL, MD, DM
Associate Professor, Department of Clinical
Immunology, Sanjay Gandhi Postgraduate
Institute of Medical Sciences, Lucknow,
Uttar Pradesh, India

CEM CALLI, MD
Professor of Radiology; and Chief of
Neuroradiology Section, Department of
Radiology, Medical Faculty, Ege University,
Bornova, Izmir, Turkey

MAURICIO CASTILLO, MD, FACR
Division of Neuroradiology, Department of
Radiology, University of North Carolina at
Chapel Hill, Chapel Hill, North Carolina

SANDEEP CHAUHAN, MD, FICP
Specialty Doctor, Department of
Rheumatology, Nobles Hospital, Isle of Man,
United Kingdom

CHI-JEN CHEN, MD
Department of Diagnostic Radiology,
Shuang-Ho Hospital, Taipei Medical
University, New Taipei City, Taiwan,
Republic of China

SWATI CHINCHURE, MD
Department of Imaging Sciences and
Interventional Radiology, Sree Chitra Tirunal
Institute for Medical Sciences and Technology,
Trivandrum, Kerala, India

**PATRICIA M. DESMOND, MSc, MD,
FRANZCR**
Director of Imaging, Department of Radiology;
Edgar Rouse Professor of Radiology,
University of Melbourne, Royal Melbourne
Hospital, Parkville, Victoria, Australia

AJAY GARG, MD
Additional Professor of Neuroradiology,
Department of Neuroradiology, Neurosciences
Centre, All India Institute of Medical Sciences,
Ansari Nagar, New Delhi, India

CHRISTINE GOH, MBBS, FRANZCR
Department of Radiology, Royal Melbourne
Hospital, Parkville, Victoria, Australia

RAKESH K. GUPTA, MD
Professor, MR Section, Department of
Radiodiagnosis, Sanjay Gandhi Postgraduate
Institute of Medical Sciences, Lucknow,
Uttar Pradesh, India

VIVEK GUPTA, MD
Associate Professor, Department of
Radiodiagnosis, Post Graduate Institute of
Medical Education and Research, Chandigarh,
India

SANJEEV KUMAR HANDIQUE, MD
Chief Consultant Radiologist, Department of
Radiology and Imaging, Institute of
Neurological Sciences, Dispur, Assam, India

YEN-LIN HUANG, MD
Department of Diagnostic Radiology,
Shuang-Ho Hospital, Taipei Medical
University, New Taipei City, Taiwan,
Republic of China

NUZHAT HUSAIN, MD
Dean RMLIMS and Head, Department of
Pathology, Dr Ram Manohar Lohia Institute of
Medical Sciences, Lucknow, Uttar Pradesh,
India

CHANDRASEKHARAN KESAVADAS, MD
Additional Professor, Department of Imaging
Sciences and Interventional Radiology, Sree
Chitra Tirunal Institute for Medical Sciences
and Technology, Trivandrum, Kerala, India

N. KHANDELWAL, MD, Dip NBE, FICR
Professor and Head, Department of
Radiodiagnosis, Post Graduate Institute of
Medical Education and Research, Chandigarh,
India

OSMAN KIZILKILIC, MD
Associate Professor of Radiology and
Neuroradiology, Department of Radiology,
Cerrahpasa Medical Faculty, University of
Istanbul, Kocamustafapasa, Istanbul, Turkey

PRAVEEN KUMAR, MSc
Department of Pathology, Dr Ram Manohar
Lohia Institute of Medical Sciences, Lucknow,
Uttar Pradesh, India

SUNIL KUMAR, MD
Professor, Department of Radiodiagnosis,
Sanjay Gandhi Postgraduate Institute of
Medical Sciences, Lucknow, Uttar Pradesh,
India

S.K. SUSHEEL KUMAR, MD
Consultant, Department of Radiology, Priyam
Zhaveri PET–CT Centre, Dr Balabhai Nanavati
Hospital, Mumbai, Maharashtra, India

PRAMIT M. PHAL, MBBS, FRANZCR
Director of MRI, Department of Radiology,
Royal Melbourne Hospital, Parkville,
Victoria, Australia

SHILPA S. SANKHE, MD
Assistant Professor, Chief of MRI Division,
Department of Radiology, King Edward
Memorial Hospital, Parel, Mumbai,
Maharashtra, India

**P. SATISHCHANDRA, DM (Neuro),
FAMS, FIAN**
Director/Vice Chancellor, Department of
Neurology, NIMHANS, Bangalore, Karnataka,
India

PARAMJEET SINGH, MD
Professor, Department of Radiodiagnosis,
Post Graduate Institute of Medical Education
and Research, Chandigarh, India

SANJIB SINHA, MD, DM
Additional Professor of Neurology, Department
of Neurology, NIMHANS, Bangalore,
Karnataka, India

**C.C. TCHOYOSON LIM, MBBS, FRCR,
MMed (DiagRadiol)**
Senior Consultant, Department of
Neuroradiology, National Neuroscience
Institute; and Adjunct Associate Professor,
Department of Neurology, Duke NUS Graduate
Medical School, Singapore

ARVEMAS WATCHARAKORN, MD
Division of Neuroradiology, Department of
Radiology, University of North Carolina at
Chapel Hill, Chapel Hill, North Carolina;
Department of Radiology, Faculty of Medicine,
Thammasat University, Pathumthani,
Thailand

Contents

> The development in neuroimaging techniques has revolutionized the way neurology
> is practiced, including neurologic disorders in tropics. Some diseases occur exclu-
> sively, whereas some are more common in tropical regions. However, some are be-
> coming increasingly prevalent in the developed world too, as a result of patterns of
> human migration and globalization. It is imperative to learn about the role of imaging
> in tropical neurology, which might assist early diagnosis and treatment and also add
> to the existing knowledge. Infections are more common in the tropics and require
> special attention in view of their potential treatability.

> Tropical diseases affecting the central nervous system include infections, infesta-
> tions, and nutritional deficiency disorders. This article discusses the commonly
> encountered diseases. The infections include bacterial, mycobacterial, fungal, par-
> asitic, and viral infections with varied clinical manifestations. Imaging sensitivity and
> specificity for the prediction of the cause of infections has improved with application
> of advanced techniques. Microbial demonstration and histology remain the gold
> standard for diagnosis. Understanding the basis of imaging changes is mandatory
> for better evaluation of images. Nutritional disorders present with generalized and
> nonspecific imaging manifestations. The pathology of commonly encountered vita-
> min deficiencies is also discussed.

> Viral infections of the central nervous system in the tropical countries of Asia and the
> Indian subcontinent are different from those of the Western and developed world.
> Many of the endemic and epidemic encephalitides that are prevalent in these
> regions, such as Japanese encephalitis, have characteristic findings on imaging,
> especially on magnetic resonance imaging, allowing a rapid diagnosis and differen-
> tiation from clinically similar syndromes. Other emerging viral infections in the region
> in recent years have posed new challenges. The contribution of neuroimaging to the
> management of these emerging infections is also discussed.

> Central nervous system (CNS) tuberculosis is frequently encountered in tropical
> countries. Imaging plays an important role in its recognition and in its differentiation

from other similar conditions. Specific magnetic resonance techniques, such as magnetization transfer imaging, proton magnetic resonance spectroscopy, diffusion, and perfusion imaging are useful in its characterization and management. This article reviews the various forms of CNS tuberculosis, including its complications and imaging features.

This article reviews the characteristic imaging appearances of parasitic diseases of the central nervous system, including cysticercosis, toxoplasmosis, cystic echinococcosis, schistosomiasis, amebiasis, malariasis, sparganosis, paragonimiasis, and American and African trypanosomiases. Routine precontrast and postcontrast MR imaging helps in localization, characterization, delineation of extension, and follow-up of the parasitic lesions. Moreover, recently developed tools, such as diffusion, perfusion, and MR spectroscopy, help to differentiate parasitic diseases of the central nervous system from simulating lesions. Combining imaging findings with geographic prevalence, clinical history, and serologic tests is required for diagnosis of parasitic diseases of the central nervous system.

The myelin sheath and oligodendrocytes in the brain may be damaged by autoimmune-mediated inflammatory processes secondary to postinfectious demyelination or nutritional and vitamin deficiency. This article describes acute disseminated encephalomyelitis, acute hemorrhagic leukoencephalitis, acute necrotizing encephalopathy, and tumefactive demyelination as well as osmotic demyelination, Wernicke encephalopathy, Marchiafava–Bignami disease, and subacute combined degeneration of the spinal cord. Although some characteristic MR imaging features allow radiologists to suggest a diagnosis, these may overlap, and images should be interpreted in light of clinical symptoms and laboratory investigations.

Fungal infections of the central nervous system range from chronic indolent forms to acute fulminant forms causing significant morbidity and mortality. They often show atypical and variable neuroradiologic findings because of the absence of typical inflammatory response. The neuroradiologist must have high degree of suspicion in immunocompromised patients regarding the possibility of central nervous system fungal infections and keep in mind the appearances of various fungi even when immune response is intact. Next is to identify the pattern of involvement whether hematogenous or direct sinonasal and then make a well-informed speculation regarding the type of the pathogen based on the clinical features and imaging appearance.

Epilepsy is a major public health problem in many tropical countries. Also, some of the tropical diseases are major contributors to the higher prevalence of epilepsy in these countries. The etiologic factors responsible for epilepsy in these countries are quite different from those in the developed world. This article discusses the etiologic factors and neuroimaging of epilepsy in light of the conditions in these tropical countries.

Craniovertebral junction (CVJ) disorders in the Occident are usually associated with systemic disorders. In contrast, in the Orient, a greater incidence of isolated CVJ anomalies is seen. Although these are developmental anomalies, they manifest late in life, with trauma and/or infection playing a promotive role. The most significant and common of these anomalies are basilar invagination and atlantodental disloca- tion, which also occur together. Accurate diagnosis of these anomalies is feasible using computed tomography and magnetic resonance imaging. Greater awareness of this subset of patients is essential for greater understanding and effective man- agement of these ailments.

Vascular pathologies of brain comprise a heterogeneous group of abnormalities such as vasculitis, dural arteriovenous malformations, carotid-cavernous fistulas, cerebral venous thrombosis, and intracerebral hemorrhage. Modern imaging tech- niques are increasingly unraveling these vascular lesions of the brain at a stage when many of them are still asymptomatic. This article focuses on acquired vascular pathologies of brain prevalent in tropical countries that are encountered in clinical practice.

Brucellosis is a multisystem infection with a broad spectrum of clinical presenta- tions. Its nervous system involvement is known as neurobrucellosis. Neurobrucello- sis (NB) has neither a typical clinical picture nor specific cerebrospinal fluid (CSF) findings. Its diagnosis is based on the existence of a neurologic picture not explained by any other neurologic disease, evidenced by systemic brucellar infection and the presence of inflammatory alteration in CSF. Imaging findings of NB is divided into four categories: (1) normal, (2) inflammation (recognized by granulomas, abnormal enhancement of the meninges, perivascular space, or lumbar nerve roots), (3) white matter changes, and (4) vascular changes.

Hirayama disease (juvenile muscular atrophy of distal upper extremity) is a cervical myelopathy. Predominantly affecting male adolescents, it is characterized by pro- gressive muscular weakness and atrophy of distal upper limbs, followed by sponta- neous arrest within several years. Although the cause of cervical myelopathy remains unclear, neuropathologic and neuroradiologic findings suggest a forward displacement of the posterior cervical dural sac during neck flexion, causing com- pression of the cervical cord, and results in atrophic and ischemic changes in the

Transverse myelitis is an acute inflammatory condition. A relatively rare condition, the diversity of causes makes it an important diagnostic challenge. An approach to the classification and work-up standardizes diagnostic criteria and terminology to facilitate clinical research, and forms a useful tool in the clinical work-up for patients at presentation. Its pathogenesis can be grouped into four categories. Imaging appearances can be nonspecific; however, the morphology of cord involvement, enhancement pattern, and presence of coexistent abnormalities on MR imaging can provide clues as to the causes. Neuroimaging is important in identifying subgroups that may benefit from specific treatment.

Pyomyositis is the primary infection of the skeletal muscle. It is common in the tropics, but is increasingly being reported worldwide. It can affect immunocompromised and immunocompetent individuals. *Staphylococcus aureus* is the most common causative organism. Muscle histology and its culture remain the gold standard for diagnosis. However, among noninvasive methods, MR imaging is highly sensitive and can image large areas of the body and detect subclinical involvement. Early diagnosis, institution of appropriate antibiotic therapy, and drainage of pus lead to favorable outcome.

Foreword
World is Flat: Globalization of Tropical Disease

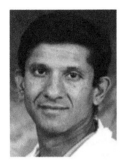

Suresh K. Mukherji, MD
Consulting Editor

I agree with Thomas Friedman that the "The world is flat!!" What were once viewed as exotic diseases isolated to distant parts of the world are now becoming more prevalent in the Western world in this era of globalization. Unfortunately, I have actually had direct experience with this phenomenon. I spent a portion of my fourth year medical school electives studying tropical diseases at the School of Tropical Medicine in Calcutta, India. Two weeks after returning to Washington, DC, I had migratory nighttime fevers associated with severe headaches. I was eventually admitted to the hospital and the differential diagnosis was Leishmaniasis, Dengue fever, or typhoid fever. Well, it turns out that I had *Salmonella parathyphic*, which I caught from eating contaminated ice cream at a cricket match and not from any exposure during my clerkship. It was also the first time this disease had been diagnosed at Fairfax Hospital. Isn't it great to be the first at something?!!

We have made a concerted effort to "globalize" *Neuroimaging Clinics* and have formally changed the name from *Neuroimaging Clinics of North America* to *Neuroimaging Clinics*. This reflects the "flattening" of our scientific community and recognizing talented individuals who have made extraordinary scientific contributions that may not have received appropriate recognition. An excellent example of this is the editor of this issue, Rakesh Gupta, MD. I have known of Dr Gupta's work for over 20 years. He has made extraordinary contributions in the imaging of tropical disorders by developing and applying advanced imaging techniques in diseases such as tuberculosis and cysticercosis that are prevalent in Southeast Asia and developing countries. He has tremendous experience and the quality of his scientific work is superb.

Dr Gupta has assembled an excellent group of collaborators who are very experienced in their selected areas. I am sure you will find this collection of these unique articles very informative. When I was a resident, one of my attending physicians (Harry Mellins, MD) would always say "You only see what you look for and you only diagnose what you know!" The information contained in this edition of *Neuroimaging Clinics* will both improve our "vision" and broaden our knowledge.

Suresh K. Mukherji, MD
Department of Radiology
University of Michigan Health System
1500 East Medical Center
Ann Arbor, MI 48109-0030, USA

E-mail address:
mukherji@med.umich.edu

Neuroimag Clin N Am 21 (2011) xi
doi:10.1016/j.nic.2011.07.016
1052-5149/11/$ – see front matter © 2011 Elsevier Inc. All rights reserved.

Preface

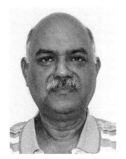

Rakesh K. Gupta, MD
Guest Editor

In this era of increased global travel and migration of people from the developing world to the developed world and vice versa, there is a need to understand diseases that were believed to be confined to the tropics. On one hand the Western world is fighting the threat of prion infections, immune inflammatory disorders, and cancer, whereas tropics are still battling hard-to-contain parasitic, mycobacterial, fungal, bacterial, and viral infections. Most of these diseases are still a major cause of morbidity and mortality in tropics.

Most of these infections result from poverty, undernutrition, overcrowded living conditions, poor hygiene, and poor accessibility to medical care. Moreover, overlapping clinical features and lack of diagnostic laboratory facilities add to the problems. Despite recent advances in science and the expanding health care system, the burden of some of these diseases is so enormous that a sea of change in the health care infrastructure is required to tackle them.

Neuroimaging techniques have undergone a major change in last two decades and have helped clinicians in better understanding and diagnosis of these conditions. In this issue of *Neuroimaging Clinics of North America*, experts from the tropical countries have shared their experiences regarding various tropical disorders. Some of these diseases are uncommon in the Western world. The pathology,

pathogenesis, and role of newer imaging tools for the diagnosis have been discussed to provide comprehensive information about these diseases.

The educational process depends upon individuals who are willing to spend their time generously to share their expertise with clinicians around the world. I express my sincere gratitude toward all the authors who have spent their time and energy in preparing their articles. The success of this issue will largely be due to the immense efforts put forth by the contributors. I would like to extend my sincere thanks to Dr Suresh Mukherji for the invitation to be the guest editor for this issue. I would also like to thank Ms Joanne Husovski, Ms Eva Kulig, and others at Elsevier for their assistance and support.

We all are hopeful that this issue will be informative and educational and will help clinicians across the globe in an improved understanding of tropical diseases of the central nervous system.

Rakesh K. Gupta, MD
Department of Radiodiagnosis
Sanjay Gandhi Postgraduate Institute of
Medical Sciences
Rae Bareli Road, Lucknow 226014
Uttar Pradesh, India

E-mail address:
rakeshree1@gmail.com

doi:10.1016/j.nic.2011.07.015
1052-5149/11/$ – see front matter

Relevance of Neuroimaging in the Diagnosis and Management of Tropical Neurologic Disorders

P. Satishchandra, DM (Neuro), FAMS, FIAN*,
Sanjib Sinha, MD, DM

KEYWORDS

- Neuroimaging • Tropical neurological disorders
- Diagnosis • Management

COMMON INFECTIONS AFFECTING THE NERVOUS SYSTEM IN THE TROPICS
Cerebral Malaria

Clinical features, natural history, and prognosis
Cerebral malaria occurs as a result of *Plasmodium falciparum* malaria that causes unconsciousness from widespread brain disease affection.[1–3] If left untreated, it is a fatal disease in 25% to 50% of patients within 72 hours. Neurologic sequelae are associated with protracted seizures, prolonged and deep coma, hypoglycemia, and severe anemia. Some of the neurologic deficits like ataxia are transient, whereas others like hemiparesis and cortical blindness may not improve incompletely. There are reports of African children with severe spastic tetraparesis and vegetative states, who usually die within a few months of discharge. Those who survive might have sequelae in the form of persistent neurocognitive defects and language and behavioral problems (especially among survivors in sub-Saharan Africa). The histopathologic signature is sequestration of cerebral capillaries and venules with parasitized red blood cells (RBCs) and nonparasitized RBCs. The specific treatment consists of chemotherapy with quinine or artemisinin (artesunate and artemether) and several adjunctive measures (ie, management of hypoxemia, hypoglycemia, hypovolemia, shock, anemia, metabolic acidosis, seizures, and neuroprotective therapy).[1,2,4]

Role of imaging in cerebral malaria
Imaging has a lesser role to play in the diagnosis and management of cerebral malaria. However, magnetic resonance (MR) imaging studies offer a better understanding of the pathogenesis of cerebral malaria.[5,6] Almost all MR imaging studies to date have involved a single case report or small series of patients. The first MR imaging study of a series of patients with malaria living in an endemic area was performed using a 0.2-T scanner, which showed that cerebral edema is not a consistent feature in living patients with cerebral malaria.[5,6] The other reported MR imaging findings noted are white matter changes and pontine signal alterations.[7] A computed tomography (CT) brain scan has poor sensitivity compared with MR imaging and is reported to reveal diffuse cerebral edema. In a CT pathologic study of 21 patients with cerebral malaria, the scan did

Conflict of Interest: Nil.
Financial disclosures: None.
Department of Neurology, NIMHANS, Hosur Road, Bangalore 560029, Karnataka, India
* Corresponding author.
E-mail address: drpsatishchandra@yahoo.com

Neuroimag Clin N Am 21 (2011) 737–756
doi:10.1016/j.nic.2011.07.002

not show features like petechial hemorrhages in any of the 7 patients on whom an autopsy was performed.[8] Newer MR imaging techniques like susceptibility sequences show diffuse petechial hemorrhages throughout the gray-white matter junction, corpus callosum, and internal capsules.[9] Techniques like diffusion-weighted imaging (DWI) and apparent diffusion coefficient (ADC) mapping might unravel restricted or free diffusion, whereas diffusion tensor imaging analysis might show additional white matter changes in patients with cerebral malaria, which might provide better understanding.[10]

Central Nervous System Amebiasis

Central nervous system (CNS) infections in humans caused by free-living amoebae of the genera Naegleria or Acanthamoeba were first described in 1965 by Fowler and Carter and in 1966 by Butt. Naegleria and Acanthamoeba organisms are responsible for causing primary Acanthamoeba meningitis (PAM) and granulomatous amoebic encephalitis (GAE), respectively, having distinctive epidemiology, pattern of presentation, clinical course, pathology, and imaging findings.[1,2] GAE is a subacute to chronic infection caused by Acanthamoeba and also Leptomyxida organisms. Acanthamoeba species are found in all types of environments. Cases have also been associated with amoebic keratitis from contaminated contact lens solutions or with hematogenous spread from a primary source of infection, either a pulmonary focus or a skin ulcer. GAE is known to occur in patients who are debilitated or immunocompromised by AIDS, chemotherapy, or steroid therapy. The clinical course is characterized by a long duration of focal neurologic symptoms unlike the rapid progression and fulminant course of patients with PAM. GAE is diagnosed by identifying Acanthamoeba trophozoites or cysts in cerebrospinal fluid (CSF)/brain biopsy. Cultures of brain tissues or CSF can also reveal Acanthamoeba organisms. The identification of amoeba requires immunofluorescence, immunohistochemistry, or DNA probes. Direct fluorescent antibody studies confirm the species type. The mainstay of treatment of PAM is amphotericin B, rifampicin, and miconazole.[1,2,11]

Role of imaging in CNS amebiasis
Imaging features of PAM are nonspecific and, to our knowledge, have rarely been described previously. Findings of CT and MR imaging may be normal early in the disease, with evidence of brain edema and basilar meningeal enhancement. Follow-up CT and MR imaging might reveal a pattern of brain edema and hydrocephalus, with rapid progression of the disease. There are reports of obliteration of the cisterns with enhancing basilar exudates. Rarely infarction of the right basal ganglia, possibly because of obliteration of the perforating vessels by the extensive exudates, has been described (**Fig. 1**).[11,12]

Neurocysticercosis

Clinical features, natural history, and prognosis
Neurocysticercosis (NCC) is an important cause of neurologic morbidity in developing countries, and is becoming increasingly prevalent in the developed world too, because of current patterns of human migration. It is the most common parasitic disease affecting the brain. Humans are the definitive host and pigs are the intermediate host for Taenia solium. If humans ingest T solium eggs, they develop cysticercosis. Larvae penetrate the intestinal wall and are carried to many tissues, where cysticerci develop. Neurologic manifestations are most common and include seizures caused by inflammation surrounding cysticerci in the brain, features of increased intracranial pressure (ICP), meningitis, and uncommonly other focal neurologic deficit. Unlike patients from Latin America and Africa, Indian patients with NCC commonly have single or a few intraparenchymal cysts with minimal recurrence of seizures. In tropical countries like India, NCC is one of the commonest causes of acute symptomatic seizures (localization related). The clinical manifestations are caused by deposition of larvae of the parasite T solium in cerebral parenchyma, meninges, spinal cord, muscles, eyes, and skin. Around 60% to 70.8% of NCC in India is in the form of solitary cerebral cysticercal lesion (SCCL). The diagnosis of cerebral NCC can be arrived at by good-quality CT and MR imaging. Serologic tests provide additional support in establishing the diagnosis. Histopathologic examination of lesion may rarely be required to prove the diagnosis. The anticysticercal drugs albendazole and praziquantel are variably effective for all forms of NCC. However, there is a controversy regarding its usage in both SCCL and malignant multiple NCC. Effective preventive health measures are safe drinking water, good hygiene, avoiding uncooked and contaminated food, and proper disposal of excreta.[1,2,13–15] The diagnosis of NCC has been greatly facilitated by the advent of reliable imaging using CT and MR imaging. Radiological descriptions assist in clinical classifications of NCC based on the topography and stage of the lesions, and determining the rational therapeutic approach for the different forms of the disease (**Fig. 2**). Imaging features of NCC are described in detail in the section on parasitic diseases.

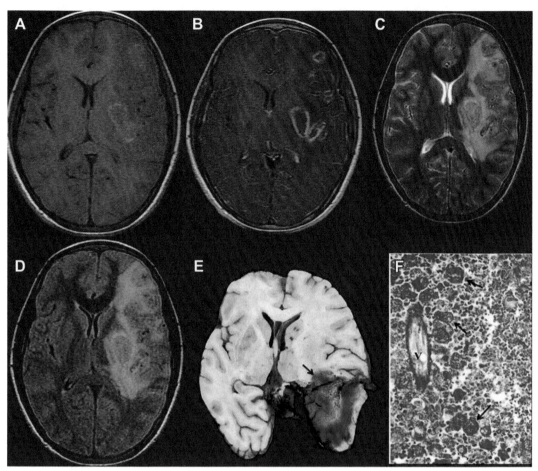

Fig. 1. *Acanthamoeba* meningoencephalitis. MR imaging (brain) axial images (*A–D*) showing ill-defined hemorrhagic lesion (*A*: T1-weighted hyperintensity) with faint but definite postgadolinium enhancement with gadolinium (*B*: postcontrast T1-weighted) in the left basal ganglionic and frontal regions with mild mass effect suggestive of hemorrhagic infarction (*C*: T2-weighted, *D*: fluid-attenuated inversion recovery [FLAIR]) in patient who died because of *Acanthamoeba* meningoencephalitis. (*E*) Axial slice of brain shows a large hemorrhagic lesion destroying the left parietooccipital lobe. (*F*) Histology of lesion revealed perivascular collections of amebic trophozoites (*arrows*) (hematoxylin-eosin, original magnification ×20). v, vessel.

Parasitic Eosinophilic Meningitis

Clinical features, natural history, and prognosis

Angiostrongylus cantonensis, also known as the rat lungworm, is the most common cause of eosinophilic meningitis worldwide. This parasitic infection is endemic in the Southeast Asian and Pacific regions. The intermediate hosts are raw fish and snails. The typical clinical presentation is acute meningitis with an eosinophilic pleocytosis frequently accompanied by encephalopathy. The pathologic findings in the CNS include the following: (1) meningitis with a predominance of eosinophils and plasma cells, (2) tortuous tracks of various sizes in the brain and spinal cord surrounded by an inflammatory reaction and degenerating neurons, (3) granulomatous response to the dead parasites, and (4) nonspecific vascular reactions including thrombosis, rupture of vessels, arteritis, and aneurysm formation.[1,2]

Role of imaging in parasitic eosinophilic meningitis

The brain CT scan can be normal or can reveal cerebral edema, ventricular dilatation, or enhancing ring or disc lesions, resembling tuberculoma. The features of the brain MR imaging scan were previously limited to a few case reports. These reports revealed vascular thrombosis, tortuous tracts in the vicinity of small vascular lesions, adjacent tissue reaction, and meningeal enhancement.

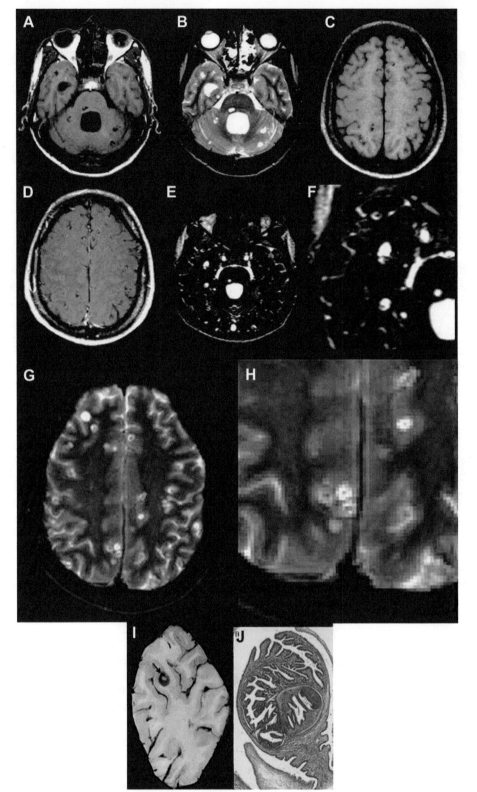

Fig. 2. (*A–H*) Various sequences of MR imaging (brain) revealing features of NCC with definite scolex observed in almost all the sequences (T1-weighted, T2-weighted, postgadolinium, fluid-attenuated inversion recovery [FLAIR], three-dimensional constructive interference in steady state [CISS-3D]); there is mild perilesional edema; in addition there is prominent ventriculomegaly. (*I*) Solitary cysticercal cyst (*arrow*) seen at gray-white junction of occipital lobe. Note invaginated scoles in center. (*J*) Microscopic view of cysticercal scolex with spiral canal, showing suckers and hooklets (hematoxylin-eosin, original magnification ×20).

MR imaging findings in CNS infection with *A cantonensis* are nonspecific, ranging from normal to leptomeningeal enhancement, ventriculomegaly, punctate area of abnormal enhancement, and hyperintense signal lesions on T2-weighted images. There seems to be a special predilection for involvement of the globus pallidus and cerebral peduncle in some patients. This finding is correlated with presence of worms in the CSF, severity of headache, CSF pleocytosis, and CSF and peripheral eosinophilia.[16,17]

CNS Tuberculosis

Clinical features, natural history, and prognosis
The various forms of CNS tuberculosis include tubercular meningitis (TBM); tuberculoma parenchymal or extraparenchymal, intraventricular, basal cisternal; tubercular cerebritis or abscess; and spinal cord tuberculosis especially spinal arachnoiditis. The clinical features of TBM differ from other bacterial meningitis in that it has a subacute course (days to weeks), high mortality, less CSF pleocytosis, and higher risk of sequelae despite treatment. The prodrome includes headache, vomiting, fever, irritability, and insomnia for 2 to 3 weeks. Then there are neck stiffness, seizures (especially in children), cranial nerve syndromes (late), stupor, and coma. Fever (which initially may be low grade), irritability, stiff neck, Kernig and Brudzinski signs, papilledema, cranial nerve abnormalities (especially third nerve palsy), and other focal signs. Later apathy, confusion, lethargy, and stupor might be observed. CSF shows increased pressure, slightly cloudy, moderate pleocytosis (100–500 cells/mm^3, mostly lymphocytes), increased protein, and decreased glucose. Growth on CSF cultures is rare. Confirmation of CSF for tuberculosis could be by (1) stained smear identifying acid-fast bacilli; (2) polymerase chain reaction (PCR) for mycobacterial DNA; or (3) mycobacterial culture. The treatment includes initiation with 4 oral drugs (rifampin, isoniazid, pyrazinamide, ethambutol) with steroids for the initial 2 months. Subsequently rifampin and isoniazid might be required for a period of another 10 months or so. Multidrug resistance tuberculosis is increasing and requires 5 or 6 drugs and a longer-term treatment regime.[1–3,18] Brain tuberculosis may occur in a variety of forms on MR imaging, including meningitis, tuberculomas, cerebritis, and frank abscesses. Tuberculous meningitis is most commonly seen as a communicating hydrocephalus with diffuse enhancement disproportionately affecting the basal cisterns (**Fig. 3**A–D). The role of imaging in CNS tuberculosis is described separately elsewhere in this issue.

Acute Bacterial Meningitis

Clinical features, natural history, and prognosis
Acute bacterial meningitis is characterized by acute onset of intense headache, fever, nausea, vomiting, photophobia, and meningism (ie, neck stiffness or Kernig sign). Neurologic signs include lethargy, delirium, coma, and convulsions. Focal deficits are uncommon in pyogenic meningitis. Acute complications include increased ICP, seizures, sepsis, paralysis, SIADH (syndrome of inappropriate antidiuretic hormone hypersecretion). The common organisms differ by age, for example, adults: *Streptococcus pneumoniae*, then *Neisseria meningitidis*, then cryptogenic (organism not identified); neonates: group B streptococci, *Escherichia coli*; children: *Hemophilus influenzae*. Acute meningeal syndrome mandates emergency neuroimaging, lumbar puncture (if not contraindicated), and emergent empiric intravenous antibiotic therapy. Initial antibiotic therapy is third-generation cephalosporin and vancomycin; ampicillin is added, if *Listeria monocytogenes* is considered. Definitive therapy is guided by organism and identification of source of infection. The mortality of acute bacterial meningitis is about 21% (depending on the organism) and occurs mostly within the first 48 hours.[1–3]

Role of imaging in acute bacterial meningitis
Neuroimaging studies have important adjunctive roles in identifying the complications of bacterial meningitis, such as hydrocephalus, subdural effusions, or subdural empyema, and in detecting parameningeal abscesses or CSF leaks. Indications for neuroimaging in acute bacterial meningitis include depressed level of consciousness, prolonged, partial, or late seizures, focal neurologic deficits, enlarging head circumference, persistent or recurrent fever during the later stages of treatment, and recurrent meningitis, sometimes before performing even lumbar punctures.[19] Neuroimaging studies can also improve clinicians' ability to prognosticate. Imaging should be considered strongly in neonates with bacterial meningitis, especially when gram-negative organisms are identified. Although noncontrast conventional MR imaging in uncomplicated infectious meningitis is usually normal, prominence of subarachnoid space or increased signal of the cisterns may occasionally be seen on proton density images. Fluid-attenuated inversion recovery (FLAIR) is the most sensitive MR imaging sequence for the evaluation of intracranial infections and has higher sensitivity than T2-weighted imaging for detecting meningitis. Abnormalities on FLAIR images include hyperintensity of the subarachnoid space and

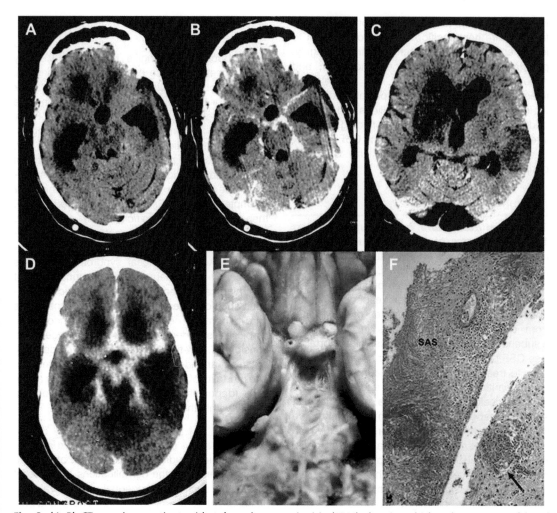

Fig. 3. (A–D) CT scan in a patient with tuberculous meningitis (TBM) showing thick enhancement of basal exudates (B) and massive hydrocephalus and arteritis involving right thalamus, basal ganglia, and right temporal regions. (E) Close-up view of base of brain reveals thick organizing exudate in optochiasmatic and prepontine cisterns entrapping optic nerves (A), the internal carotids, and oculomotor nerves. Histologic examination shows necrotizing exudate in subarachnoid space (F, SAS) with epithelioid granulomas in subpial zone (arrow). (F: hematoxylin-eosin, original magnification ×10.)

hyperintense vessels. On postcontrast MR imaging scans, homogeneous leptomeningeal enhancement of the falx, tentorium, convexities, and basal cisterns may be noted. Intravascular enhancement may also be seen. Abnormal meningeal or intravascular enhancement, or FLAIR subarachnoid hyperintensity on MR imaging, may occur in a variety of conditions other than infectious meningitis. Conventional MR imaging and CT are more useful tools for the diagnosis of the complications of meningitis, such as ventriculitis, hydrocephalus, infarction, cerebritis/abscess, myelitis, and subdural empyema. The use of DWI and magnetization transfer may increase the sensitivity of MR imaging in diagnosing infectious meningitis

and its ischemic complications.[1,3,20] Newer techniques like three-dimensional constructive interference in steady state and MR cisternography could be used to delineate CSF leakage in patients with recurrent meningitis (Fig. 4A–D).[21]

Brain abscess

Neuroimaging studies are essential for making a diagnosis of brain abscess. They reveal a focal process that rapidly assumes the character of a mass lesion with a contrast-enhancing margin. If MR imaging is not available, CT is the preferred procedure. Perilesional mass effect and even midline shift are often noted. Hyperintensity on DWI with a reduced ADC is characteristic of brain

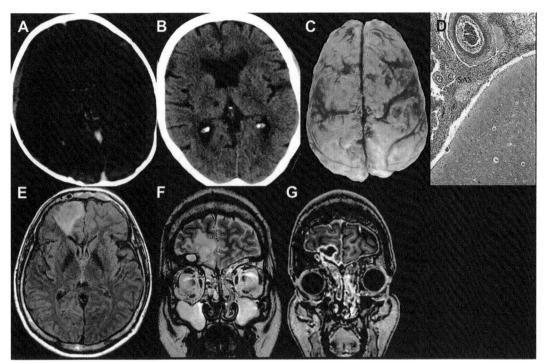

Fig. 4. CT scan showing subdural empyema (*A*) and infarct in left thalamus (*B*) in a patient with acute bacterial meningitis. Histopathology of bacterial meningitis: (*C*) thick purulent exudates is seen covering the superolateral surface of the brain, entrapping congested cortical veins; (*D*) acute inflammatory exudate is seen expanding the subarachnoid space (SAS) (hematoxylin-eosin, original magnification ×10). (*E–G*) Right basifrontal posttraumatic bacterial abscess caused by fracture of orbital roof plate.

abscess. In the absence of restricted diffusion on DWI, in vivo proton MR spectroscopy can distinguish brain abscesses from cystic tumors. In patients with cyanotic congenital heart disease, brain abscess must be differentiated from intracranial vascular accidents and hypoxic attacks (see **Fig. 4E–G**).[22]

Neurosyphilis

Clinical features, natural history, and prognosis
Syphilis, a potentially treatable condition, involves the nervous system at multiple neuraxes and thereby has protean manifestations. It was common in the first half of the 20th century, but after effective use of penicillin, its incidence has decreased considerably. However, in the last decade, there has been a 50-fold increase in its incidence in Eastern Europe. Further, in the human immunodeficiency virus (HIV) era, besides an increased incidence, it has acquired a fulminant course. According to a World Health Organization estimate, the total number of new cases of syphilis in the world in 1999 was 12 million, of which 90% were from developing countries. The classically described phases of the illness are asymptomatic,

meningovascular syphilis, tabes dorsalis, general paralysis of insane, and gummata.

The spectrum of neurologic manifestations includes meningitis, stroke, myelopathy, cranial nerve involvement, symptoms of demyelination, seizures, and headache, which can be confused with many neurologic diagnoses. A high index of suspicion and the clinician's awareness are thus important in diagnosis of neurosyphilis. CSF Venereal Disease Research Laboratory test is the most widely used, whereas the FTA-abs (fluorescent treponemal antibody absorption) test in the CSF is a highly sensitive marker for the presence of neurosyphilis.[23]

Role of imaging in neurosyphilis
Neuroradiological findings in neurosyphilis may vary with the stage of the disease and meningitis, cranial neuritis, cerebrovascular disease, cerebral atrophy, or parenchymal gumma. Orbital involvement may also occur, particularly of the roof and supraorbital rim. The cerebrovascular disease is characterized by endarteritis, with neuroimaging studies typically revealing multiple areas of ischemia and infarction. Syphilitic gummas appear as discrete masses, ranging

from a few millimeters to several centimeters in diameter and typically involving the cerebral cortex. Single-photon emission computed tomography (SPECT) studies reveal thalamic hyperperfusion in the acute stage, which is replaced by hypoperfusion in subacute or chronic stage.[24] Rao and colleagues[25] reviewed 35 MR images in patients with neurosyphilis. MR imaging of the brain was abnormal in 27 and revealed cerebral atrophy and signal changes in 18 each (Table 1). MRA revealed basilar artery occlusion in one. In the myelopathy group, MR imaging of the spine showed signal changes, involving more than 3 vertebral segments, in thoracic cord in 7 patients. One of the 3 patients with normal MR spine imaging had medial temporal involvement, and 1 each with cord abnormalities had multiple lacunes and temporal lobe changes.[25] In a proper clinical context, presence of signal changes in medial temporal and posterior column of spinal cord, especially with unexplained CSF pleocytosis, might suggest the diagnosis (Fig. 5).

Nervous System Involvement in HIV

Clinical features, natural history, and prognosis
Involvement of the nervous system at autopsy is noted in about 80% to 90% of HIV-seropositive patients. There are reports of neurologic disorders as the presenting initial manifestation in 5% to 10% of patients with AIDS.[26] Although seizures could be caused by HIV infection per se, they are more commonly observed in underlying opportunistic infections (OIs), systemic illness, drug or alcohol abuse, and even antiretroviral usage.[27–29]

Role of imaging in HIV
The imaging changes in HIV-seropositive patients in tropical countries, although similar to those described elsewhere, are complicated by the presence of OIs more often than elsewhere.[27–31] However, often imaging shows evidence of both HIV-related and OI- related changes. Progressive multifocal leucoencephalopathy (PML) does cause white matter signal alterations suggestive of demyelination (Fig. 6) and often causes diagnostic difficulties, especially when associated with OIs.

Toxoplasmosis
Acquired cerebral toxoplasmosis is a parenchymal infection caused by *Toxoplasma gondii*, which occurs in the population with HIV and in other immunocompromised hosts. In addition to being one of the common opportunistic CNS infection in patients with AIDS, it is the most common cause of focal brain lesion. Typically presenting with fever, headache, confusion, and focal neurologic signs with focal seizures, cerebral toxoplasmosis is often encountered in the emergency setting. For this reason, CT is frequently used as an initial diagnostic modality, although MR imaging is more sensitive in detecting the disease. On non-contrast CT scans, acute or subacute lesions typically appear hypodense with surrounding vasogenic edema. Chronic lesions might appear calcified, especially after treatment. Lesions are most commonly multiple and affect the deep central gray nuclei in the basal ganglia and lobar gray-white junction. Other common locations include the posterior fossa, cerebral cortex, and periventricular white matter. Toxoplasmosis lesions typically appear isointense to hypointense on T1-weighted images and hypointense to hyperintense on T2-weighted images. Prominent edema and mass effect are typically seen. The edema is often disproportionately large relative to the lesion size. However, rarely, nonedematous lesions without mass effect may be seen, especially in non-AIDS cases. On T2-weighted images, the masses may be difficult to distinguish from the surrounding edema, or a central isointense or

Table 1
MRI abnormalities in patients with neurosyphilis

MRI Abnormalities	N (35)
Abnormal	27
Neuropsychiatric manifestations	**17**
Cerebral atrophy	15
Diffuse	13
Fronto-temporal	02
Signal changes	11
Medial temporal	03
Fronto-temporal	03
Multifocal	03
Parietal	01
Basal-ganglion	01
Cerebellum	01
Meningo-vascular manifestations	**08**
Diffuse Cerebral atrophy	03
Signal changes	06
Medial temporal	01
Multifocal	05
MRA – basilar occlusion	01
Myelopathy manifestations	**10**
Hyperintense signal changes	09
>3 vertebral segments	07
<3 vertebral segments	02

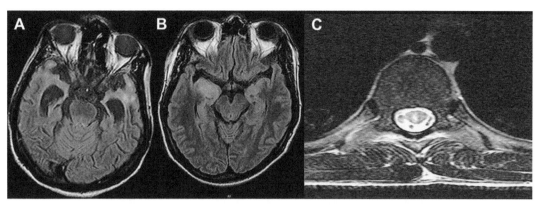

Fig. 5. Characteristic imaging features of neurosyphilis: (*A, B*) medial temporal signal changes as noted in axial FLAIR sequence and with evidence of atrophy in the temporal lobe (*A*); (*C*) another patient with subacute myelopathy and mild CSF pleocytosis showing signal change in the thoracic cord on the right side.

hypointense core may be noted on T2-weighted images, giving a target appearance. The optimal conventional imaging study for toxoplasmosis is MR imaging with intravenous gadolinium contrast administration, because the lesions characteristically enhance. MR imaging plays a central role in

monitoring the response to antibiotic therapy and for prognosis. MR imaging improvement is typically noted 14 to 28 days after treatment (**Fig. 7**).[28,29]

The imaging observations of some of the OIs (ie, CNS tuberculosis and fungal infections) are dealt with in separate sections.

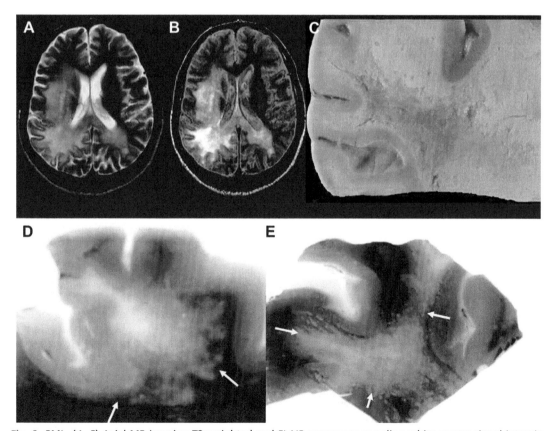

Fig. 6. PML. (*A, B*) Axial MR imaging T2-weighted and FLAIR sequences revealing white matter signal intensity changes in the parietal and frontal (right) and occipital (both sides) without any mass effect; (*C*) demyelination of the white matter; (*D, E*) Luxol fast blue stain showing demyelination; these features are consistent with PML.

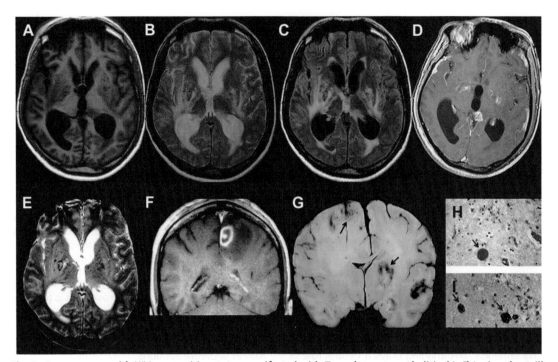

Fig. 7. A young man with HIV-seropositive status manifested with *Toxoplasma* encephalitis. (*A–E*) Lesions have ill-defined margins with mild perilesional edema; it is slightly hyperintense on T1-weighted and hiplines on T2-weighted images with postgadolinium enhancement. (*F*) The path gnomonic eccentric nodular enhancement. (*G*) Coronal slice of brain shows hemorrhagic lesions involving basal ganglia and frontal and temporal cortex; in addition, there is ventriculomegaly. (*H*) Histology shows characteristic *Toxoplasma bradyzoites* close to microglial nodules. (*I*) Immunostaining highlights bradyzoite and tachyzoite forms of *T gondii*.

Viral Encephalitis

Viral encephalitides are common in developing and tropical countries, including the Indian subcontinent. The common viruses producing encephalitis are Japanese encephalitis virus (JEV), dengue, West Nile, mumps, measles, polio, Coxsackie, enteric cytopathic human orphan, enterovirus 70, rabies, and Kyasanur forest disease.[1,2,32,33]

Japanese B encephalitis

Clinical features, natural history, and prognosis Japanese encephalitis (JE) is one of the most important endemic encephalitis in the world especially in Eastern and Southeastern Asia. JE affects more than 50,000 patients and results in 15,000 deaths annually. JEV is a single-stranded positive-sense RNA virus belonging to the family Flaviviridae. JEV is transmitted through a zoonotic cycle between mosquitoes, pigs, and water birds. Humans are accidentally infected and are a dead-end host because of low-level and transient viremia. Symptomatic JEV infection manifests with nonspecific febrile illness, aseptic meningitis, or encephalitis. Encephalitis manifests with altered

sensorium, seizures, and focal neurologic deficit. Acute flaccid paralysis may occur as a result of anterior horn cell involvement. A wide variety of movement disorders, especially transient parkinsonism and dystonia (limb, axial, orofacial), are reported in 20% to 60% of patients. JE mainly affects the thalamus, corpus striatum, brainstem, and spinal cord, as revealed by MR imaging and on autopsy studies.[33] Laboratory diagnosis of JE is by IgM capture enzyme-linked immunosorbent assay, which has high sensitivity and specificity. Patients require symptomatic and supportive therapies and preventive measures. Purified formalin inactivated mouse brain derived vaccine and live attenuated vaccine is available; the latter is reported to be safe, effective, and cheap. Control of JE is related to the wider issues of hygiene, environment, education, and economy.[1,2,32–34] On MR imaging, thalamus, basal ganglia, and brainstem involvement are common, and thalamic involvement has been reported to be suggestive of JE in an endemic area, especially in the postmonsoon period (**Fig.** 8A–E). The details of imaging observations of JE are described in the relevant section.

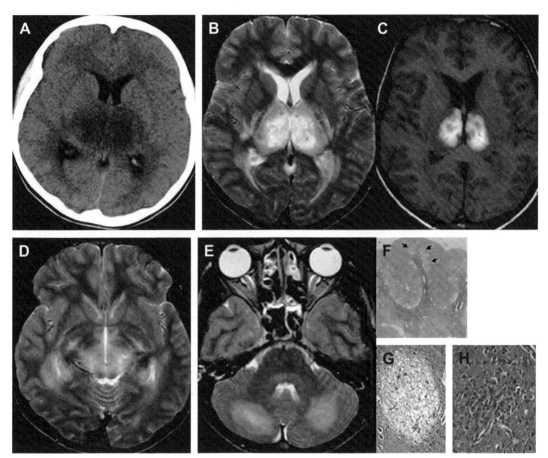

Fig. 8. (*A–E*) CT brain showing hypodensity in bilateral thalami and MR imaging showing signal changes in the thalami, midbrain, and cerebellum characteristic of JE; hemorrhagic lesions are seen in the thalami. (*F*) Whole mount preparation of cerebral cortex showing multiple round rarefied necrolytic lesions along the cortical ribbon along gray-white junction (*arrows*) (Luxol fast blue original magnification ×4). (*G*) Higher magnification of necrolytic lesion shows depletion of axons and minimal inflammation (hematoxylin-eosin, original magnification ×10). (*H*) Microglial nodule in gray matter (hematoxylin-eosin, original magnification ×40).

Other viral encephalitis in the tropics

Nipah viral encephalitis Nipah virus has recently caused an outbreak of encephalitis in Malaysia and Singapore. The causative agent was a new paramyxovirus named Nipah, closely related to the Hendra virus described in Australia, and potentially a new genus. The Nipah virus is a zoonosis infecting pigs, and almost all patients infected in this outbreak had direct contact with pigs. There is no specific treatment. MR imaging might show multiple small (<1 cm in maximum diameter) bilateral abnormalities within the subcortical and deep white matter; in some patients, the cortex, brainstem, and corpus callosum were also involved. Many of these lesions were detected on DWI, which was advantageous in increasing lesion conspicuously, as well as providing additional information and characterizing pathologic processes in the brain. DW MR imaging is capable

of depicting acute cytotoxic edema in the clinical assessment of acute cerebral infarction. In patients with Nipah virus with acute infection, DWI changes, supported by contrast enhancement, were helpful in confirming that the effects of acute viral infection were responsible for these lesions, and that they were not preexisting abnormalities caused by aging or other nonvirus-related causes. Recognition of the MR imaging pattern may be useful in differentiating it from JE, particularly at the height of an epidemic before serologic confirmation is available.[35,36]

Dengue hemorrhagic encephalitis Dengue virus belongs to the family Flaviviridae, which also includes yellow fever, and JE and West Nile encephalitis viruses. The dengue virus infection may manifest with both hepatic and neurologic involvement; the latter is attributed to metabolic alterations, hypotension, and hemorrhagic manifestations. Lately, there have been reports of neurologic complications of dengue virus infection. In patients with dengue encephalitis, CSF pleocytosis, and positive IgM and PCR tests have also been reported, suggesting neuroinvasion. The neurologic manifestations could be categorized into encephalopathy, encephalomyelopathy, and flaccid quadriparesis. The MR imaging abnormalities include cerebral edema, scattered focal lesions, and thalamic and basal ganglia (Fig. 9).[37,38]

Subacute Sclerosing Panencephalitis

Clinical features, natural history, and prognosis

Subacute sclerosing panencephalitis (SSPE) is a rare but fatal disease of the CNS caused by persistent infection of a mutant measles virus. It has a progressive course and results in premature death, within 2 to 4 years of onset.[39] Because of its varied manifestations at presentation, early diagnosis and clinical staging are not always easy. The electroencephalography (EEG) pattern in SSPE is one of the most characteristic and disease-specific of all EEG patterns. Periodic complexes, the hallmark of the disease, do occur in a wide variety of neurologic conditions like Creutzfeldt-Jakob disease, anoxic encephalopathy, metabolic encephalopathy, hepatic failure, drug toxicity, thyrotoxicosis, and progressive myoclonic epilepsy.[40] In most instances either periodicity is lacking or sharp waves/triphasic waves form the complexes.

Role of imaging in SSPE

MR imaging of the brain might be normal (9%) or else reveal changes in cerebral atrophy (78%), white matter (parietooccipital) (76%), and basal ganglia (6%). Restricted diffusion in the periventricular/subcortical region is rarely reported. A CT scan might show similar observations in a lesser degree of patients in view of its poor resolution. MR spectroscopy might show decreased N-acetyl aspartate peaks and increased choline peaks. Imaging findings in SSPE might show some degree of correlation with the clinical stage of illness and EEG (Fig. 10).[40–43]

Rabies

Clinical features, natural history, and prognosis

Rabies is a viral zoonosis. Infection of humans usually follows bites by rabid animals and is almost invariably fatal once the signs of the disease manifest. It is estimated that each year at least 55,000 people die from rabies, of which 20,000 are from India. Human rabies continues to be endemic in India except for the islands of Andaman, Nicobar, and Lakshadweep. The annual incidence of rabies in India is 2/100,000 population. Atypical/paralytic cases constitute about 20% of these cases. The animal responsible for most bites in India is the dog (96.2%), followed by several other species. Two distinct clinical syndromes, furious and paralytic rabies, have been recognized in humans. Rabies is well recognized in its classic furious form, with predominant limbic symptoms, hydrophobia,

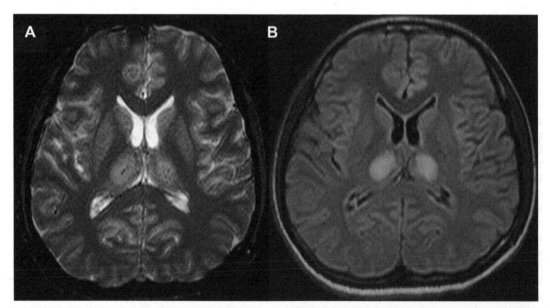

Fig. 9. (A) MR imaging showing bilateral thalamic signal changes in a patient with dengue hemorrhagic fever in both T2-weighted and FLAIR sequences. (B) T2-weighted sequences showing hypointensities in addition to hyperintensities, suggesting hemorrhages.

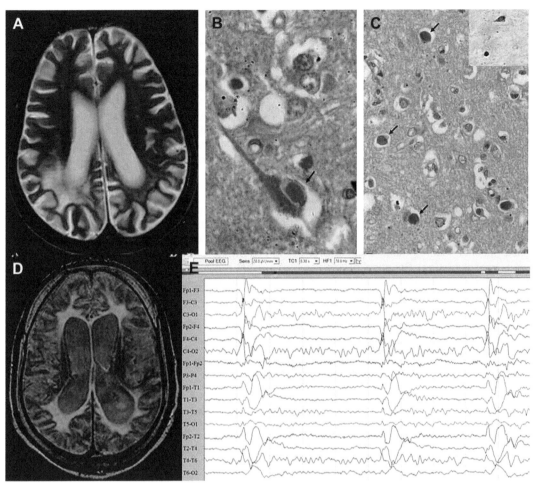

Fig. 10. The characteristic MR imaging (*A, D*), EEG (*E*), and pathologic (*B, C*) changes in SSPE. (*A*) T2-weighted axial MR imaging showing parietal periventricular white matter hyperintensity (right >left) and (*D*) FLAIR imaging showing diffuse atrophy with periventricular hyperintensity and (*D*) EEG showing classic periodic high-voltage slow-wave discharges (every 4 seconds). (*B, C*) Characteristic intranuclear eosinophilic inclusions seen in neuron (*B, arrow*) and oligodendroglial cells (*C, arrows*) containing measles viral antigen confirmed by immunohistochemsitry (*C, inset*). [*B*: hematoxylin-eosin, original magnification ×40; *C*: hematoxylin-eosin, original magnification ×20; *C*: immunostaining, original magnification ×10].

aerophobia, and phobic or inspiratory spasms.[44] There is a paucity of information on the clinical features of rabies presenting in the paralytic form. These cases are often clinically, electrophysiologically, and pathologically indistinguishable from Guillain-Barré (GB) syndrome. The situation is further compounded by the unavailability of a definitive diagnostic test for GB syndrome and limited availability of antemortem tests for rabies. Rapid diagnosis of rabies is important for appropriate infection control and public health measures to be instituted. Although no well-documented cases of transmission between humans after a bite from an infected individual have been reported (with the exception of organ transplants), barrier nursing is used, and preexposure prophylactic vaccination is offered to the relatives and treating clinical and nursing staff. In addition, specimens sent to nonspecialist laboratories may need to be tracked down for accurate case detection and epidemiologic data.[44,45]

Role of imaging in rabies
A CT scan is frequently normal but may show focal or diffuse areas of decreased attenuation in the basal ganglia, periventricular matter, hippocampus, and brain stem. Pontine hemorrhages have also been reported. Murthy had reported[46] findings of multiple areas of white matter on MR images, including the brain stem, cerebellar peduncles, and both cerebral hemispheres in a case of vaccine-induced acute demyelinating

encephalomyelitis (ADEM). This condition was postulated to be caused by transient arterial spasm induced by the viral infection. MR imaging of the brain might show signal intensity changes in bilateral basal ganglia, thalami, and cerebral peduncles.[45,47–49] Postprophylaxis with Semple vaccine could cause a clinical and radiological picture similar to ADEM (**Fig. 11**).[46,50]

Fungal Infections of the Nervous System

Clinical features, natural history, and prognosis

Fungal infections of the CNS are rare and are invariably secondary to primary focus elsewhere, usually in the lung or intestine. Except for people with long-standing diabetes, these infections are most frequently encountered in immunocompromised patients such as those with AIDS or after organ transplantation. Because of the lack of inflammatory response, neuroradiologic findings are often nonspecific and are frequently mistaken for tuberculous meningitis, pyogenic abscess, or brain tumor. Intracranial fungal infections are being identified more frequently because of the increased incidence of AIDS, better radiological investigations, more sensitive microbiological techniques, and better critical care of moribund patients. Although almost any fungus may cause encephalitis, cryptococcal meningoencephalitis is most frequently seen, followed by aspergillosis and candidiasis.[51]

Role of imaging in fungal infections of the nervous system

Fungal brain infections in the population with HIV and in other immunocompromised hosts display a myriad of manifestations on MR imaging. Fungi that proliferate in hyphal or pseudohyphal forms, such as *Aspergillus* and Mucorales, are associated

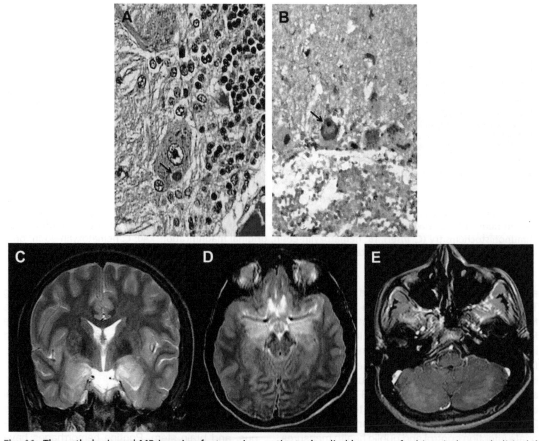

Fig. 11. The pathologic and MR imaging features in a patient who died because of rabies viral encephalitis. (*A*) intracytoplasmic eosinophilic inclusions (Negri bodies) seen within Purkinje neurons of cerebellum (*arrow*) (hematoxylin-eosin, original magnification ×40); (*B*) immunostaining with rabies viral nucleocapsid shows accumulation of viral antigen within Purkinje neurons (*arrow*) with dendritic spread along molecular layer (Immunoperoxidase, original magnification ×20); (*D–E*) MR imaging showing medial temporal and cerebellar signal changes on T2-weighted/FLAIR sequences.

with hemorrhage, cerebritis, and ischemia/infarction because of their angioinvasive potential (Fig. 12A–I). These fungi also commonly involve the orbits and paranasal sinuses. Fungi that reproduce in yeast forms, such as *Cryptococcus* and *Histoplasma*, typically manifest as leptomeningitis with or without parenchymal involvement (Fig. 13). Fungal meningitis is most commonly seen on MR imaging as a communicating hydrocephalus with diffuse nodular enhancement of the basal cisterns. Spinal involvement may occur because of fungal infection in the population with HIV with involvement of the leptomeninges, spinal cord, or both, because of hematogenous spread.[28,29,51,52]

Rheumatic Chorea and PANDAS

Rheumatic chorea and PANDAS (pediatric autoimmune neuropsychiatric disorders associated with streptococcal infection) are the manifestation of rheumatic fever. Rheumatic chorea is said to be autoimmune after infection with group 1A hemolytic *Streptococcus*. Chorea may be delayed for months. It is caused by presumed cross-reaction of streptococcal antibodies with neurons in caudate, subthalamic nuclei. PANDAS have a possible relationship between infection with group 1A hemolytic *Streptococcus*. It manifests with tic disorders and obsessive-compulsive disorder. Most individuals infected (80%) are between 5 and 15 years of age. The male/female ratio is 1:2. The disease is rare in developed countries. The laboratory tests include tests for rheumatic fever, antinuclear antibodies, antistreptolysin titers, and CSF oligoclonal bands. Complete recovery occurs in almost all patients in 3 to 6 weeks. However, recurrence has been noted in 35%. The complications are cardiac, usually endocarditis, in 20% of patients. Psychiatric/behavioral abnormalities may persist in some patients. Treatment includes bed

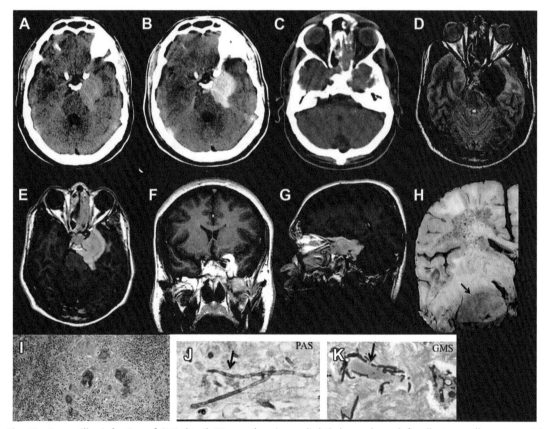

Fig. 12. *Aspergillus* infection of CNS. (*A–C*) CT scan showing a slightly hyperdense left sellar/parasellar extra-axial lesion extending into the middle cranial fossa with brilliant enhancement and bone destruction. (*D–G*) MR imaging delineating the same lesion with postgadolinium enhancement with the remarkable FLAIR hypointensity (*D*). (*H*) A large circumscribed, firm, solid lesion seen infiltrating basitemporal region (*arrow*). (*I*) Histology of the lesion revealed giant cell rich granulomas (hematoxylin-eosin, original magnification ×10). (*J*) Septate, acute angled branching fungal hyphae of *Aspergillus* spp seen within the lesion (periodic acid-Schiff stain, original magnification ×40, *arrow*). (*K*) Methenamine silver stain highlights septate branching hyphae within giant cells (*J, K, arrow*) (Grocott methenamine silver stain, original magnification ×20).

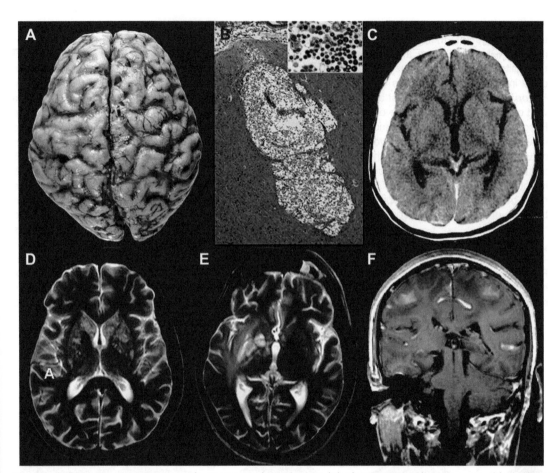

Fig. 13. An HIV-seropositive man with cryptococcal meningitis. (*A*) Characteristic glistening mucoid exudates covering surface of the brain. (*B*) Histologic examination shows *Cryptococci* extending into parenchyma from the meninges along pial vessels distending the Virchow Robin spaces. Inset shows periodic acid-Schiff–positive capsule of budding yeast forms of *Cryptococci* in subarachnoid space (hematoxylin-eosin, original magnification ×5, *inset*: periodic acid-Schiff, original magnification ×40). (*C*) CT showing mild atrophy. (*D–E*) Prominent signal alterations in the V-R spaces of the basal ganglionic region. (*F*) Postcontrast T1-weighted images of another patient with cryptococcal meningitis showing ill-defined enhancing parenchymal lesions.

rest, sedation, and dopamine-depleting agents (tetrabenazine) for chorea. Prophylactic penicillin is recommended for preventing rheumatic fever.[1,2]

Role of imaging in rheumatic chorea and PANDAS

Routine CT and MR imaging are often normal and have a limited role in the diagnosis. An [18F]fluoro-deoxyglucose positron emission tomography scan might show striatal hypermetabolism.

NONINFECTIVE DISORDERS AFFECTING THE NERVOUS SYSTEM IN THE TROPICS
Tropical Spastic Paraparesis

Clinical features, natural history, and prognosis
Tropical spastic paraparesis (TSP), a myeloneuropathy, has been reported in the last few decades from different parts of the world, including Jamaica, Martinique, Seychelles, Colombia, and Japan, and the clinical features seem to be uniform in these reports. TSP predominates in 2 races (Japanese and Black Africans), although Whites, Hindus, and Orientals are also affected. Human T-cell lymphotropic virus (HTLV) might have been brought to Japan by Portuguese traders who came with African slaves and monkeys. The causes of TSP-like illness are lathyrism, chronic cyanide intoxication caused by consumption of cassava, malnutrition, and infections. The association between HTLV type I (HTLV-1) and TSP opened new vistas in its cause and epidemiology. HTLV-I and II are human retroviruses that were first described in the early 1980s. HTLV-I is the causative agent of HTLV-associated myelopathy (HAM; also known as TSP), a progressive neurologic

disorder characterized by leg weakness, diffuse hyperreflexia, clonus, loss of vibration sense, and detrusor insufficiency leading to bladder dysfunction. Of the millions of individuals infected with HTLV-I worldwide, it is estimated that approximately 4% develop HAM during their lifetime. Although the role of HTLV-II in HAM is controversial, there is increasing evidence that supports an association, and a recent critical review has recognized this entity clearly.[1,2,53,54]

Several studies suggest that HTLV may be associated with a wider spectrum of neurologic manifestations that do not meet diagnostic criteria for HAM. These symptoms and conditions may later progress to HAM or constitute isolated neurologic syndromes associated with HTLV infection. Sensory neuropathy, gait abnormalities, bladder dysfunction, erectile dysfunction, amyotrophic lateral sclerosis, mild cognitive deficits, and rarely, motor neuropathies have all been reported among HTLV-I–infected individuals without HAM. Although little research has focused on HTLV-II, sensory neuropathy has been observed with HTLV-II alone and with HIV coinfection. A spinocerebellar syndrome has also been documented in a few case reports of HTLV-I–infected and HTLV-II–infected patients.[1,2,53,54]

Role of imaging in TSP

MR imaging has been proposed as a tool to aid in the diagnosis of HAM/TSP, to follow the response to therapy, or to distinguish HAM/TSP from multiple sclerosis (MS). Although the typical clinical presentation of HAM/TSP involves lower extremity paralysis and urological symptoms, which localize to a lesion in the thoracic spine, corresponding MR imaging lesions are seen in some patients. The incidence of spinal cord atrophy varies from 6% to 74% because no validated radiological criteria exist. In contrast, small white matter lesions are frequently seen in subcortical and periventricular areas in patients with HAM/TSP at a higher frequency than seen in noninflammatory neurologic diseases. A cross-sectional study using HTLV-I carriers without other neurologic disease showed that cerebral white matter lesions occur in a large percentage of all HTLV-I–infected individuals. A large proportion of HTLV-I carriers have neurologic and urological manifestations similar to those observed in HAM/TSP.[53–55]

Lathyrism-induced Myelopathy

Clinical features, natural history, and prognosis

Lathyrism is a neurodegenerative disease characterized by spastic paraplegia after chronic ingestion of *Lathyrus sativus* (LS). LS is a hardy plant that grows easily. Grains of LS are boiled in water to make gruel (dal), and its flour is used to prepare bread. During periods of scarcity of food such as famine or droughts, LS is used as the staple food, especially by economically deprived villagers. Three modes of presentation of neurolathyrism have been reported, the commonest being a sudden onset of leg weakness when going to sleep or when awakening from sleep. Some patients complain of a subacute onset of walking difficulty, whereas others experience an insidious progression of spastic paraparesis extending over months. Lathyrism has been reported in Asia, Africa, and Europe: its current foci are in Bangladesh, China, Ethiopia, Greece, Israel, India, Spain, and West Germany. Lathyrism is still common in certain developing countries such as Bangladesh, Ethiopia, India, and Nepal. In India, lathyrism is mainly reported from the states of Uttar Pradesh, Bihar, and Madhya Pradesh. Most of the clinical studies on lathyrism highlight the epidemiologic aspects of the disease. The toxin from the pulse, β_3-N-oxalylamino-L-alanine, caused neurolathyrism characterized by spastic paraplegia. Autoclaving the seeds of LS with lime removes the toxin.

The clinical picture of lathyrism in a study on 41 patients regularly consuming LS from Unnao was studied.[56] Their mean age was 42.9 years and the mean duration of the illness was 17.1 years. The patients complained of walking difficulty as a result of weakness and leg stiffness (32 each) and of frequency of micturition (4). Gait abnormalities included spastic gait (24), toe walking (15), and the necessary use of walking sticks (13). Weakness was mild to moderate, and was less prominent than was spasticity. In 8 patients the physical signs were asymmetrical. Peripheral neuropathy was present in only 1 patient, but muscle atrophy and widespread fasciculation were not found. A higher frequency of peripheral neuropathy and lower motor neuron involvement has been reported in other studies.[57] Severe spasticity in the absence of prominent weakness in lathyrism may be caused by the involvement of certain specific groups of corticospinal fibers.[56] There are no reports of MR imaging findings in neurolathyrism in the literature.

Postpartum Cerebral Venous Thrombosis

Cerebral venous thrombosis (CVT) is caused by clots in the dural venous sinuses and cerebral veins and accounts for 0.5% to 1% of all strokes. It disproportionally affects women who are pregnant or taking oral contraceptives and people 40 years and younger. CVT, an important cause of stroke in puerperium, is frequently observed in south and eastern India. The common clinical features are headache and other features of increased ICP, seizures, altered sensorium, and neurologic deficits. Treatment of CVT has been controversial and methods include decongestive measures, anticoagulants, decompressive surgery, and interventional thrombolysis. Antiepileptic drugs are required in almost all patients with parenchymal changes.[58,59]

Role of imaging in postpartum CVT

A CT scan (noncontrast) shows the classic finding as the delta sign, which is observed as a dense triangle (from hyperdense thrombus) within the superior sagittal sinus. On a contrast-enhanced CT scan, the reverse delta sign (ie, empty delta sign) can be observed in the superior sagittal sinus from enhancement of the dural leaves surrounding the comparatively less dense thrombosed sinus. The presence of both the delta and reverse delta signs increases the likelihood of the diagnosis of CVT. Hemorrhagic infarctions in a nonarterial distribution in the white matter or cortical white matter junction, with disproportionate mass effect, should suggest the possible diagnosis of venous thrombosis. Bilateral cerebral involvement can occur, including the superior cerebral white matter of the convexities from superior sagittal sinus thrombosis, or the basal ganglia and thalami from internal cerebral vein thrombosis in which the internal cerebral veins appear hyperdense in the noncontrast scan. MR imaging with MR venography without intravenous gadolinium contrast aid in confirming the diagnosis. A thrombus can be directly visualized within a vessel. Secondary venous infarctions and foci of hemorrhage can be seen with gradient-echo images. Susceptibility-induced signal loss from deoxyhemoglobin provides a basis for detection of even small foci of hemorrhage, which tend to occur in the subcortical white matter, thalami, and basal ganglia. Parenchymal regions of T2-hyperintense signal abnormality in the distribution of the draining sinus are often observed and may be reversible, even when large. The appearance of intravenous thrombus on conventional MR imaging depends on the age of the blood clot within the vessel. In acute venous thrombosis, loss of flow void on T1-weighted images occurs along with hypointensity on T2-weighted images, making the determination of sinus occlusion difficult. In the subacute phase, blood clot can result in loss of normal flow void on T1-weighted images and T1 hyperintensity; conversely, on T2-weighted images, blood clot can be of low signal intensity, thus mimicking flowing blood. In this instance, blood is in the intracellular methemoglobin stage. Flow-related enhancement phenomena created by slow flow can occur in veins and cause T1 hyperintensity. To circumvent this problem, flow-sensitive imaging techniques can be used (ie, two-dimensional time-of-flight or phase-contrast MR venography) to accurately assess the venous sinuses. Restricted diffusion may or may not be seen in CVT and, when present, may occasionally be reversible (**Fig. 14**).[3,58,59]

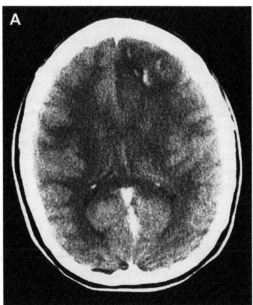
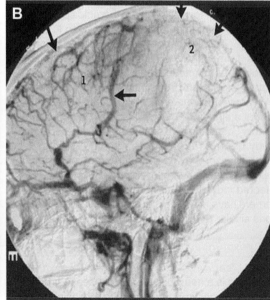

Fig. 14. (A, B) CT scan showing a large nonarterial territory hemorrhagic infarct with hyperdense venous sinuses (cord sign) and MR venography (MRV) showing absence of flow in the superior sagittal sinus.

ACKNOWLEDGMENTS

We thank Dr J Saini, Department of Neuroradiology, and Human Brain Tissue Repository (Brain Bank), Department of Neuropathology, NIMHANS, Bangalore for providing some of the figures and photomicrographs.

REFERENCES

1. Fauci AS, Braunwald E, Kasper DL, et al, editors. Harrison's principles of internal medicine. 17th edition. New York: McGraw-Hill; 2007.

2. Eddleston M, Stephen P, Robert W, et al, editors. Oxford handbook of tropical medicine. 2nd edition. Oxford University Press; 2005.

3. Scott AW, editor. Magnetic resonance imaging of the brain and spine. 4th edition. Lippincott Williams & Wilkins; 2008.

4. Newton RJ, Hien TT, White N. Cerebral malaria. J Neurol Neurosurg Psychiatry 2000;69:433–41.

5. Cordoliani YS, Sarrazin JL, Felten D, et al. MR of cerebral malaria. AJNR Am J Neuroradiol 1998;19: 871–4.

6. Looareesuwan S, Laothamatas J, Brown TR, et al. Cerebral malaria: a new way forward with magnetic resonance imaging (MRI). Am J Trop Med Hyg 2009; 81(4):545–7.

7. Kampfl AW, Birbamer GG, Pfausler BE, et al. Isolated pontine lesion in algid cerebral malaria: clinical features, management, and magnetic resonance imaging findings. Am J Trop Med Hyg 1993;48: 818–22.

8. Patankar TF, Karnad DR, Shetty PG, et al. Adult cerebral malaria: prognostic importance of imaging findings and correlation with postmortem findings. Radiology 2002;224(3):811–6.

9. Nickerson JP, Tong KA, Raghavan R. Imaging cerebral malaria with a susceptibility-weighted MR sequence. AJNR Am J Neuroradiol 2009;30:85–6.

10. Sakai O, Barest GD. Diffusion-weighted imaging of cerebral malaria. J Neuroimaging 2005;15:278–80.

11. Walker M, Kublin JG, Zunt JR. Parasitic central nervous system infections in immunocompromised hosts: malaria, microsporidiosis, leishmaniasis, and African trypanosomiasis. Clin Infect Dis 2006;42(1): 115–25.

12. Singh P, Kochhar R, Vashishta RK, et al. Amebic meningoencephalitis: spectrum of imaging findings. AJNR Am J Neuroradiol 2006;27:1217–21.

13. White AC Jr. Neurocysticercosis: a major cause of neurological disease worldwide. Clin Infect Dis 1997;24:101–15.

14. Garcia HH, Pretell EJ, Gilman RH, et al. A trial of antiparasitic treatment to reduce the rate of seizures due to cerebral cysticercosis. N Engl J Med 2004; 350:249–58.

15. Ng SH, Tan TY, Fock KM. The value of MRI in the diagnosis and management of neurocysticercosis. Singapore Med J 2000;41:132–4.

16. Nye SW, Tangchai P, Sundarakiti S, et al. Lesions of the brain in eosinophilic meningitis. Arch Pathol Lab Med 1970;89:9–19.

17. Hung-chin Tsai, Liu YC, Kunin CM, et al. Eosinophilic meningitis caused by *Angiostrongylus cantonensis* associated with eating raw snails: correlation of brain magnetic resonance imaging scans with clinical findings. Am J Trop Med Hyg 2003;68(3): 281–5.

18. Thwaites G, Fisher M, Hemingway C, et al, British Infection Society. British Infection Society guidelines for the diagnosis and treatment of tuberculosis of the central nervous system in adults and children. J Infect 2009;59(3):167–87.

19. van Crevel H, Hijdra A, de Gans J. Lumbar puncture and the risk of herniation: when should we first perform CT? J Neurol 2002;249:129–37.

20. Hughes DC, Raghavan A, Mordekar SR, et al. Role of imaging in the diagnosis of acute bacterial meningitis and its complications. Postgrad Med J 2010; 86(1018):478–85.

21. Vanopdenbosch LJ, Dedeken P, Casselman JW, et al. MRI with intrathecal gadolinium to detect a CSF leak: a prospective open-label cohort study. J Neurol Neurosurg Psychiatry 2011;82(4):456–8.

22. Shetty P, Moiyadi A, Pantvaidya G, et al. Cystic metastasis versus brain abscess: role of MR imaging in accurate diagnosis and implications on treatment. J Cancer Res Ther 2010;6(3):356–8.

23. Sinha S, Harish T, Taly AB, et al. Symptomatic seizures in neurosyphilis: experience from a university hospital in south India. Seizure 2008;17:711–6.

24. Ortego NJ, Miller BL, Mena I, et al. SPECT in neurosyphilis. Clin Nucl Med 1995;20(3):272.

25. Sudhanva HS, Sinha S, Taly AB, et al. MR imaging profile in neurosyphilis: experience from a south Indian tertiary care centre in last decade. Ann Indian Acad Neurol 2009;12(1):19.

26. Rachlis AR. Neurologic manifestations of HIV infection. Postgrad Med 1988;103:1–11.

27. Dal Pan GJ, McArther JC, Harrison MJG. Neurological symptoms in HIV infection. In: Berger JR, Levy RM, editors. AIDS and nervous system. 2nd edition. Philadelphia: Lippincott-Raven; 1997. p. 141–72.

28. Sinha S, Satishchandra P, Nalini A, et al. New-onset seizures among HIV infected drug naïve patients from south India. Neurology Asia 2005;10:29–33.

29. Satishchandra P, Sinha S. Seizures in HIV seropositive individuals: NIMHANS experience and review. Epilepsia 2008;49(S6):33–41.

30. Satishchandra P, Sinha S. Seizures in HIV seropositive individuals. In: Shorvon S, Guerrini R, Andermann F, editors. The causes of epilepsy. 1st edition. Cambridge University Press; 2011. p. 520–7.

31. Provenzale JM, Jinkins JR. Brain and spine imaging findings in AIDS patients. Radiol Clin North Am 1997;35:1127–66.

32. Kalita J, Misra UK. Comparison of CT scan and MRI findings in the diagnosis of Japanese encephalitis. J Neurol Sci 2000;174:3–8.

33. Kalita J, Misra UK, Pandey S, et al. A comparison of clinical and radiological findings in adults and children with Japanese encephalitis. Arch Neurol 2003; 60:1760–4.

34. Shankar SK, Rao TV, Mruthyunjayanna BP, et al. Autopsy study of brains during an epidemic of Japanese encephalitis in Karnataka. Indian J Med Res 1983;78:431–40.

35. Rumboldt Z. Imaging of topographic viral CNS infections. Neuroimaging Clin N Am 2008;18(1):85–92.

36. Lim CC, Lee KE, Lee WL, et al. Nipah virus encephalitis: serial MR study of an emerging disease. Radiology 2002;222(1):219–26.

37. Solomon T, Dung NM, Vaughn DW, et al. Neurological manifestations of dengue infection. Lancet 2000;355(9209):1053–9.

38. Misra UK, Kalita J, Syam UK, et al. Neurological manifestations of dengue virus infection. J Neurol Sci 2006;244(1–2):117–22.

39. Cobb WA, Marshall J, Scaravilli F. Long survival in SSPE. J Neurol Neurosurg Psychiatry 1984;47: 176–83.

40. Praveen-kumar S, Sinha S, Taly AB, et al. Electroencephalographic and imaging profile in a subacute sclerosing panencephalitis (SSPE) cohort: a correlative study. J Clin Neurophysiol 2007;118: 1947–54.

41. Anlar B, Saatçi I, Köse G, et al. MRI findings in subacute sclerosing panencephalitis. Neurology 1996;47:1278–83.

42. Praveen-kumar S, Sinha S, Taly AB, et al. The spectrum of MR Imaging findings in subacute sclerosing pan encephalitis (SSPE) with clinical and EEG correlates. J Pediatric Neurology 2011, in press.

43. Sener RN. Subacute sclerosing panencephalitis findings at MR imaging, diffusion MR imaging, and proton MR spectroscopy. AJNR Am J Neuroradiol 2004;25:892–4.

44. Gadre G, Satishchandra P, Anita Mahadevan A, et al. Rabies viral encephalitis: clinical determinants in diagnosis with special reference to paralytic form. J Neurol Neurosurg Psychiatry 2010;81: 812–20.

45. Laothamatas J, Hemachudha T, Mitrabhakdi E, et al. MR imaging in human rabies. Am J Neuroradiol 2003;24:1102–9.

46. Murthy JM. MRI in acute disseminated encephalomyelitis following Semple antirabies vaccine. Neuroradiology 1998;40(7):420–3.

47. Awasthi M, Parmar H, Patankar T, et al. Imaging findings in rabies encephalitis. Am J Neuroradiol 2001; 22:677–80.

48. Mani J, Reddy BC, Borgohain R, et al. Magnetic resonance imaging in rabies. Postgrad Med J 2003;79: 352–4.

49. Desai RV, Jain V, Singh P, et al. Radiculomyelitic rabies: can MR imaging help? Am J Neuroradiol 2002;23:632–4.

50. Swamy HS, Shankar SK, Chandra PS, et al. Neurological complications due to beta-propiolactone (BPL)-inactivated antirabies vaccine. Clinical, electrophysiological and therapeutic aspects. J Neurol Sci 1984;63:111–28.

51. Murthy J. Fungal infections of the central nervous system: the clinical syndromes. Neurol India 2007; 55:221–5.

52. Satishchandra P, Mathew P, Gadre G, et al. Cryptococcal meningitis: clinical, diagnostic and therapeutic overviews. Neurol India 2007;55:226–32.

53. Biswas HH, Engstrom JW, Kaidarova Z, et al. Neurologic abnormalities in HTLV-I– and HTLV-II–infected individuals without overt myelopathy. Neurology 2009;73(10):781–9.

54. Araujo AQ, Silva MT. The HTLV-1 neurological complex. Lancet Neurol 2006;5:1068–76.

55. Morgan DJ, Caskey MF, Abbehusen C, et al. Brain magnetic resonance imaging white matter lesions are frequent in HTLV-I carriers and do not discriminate from HAM/TSP. AIDS Res Hum Retroviruses 2007;23:1499–504.

56. Misra UK, Sharma VP, Singh VP. Clinical aspects of neurolathyrism in Unnao, India. Paraplegia 1993; 31(4):249–54.

57. Misra UK, Sharma VP. Peripheral and central conduction studies in neurolathyrism. J Neurol Neurosurg Psychiatry 1994;57(5):572–7.

58. Mehndiratta MM, Garg S, Gurnani M. Cerebral venous thrombosis–clinical presentations. J Pak Med Assoc 2006;56(11):513–6.

59. Nagaraja D, Haridas T, Taly AB, et al. Puerperal cerebral venous thrombosis: therapeutic benefit of low dose heparin. Neurol India 1999;47(1):43–6.

Pathology of Tropical Diseases

Nuzhat Husain, MD*, Praveen Kumar, MSc

KEYWORDS

• Tropical diseases • Pathology • Infection • Nutrition

Tropical diseases affecting the central nervous system (CNS) include a wide array of infections and infestations as well as nutritional deficiency disorders. It is a vast subject, so in this article the description is limited to the commonly encountered diseases. The infections include bacterial, mycobacterial, fungal, parasitic, and viral infections with varied clinical manifestations. Imaging sensitivity and specificity for the prediction of the cause of the infection has improved with application of advanced techniques. Microbial demonstration and histology remain gold standard for diagnosis. Understanding the pathology basis of imaging changes is mandatory for better evaluation of images. Nutritional disorders present with generalized and nonspecific imaging manifestations. The pathology of commonly encountered vitamin deficiencies, like thiamine and B_{12} deficiency, are also discussed.

BACTERIAL INFECTIONS

Bacterial infections of the CNS include suppurative acute, subacute, and chronic infections. Mycobacterial CNS disease forms a large proportion of cases and is discussed separately. Bacterial infections may manifest as meningoencephalitis, brain abscess, and subdural empyemas.

Brain Abscess

Brain abscess is a capsulated focal suppurative lesion within the brain parenchyma that begins as a localized area of cerebritis.[1–3] The incidence of brain abscess in the developed world is as low as 1% to 2%, whereas in the developing countries it is up to 8% of all intracranial space-occupying lesions.[2–4]

Infection may be direct from the contiguous site, such as otitis media or sinusitis, after trauma or neurosurgical procedures, or may be caused by a bacteremia from a distant primary source such as bacterial endocarditis.[2,5,6] Patients with pulmonary arteriovenous shunts or hereditary hemorrhagic telangiectasias are also prone to develop cerebral abscesses. Pyogenic abscesses of hematogenous origin are solitary in more than 50% of cases and are usually located at the gray-white matter junction in the anterior or middle cerebral artery distribution.[7,8]

Most abscesses are produced by pyogenic bacteria. In one-third of patients, more than 1 type of organism is found. Frequently isolated microbes include streptococci (both aerobic and anaerobic) and staphylococci.[9] Both aerobic and facultative anaerobes may be present.

Pathogenesis

When bacteria attach to the parenchyma vessel wall and pass into the parenchyma, they cause disruption of the blood-brain barrier and facilitate brain invasion.

Brain abscess evolves through 4 stages initiating with early cerebritis, and progressing to late cerebritis, early capsule formation, and late capsule formation. Early cerebritis stage is the initial stage of cerebritis occurring during the first 4 to 5 days of infection. During this stage, the brain reacts by developing an area of local inflammation with vascular congestion, petechial hemorrhage, and edema. By the end of first week during the late cerebritis stage, 1 or more microabscesses with acute inflammation and surrounding edema are evident. Granulation tissue with proliferating new vessels and fibroblasts starts developing

Department of Pathology, Dr Ram Manohar Lohia Institute of Medical Sciences, Vibhuti Khand, Gomti Nagar, Lucknow 226010, Uttar Pradesh, India
* Corresponding author.
E-mail address: drnuzhathusain@hotmail.com

Neuroimag Clin N Am 21 (2011) 757–775
doi:10.1016/j.nic.2011.07.003

around the abscess in the early capsule stage by the end of the second week and is characterized by the formation of a collagenous capsule surrounding the liquefied necrotic core. During the late capsular stage, a thick capsule consisting of 3 layers develops: an inner layer of granulation tissue infiltrated by lymphocytes and macrophages, a middle collagenous layer, and an outer gliotic layer with reactive astrocytes and proliferating blood vessels. It is not always possible to separate these layers on histopathology.[10,11] The wall is lined by necrotic material with an inner polymorphonuclear infiltrate (Fig. 1). Organisms may be detected by special staining techniques. Identification of the causative organism requires a battery of special stains in histology including Gram stain; Gomori methenamine silver (GMS) for fungus, actinomycosis, and nocardia; Ziehl Neilson stain for acid-fast bacilli (AFB); and Warthin-Starry for spirochetes. The sensitivity of tissue staining methods in the identification of organisms is low. On magnetic resonance (MR) images, mature pyogenic abscesses show an isointense to slightly hyperintense rim on T1-weighted images that appears hypointense on T2-weighted images, a feature that could relate to coagulative necrosis; increased accumulation of hemorrhagic products and paramagnetic materials such as iron, magnesium, and manganese; and production of free radicals, secondary to bacterial metabolism.[12]

As the abscess heals, the cavity gradually shrinks. Complications of cerebral abscesses include ventriculitis, choroid plexitis, subdural empyema, and purulent leptomeningitis.[11] Remnant fibrogliotic scars may result in epileptic foci.

Meningitis

Bacteria may cause an acute meningitis with neutrophilic pleocytosis or a subacute or chronic meningitis with a predominantly lymphocytic pleocytosis. Frequent causative pathogens are *Streptococcus pneumoniae* and *Neisseria meningitidis* in children and young adults,[3] group B streptococci in newborns, and *Listeria monocytogenes* in newborns and the elderly. *Haemophilus influenzae* has shown a vaccine-related decline. The cornerstone in the diagnosis of bacterial meningitis is cerebrospinal fluid (CSF) examination. The CSF in meningitis shows hundreds, even thousands, of neutrophils and is teeming with organisms. CSF protein is increased and glucose is low. Staining and culture on appropriate media

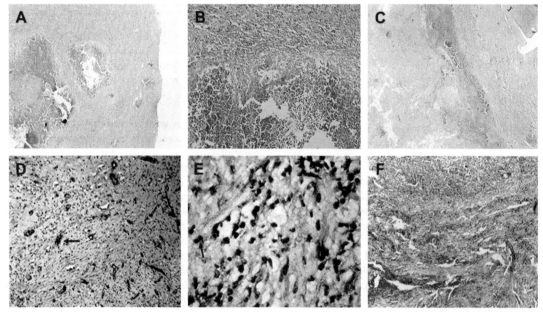

Fig. 1. Brain abscess in different stages of evolution. (*A–C*) Phases in evolution of brain abscess with cerebritis and microabscesses (*A*), large abscess with liquefaction necrosis (*B*) in the lumen, intense neutrophil infiltrate and early fibrosis, and (*C*) well-formed abscess showing, from left to right, necrotic center, granulation tissue, fibrosis, and gliosis (*A–C*: hematoxylin-eosin [H&E], ×40 digital magnification). (*D*) CD34 immunostaining highlighting neovascularization (*arrow*) (diaminobenzidine [DAB], ×100 digital magnification) (*E*) vascular endothelial growth factor (VEGF) expression (*arrow*) in macrophages, fibroblasts, and glial cells (DAB, ×400 digital magnification). (*F*) Prussian blue stain shows intense iron staining in the abscess wall (Prussian blue, ×100 digital magnification).

and other tests, including antigen detection in CSF and bacterial polymerase chain reaction (PCR), help clinch the diagnosis.

The exudates cover the cerebral hemispheres and settle along the base of the brain, around cranial nerves and the openings of the fourth ventricle. MR imaging shows enhancement and high fluid-attenuated inversion-recovery (FLAIR) signal intensity in the meninges, corresponding with the pathology. Brain damage in meningitis is caused not only by bacteria but probably more by host responses. These responses have a protective purpose (to eliminate bacteria) but are excessive and indiscriminate and set in motion destructive cascades that damage mostly host tissues. The results of inflammation are tissue and vascular injury (vasculitis) and increased intracranial pressure. Increased intracranial pressure is caused by increased vascular permeability and leakage of proteins in the interstitial space (cerebral edema) and CSF. Vasculitis causes infarcts, and increased intracranial pressure aggravates hypoxic-ischemic insult. The late complications of meningitis include cranial nerve deficits and ischemic infarction. The thick fibrinopurulent exudate in the subarachnoid space organizes into fibrous tissue that blocks the exits of the fourth ventricle and impairs CSF circulation around the cerebral convexities, causing hydrocephalus.

The infection is limited by a thick, tight mesh of astrocytic processes, joined by dense junctions and covered by basement membrane that resists penetration by bacteria and neutrophils. It provides an effective barrier that prevents the infection from spreading into brain tissue.

The commonest bacterial cause of chronic meningitis in the tropics is tuberculosis. Other pathogenic conditions and bacteria resulting in chronic meningitis include brucellosis, spirochetes (increasingly being encountered in human immunodeficiency virus [HIV] infection), borreliosis or relapsing fever (*Borrelia recurrentis*, louse-borne; *Borrelia duttonii*, tick borne), and Lyme disease (*Borrelia burgdorferi*, tick borne). The neural manifestations include meningitis, encephalitis, focal cranial neuropathies, radiculitis neuropathy, and encephalopathy. The pathology of chronic meningitis is discussed in detail later.

TUBERCULOSIS

Tuberculosis is a major cause of morbidity resulting in 8 million deaths annually in the world.[13] CNS tuberculosis has diverse manifestation as well as serious complications with a high mortality and morbidity. *Mycobacterium tuberculosis* is responsible for almost all cases of the tubercular infection in CNS.[14] Granulomatous inflammation is the hallmark of tubercular disease and may involve the meninges, brain, spinal cord, bones covering the brain, and spinal cord.

Pathology and Pathogenesis

CNS tuberculosis is secondary to a primary lesion in the lung, gastrointestinal tract, or other sites. Occasionally a contiguous spread from vertebrae, inner ear, or mastoid sinus may occur.[15] Chemotherapy, immune-compromised states, and uncontrolled diabetes mellitus may reactivate a primary quiescent focus and cause secondary hematogenous spread to neural sites. Infection starts in a subpial or subependymal cortical focus called Rich focus. The bacilli evoke a nonspecific inflammatory reaction that may be termed tubercular cerebritis. Once sensitized, the inflammatory response results in a granuloma that erodes into the subarachnoid space and CSF, causing basal leptomeningitis. The meningitis usually causes communicating hydrocephalus, but it may also cause obstruction of the foramina of Luschka and Magendie, resulting in obstructive hydrocephalus. Vasculitis involving the lenticulostriate and thalamoperforating arteries may occur and cause small infarcts in the deep gray matter nuclei and deep white matter.[16]

CSF analysis shows a lymphocytic pleocytosis, with increased CSF protein and decreased CSF sugar and chloride concentration.[17] CSF culture for AFB and CSF PCR examination are confirmatory tests for diagnosis of tubercular meningitis (TBM). Tubercular infections in the CNS may involve the meninges, brain, spinal cord, and the bones covering the brain and spinal cord, and may manifest in these various forms:

TBM

TBM manifests as chronic meningitis. The commonly involved sites are interpeduncular fossa, pontine cistern, and perimesencephalic and suprasellar cisterns. Involvement of sulci over the convexities and in the sylvian fissures can also be seen.[18–20] Cerebellar meningeal and tentorium involvement is uncommon.

In initial phases, TBM present with neutrophilic pleocytosis that evolves into chronic lymphocytic meningitis in the second week of infection. Granulomas develop in the meninges as the disease progresses. Histologic findings in TBM are the same as those of mycobacterial infections elsewhere, namely epithelioid cell granulomas with Langhans giant cells, lymphocytic infiltrates, and caseous necrosis. Epithelioid cells are macrophages engaged in mycobacterial killing. They aggregate in clusters (granulomas) or fuse, forming giant cells. These changes involve the arachnoid membrane and subarachnoid space diffusely (Fig. 2B). Acid-fast organisms can be shown in necrotic tissue and in the granulomas (see Fig. 2C). Unlike suppurative meningitis, in which the exudates are usually confined to the subarachnoid space, epithelioid cell granulomas destroy the pia and invade the brain (see Fig. 2A). The sequelae associated with TBM are more serious than pyogenic meningitis and include hydrocephalus and vasculitis.

Hydrocephalus may be the communicating type, secondary to the blockage of the basal cisterns by the inflammatory exudates, obstructive type secondary to a focal parenchymal lesion with mass effect, or caused by entrapment of the ventricle by granulomatous ependymitis. Chronic hydrocephalus may result in atrophy of brain parenchyma. Endoscopic third ventriculostomy is gaining acceptance in its management, and patency of the stoma can be shown by CSF flow dynamics.[21] The procedure is also diagnostic and characteristically shows cloudy intraventricular exudates and nodular ventriculitis that shows granulomas in histology (Fig. 3).

Vasculitis in TBM usually involves small and medium-sized vessels. The adventitial layer of the vessels develops changes similar to those of the adjacent tubercular exudates. The intima of the vessels may eventually be affected or eroded by a fibrinoid degeneration. In later stages, the lumen of the vessel may be completely occluded by reactive subendothelial cellular proliferation.[22] Ischemic cerebral infarction resulting from the vascular occlusion is thus a common sequela of tubercular arteritis.

Intracranial Tuberculoma

Brain tuberculoma forms a large percentage of intracranial mass lesions in developing countries and is responsible for high morbidity and mortality.[14] It accounts for between 15% and 50% of all intracranial lesions in the developing world.[23] Intracranial tuberculomas may be solitary or multiple. The size varies between 1 mm and 12 cm. Common locations of tuberculomas include

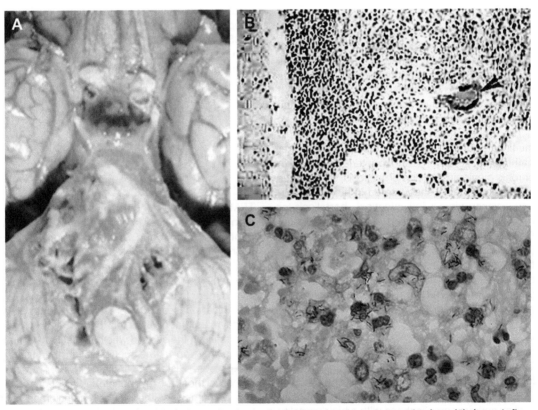

Fig. 2. TBM. (A) Gross specimen of the brain shows exudates in the basal meninges. Histology (B) shows inflammation in the meninges with lymphocytic infiltration. Note the presence of Langhan giant cell (arrow). Ziehl Neilson–stained sections (C) show pink AFB.

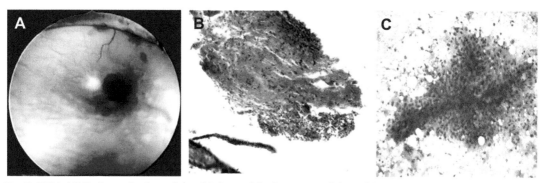

Fig. 3. TBM. (A) Endoscopic view of the third ventricle showing nodular infiltrate that, on (B) biopsy (H&E, ×40 digital magnification) and (C) squash smear, represent granulomatous inflammation (methylene blue, ×40 digital magnification).

cerebral hemispheres, basal ganglia, cerebellum, and brainstem. Rarely, ventriculitis may occur in tuberculomas communicating with the ventricles.[23]

Histopathologic evolution of tuberculomas may be empirically divided into an initial nonspecific focal cerebritis followed by noncaseating granulomas that evolve into tuberculomas with solid caseation and subsequently into tuberculomas with liquefaction of caseation. Hemorrhage and calcification may occur in some cases. The initial lesion is a tubercle consisting of a central area of incipient caseous necrosis surrounded by epithelioid and Langhans giant cells with a lymphocytic infiltrate, with an encircling zone of rich vascularity.[24] These lesions originate as a conglomerate of microgranulomata in an area of tubercular cerebritis that join to form a noncaseating tuberculoma.[25] A caseous necrosis develops that is mostly solid but, in some instances, may eventually liquefy. Granulomatous inflammation comprising epithelioid cells, multinucleated giant cells, and mononuclear inflammatory cells surround this solid caseation. Bacilli are scarce. Liquefaction commences from the center. Astrocytic gliosis and fibrosis is evident in the surrounding brain parenchyma.[26]

The well-formed tuberculomas have a rim of granulomatous infiltrate of variable thickness around the solid caseating center (Fig. 4). This rim shows enhancement on contrast-enhanced T1 images with no enhancement of the solid caseation. On MR images, the center of tuberculomas with solid caseation shows hypointensity and the rim shows hyperintensity.

Molecular Pathology of Tuberculosis

Vascular endothelial growth factor (VEGF) expression and microvascular density in tuberculomas is comparable with that in grade 2 gliomas. VEGF is strongly expressed in the Langhans cells, epithelioid cells, and also in the surrounding fibrocytes

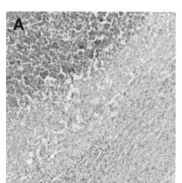
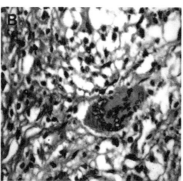
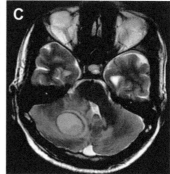

Fig. 4. Low-cellularity tuberculoma with large area of caseous necrosis. (A) H&E stain of the lesion shows necrosis surrounded by a thin layer of granulomatous infiltrate, fibrosis, and gliosis from right to left (40× digital magnification). (B) High-power view of the cellular region shows granuloma with Langhans giant cells (400× digital magnification). (C) T2-weighted axial image shows a hyperintense lesion with a hypointense rim in the right cerebellum.

and astrocytes (**Fig. 5**). Recently, Gupta and colleagues[27] performed dynamic contrast-enhanced MR imaging in 13 patients with brain tuberculoma and correlated the relative cerebral blood volume (rCBV) values with its cellular component, necrotic component, and also with expression of immunohistochemical markers, microvascular density (MVD), and VEGF. rCBV of the cellular portion significantly correlated with cellular fraction volume, MVD, and VEGF of the excised tuberculomas. In a recent perfusion MR imaging study in brain tuberculoma, the investigators reported a significant positive correlation between physiologic indices (k^{trans} and v_e) and matrix metalloproteinase 9 (MMP-9) expressions (a marker of blood-brain barrier disruption) in excised tuberculoma.

Tubercular Brain Abscess

Tubercular brain abscess is a rare condition caused by *M tuberculosis* infection. It constitutes approximately 4% to 7% of the total CNS tuberculosis in developing countries. According to the diagnostic criteria of Whitener,[28] tubercular abscesses show macroscopic evidence of abscess formation within the brain parenchyma, and histology will confirm that the abscess wall is composed of vascular granulation tissue containing both acute and chronic inflammatory cells and isolation of *M tuberculosis*. Histologically the tubercular abscess, by strict definition, has a nongranulomatous infiltrate and, in hematoxylin and eosin (H&E)–stained slides, cannot be differentiated from pyogenic abscesses and fungal lesions. However, the demonstration of *M tuberculosis* in the pus as well as the wall of the abscess is diagnostic of the tubercular abscess (**Fig. 6**). Granulomas with central liquefaction should not be categorized as abscess.

SPINAL TUBERCULOSIS
Intraspinal Tuberculosis

Spinal diseases caused by *M tuberculosis* may manifest as spinal meningitis and spinal arachnoiditis. The pathophysiology of the spinal meningitis is similar to that of TBM: during primary infection a submeningeal tubercle forms that ruptures into the subarachnoid space and elicits the mediators of delayed hypersensitivity.[29] Similar to intracranial lesions, granulomatous inflammation, areas of caseation, and tubercles with fibrosis are evident. Secondary involvement of the spinal cord may cause parenchymal infarction and syringomyelia. Parenchymal tuberculosis myelitis and tuberculoma formation may also occur.

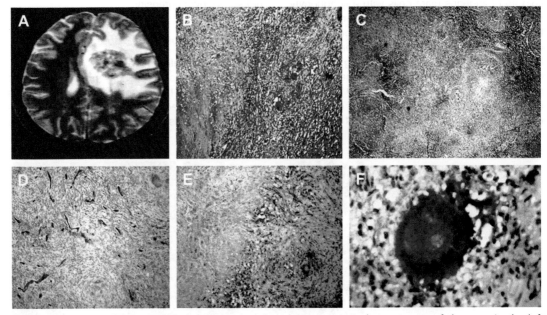

Fig. 5. Tuberculoma. (*A*) T2-weighted axial MR imaging shows variegated appearance of the mass in the left frontal region. The lesion was biopsied. (*B*) Histology of the lesion on H&E staining shows well-formed cellular tuberculoma with a thick layer of granulomatous infiltrate and areas of caseous necrosis (40× digital magnification). (*C*) Matrix metalloproteinase 9 (MMP-9) staining showed upregulated expression in granulomas (40× digital magnification). (*D*) CD34 immunostain highlighted neovascularization (100× digital magnification). (*E*) VEGF immunostain showed upregulated expression in the granuloma (100× digital magnification) that, on (*F*) high-power view, showed high cytoplasmic VEGF in the Langhans giant cell (400× digital magnification).

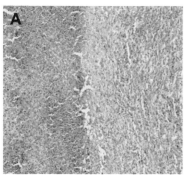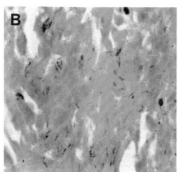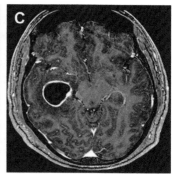

Fig. 6. (A) Chronic nongranulomatous inflammation in the abscess wall (H&E 40× digital magnification) that shows (B) strong AFB positivity in Ziehl Neilson stain for mycobacteria confirming TBM (400× digital magnification). (C) MR showing a cystic lesion with thick wall.

Tubercular Spondylitis

Tubercular spondylitis involves 1 or more extra-dural components of the spine. Vertebral bodies are most frequently affected. In addition, posterior osseous elements, epidural space, paraspinal soft tissue, and intervertebral discs can be seen primarily or secondarily.[30] The dorsal and lumbar spine are frequently affected.

FUNGAL INFECTIONS

Fungi are organisms of low pathogenicity, emerging as opportunistic organisms in an immunocompromised host; however, some infect even normal hosts. Intracranial fungal infections seem to be increasing because of increased incidence of patients with acquired immune deficiency syndrome (AIDS), better radiological investigations, sensitive microbiological techniques, and improved critical care of debilitated patients. Fungal infections of the CNS may result in granulomatous disease with variable degree of suppuration that may be acute and fulminant or chronic and indolent.[31]

Fungal pathogens are acquired through inhalation or hematogenous dissemination from foci of fungal osteomyelitis or lymphadenitis. Meningeal involvement, either isolated or associated with widely disseminated infection, results from hematogenous dissemination from the lungs. Yeastlike fungi including Cryptococcus and Histoplasma, spread hematogenously, reach the microvasculature of the meninges, penetrate the vessel walls, and result in an acute or chronic leptomeningitis. The source of infection is frequently sinuses or orbits. Hyphae from mycelia colonies are also capable of vascular invasion and obstruction of large, medium, and small arteries, resulting in infarction and cerebritis. CNS infection with Candida often results in scattered parenchymal microabscesses secondary to small-vessel (arteriole)

occlusion and tissue breakdown. Granulocytopenia, cellular-mediated, and humoral-mediated immune dysfunctions are predisposing factors to the development of CNS infections in immunosuppressed patients.

Absolute diagnosis can be established only on periodic acid-Schiff (PAS) and GMS stains.

Aspergillosis

Aspergillus fumigatus is the most common human pathogen. Other species, including Aspergillus flavus, Aspergillus niger, and Aspergillus Oxyzae, are also frequently seen. They have septate hyphae that show dichotomous branching, and produce numerous spores. Humans are infected by inhaling these spores, making the lungs the primary site of infection.[32]

CNS aspergillosis may manifest in 3 forms: infarction, granulomas, and meningitis.[33] Fungal hyphae block intracerebral blood vessels, causing thrombosis, infarction, and hemorrhage.[32,34] Invasion beyond vessel walls results in abscesses in the adjacent brain parenchyma.[34] Acute lesions show purulent exudates with neutrophilic infiltrate, macrophages, and necrosis. Chronic lesions result in a granulomatous reaction and fibrosis. Microscopically, the most characteristic features are the presence of vascular invasion, thrombosis, and vasculitis. Erosion of a vessel wall in the CNS leads to mycotic aneurysms.[34] Granulomas comprise lymphocytes, plasma cells, and multinucleated foreign body–type giant cells with fungal hyphae. Large areas of necrosis are present with prominent breakdown of leucocytes and hemorrhage. Liquefaction necrosis leads to abscesses lined by granulation tissue rich in fungi. The organism is seen as branched septate hyphae that are homogeneous, a uniform 3 to 6 μm wide, and have a progressive arboreal pattern of branching (Fig. 7).

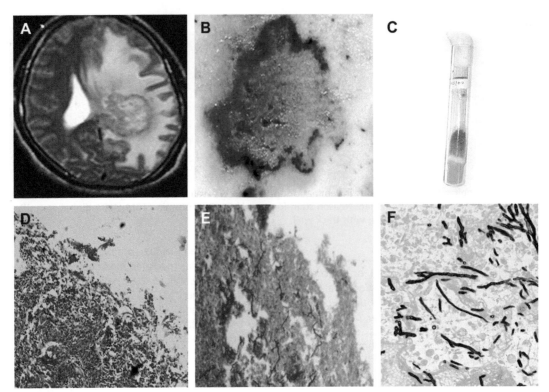

Fig. 7. Intraparenchymal aspergillosis. (*A*) MR image showing a mixed-intensity irregular lesion with white matter edema. (*B*) Gross evaluation showing hemorrhagic and necrotic lesion with surrounding infarct and punctate hemorrhages. (*C*) Culture shows growth of *A fumigatus*. (*D*) H&E stain showing diffuse inflammation in the abscess wall, and (*E*) GMS stain at low (40× digital magnification) and (*F*) high magnification showing thin hyphae branching at acute angles (100× digital magnification).

Cryptococcosis

Cryptococcus neoformans is a ubiquitous organism found in mammal and bird feces, particularly in pigeon droppings. Cryptococcal CNS disease occurs primarily in patients with impaired immunity.[35] In 30% of cases, infections have been reported with no predisposing condition.[36] Primary focus is frequently present in the lung, from where it spreads by hematogenous route to the CNS. The absence of soluble anticryptococcal factors in CSF, as well as the decreased host response caused by the polysaccharide capsule of the fungus, results in the neurotrophic tendency of crytococci. CNS infection can be either meningeal or parenchymal.[37] Meningitis is often the primary manifestation and is most pronounced at the base of the brain. The clinical course is typically fulminant if untreated. The cryptococci can be shown directly in India ink preparations of CSF, in which the thick capsule is seen as a clear halo around the round and budding cells. Latex agglutination detection of the cryptococcal antigen in CSF is a sensitive test for diagnosis.

In histologic section, the fungus shows round bodies 4 to 7 μm across surrounded by a capsule 3 to 5 μm in thickness. Budding with a thin attachment is evident. Clusters of organisms give a soap-bubble appearance in the leptomeninges and Virchow-Robin spaces and are highlighted by GMS, PAS, or mucicarmine stains (**Fig. 8**). Parenchymal involvement, also known as cryptococcomas, is characterized by dilated Virchow-Robin spaces or cortical nodules. Common parenchymal sites are the midbrain and the basal ganglia. Parenchymal lesions show a chronic granulomatous reaction composed of macrophages, lymphocytes, and foreign body–type giant cells. Cryptococcomas may also arise within the choroid plexus leading to obstructive hydrocephalus. Cerebral infarctions, usually located in the basal ganglia, internal capsule, and thalamus, may occur in 4% of cases with cryptococcal meningitis.[36]

Mucormycosis

Mucormycosis is a rare but life-threatening opportunistic fungal infection caused by one of the

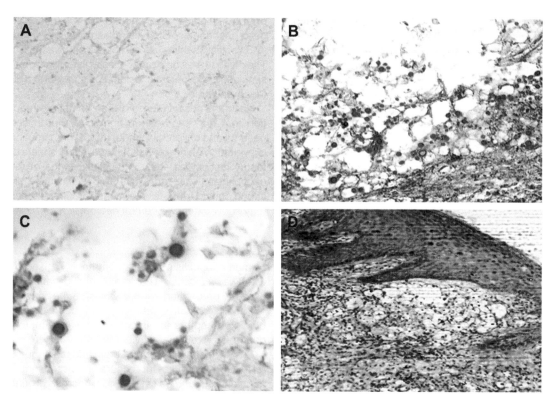

Fig. 8. A case of disseminated cryptococcosis presenting with cryptococcal meningitis. (A) Low-power view showing microbes with lymphocytic infiltrate and proteinaceous exudates in meninges (H&E, 100× digital magnification) highlighted in (B) mucicarmine stain (100× digital magnification). (C) High-power view of round, capsulated budding cryptococci in lung (mucicarmine, 400× digital magnification). (D) Section from a skin biopsy also showing dermal cryptococci (H&E, 100× digital magnification).

members of the Mucoraceae family, including *Absidia*, *Mucor*, and *Rhizopus*, with *Rhizopus oryzae* (*Rhizopus arrhizus*) being the most common cause of infection.[38] The hyphae are broad and nonseptated, with right-angle branching, and are distinct from *Aspergillus*. The hyphal forms are invasive, involve blood vessels, and disseminate hematogenously or may spread through the paranasal sinuses into the brain and orbits.[33,39] At least 70% of the reported cases have diabetes. Other susceptible groups include intravenous drug abusers; cases of anemia, leukemia, uremia, and severe burns; and patients receiving corticosteroids or chemotherapy.[40] A characteristic feature of mucormycosis is vascular invasion resulting in hemorrhage, thrombosis, infarction, and necrosis of tissue.[39]

Sinus infection from rhinocerebral mucormycosis spreads through the cribriform plate along the vessels or via extension into the orbit and then through the optic canal or superior orbital fissure into the cavernous sinus.[33] Isolated CNS mucormycosis in the absence of sinus involvement is rare and is observed in drug abusers, having

been contracted through the spores in the injected substances. Infarcts and abscesses are found on imaging studies, most commonly in the basal ganglia.[39] Involvement of basal ganglia has been observed in 82% of drug abusers whereas non–drug abusers showed involvement in only 9% of cases.[41]

The typical hyphae are broad, 5 to 20 μm wide, nonseptate, irregular in contour, and pleomorphic. The walls appear amphophilic in H&E sections and stain weakly with GMS. The angioinvasive nature of the fungus gives rise to pathologic lesions similar to aspergillosis.

Blastomycosis

Blastomycosis is caused by *Blastomyces dermatitidis*, a thermally dimorphic fungus producing mycelia with 2-mm to 10-mm round to oval or pear-shaped conidia at 25.8°C and broad-based budding yeasts with thick refractile walls varying in size from 8 to 30 mm in diameter at 37.8°C.[42,43] The yeast form disseminates by a hematogenous route, causing systemic disease.

Blastomycosis is primarily a disease of the lung. Infection is acquired through inhalation of aerosolized conidia or by direct extension from sinus or orbits. It usually presents with meningitis, subdural focal leptomeningeal abscess, or intraparenchymal abscess.[42]

Pathologic manifestations include meningitis, granulomas, or abscess. The yeast cell of *Blastomyces* undergoes broad-based budding. Isolating the organism is required for a diagnosis of blastomycosis. Serologic tests for antibodies are not useful for diagnosis of blastomycosis.[43]

Coccidioidomycosis

Coccidioidomycosis is a systemic infection caused by the dimorphic fungus *Coccidioides immitis*. Infection occurs through airborne arthrospore inhalation. The heavier the inoculation, the more serious the resulting infection. Coccidioidomycosis has been observed in endemic areas after severe dust storms, and in members of archaeological expeditions who have disturbed the soil.

In most cases, the infection is asymptomatic or causes mild illness. Approximately, 4% to 5% of symptomatic patients may develop disseminated disease with associated significant morbidity and, occasionally, mortality. CNS meningeal involvement is secondary to hematogenous dissemination from the lungs.[44]

The disease may manifest as meningitis and ependymitis, hydrocephalus, solitary or multiple granulomas, white matter disease, vasculitis, or spinal arachnoiditis. Vasculitis involves the small penetrating branches of the major cerebral vessels, resulting in deep ischemic infarction. Subarachnoid hemorrhage is a rare and fatal complication secondary to rupture of mycotic aneurysm.[45]

Histologic sections show a granulomatous necrotic response. Organisms are observed as large, round spherules or spore-forming structures, 20 to 35 μm in diameter, and have a thick refractile capsule. The spherules have endospores 2 to 5 μm in diameter.

Histoplasmosis

Histoplasmosis, caused by the dimorphic fungus *Histoplasma capsulatum*, can produce a spectrum of illness, from subclinical infection to progressive disseminated disease.[46] CNS involvement is clinically recognized in 5% to 10% of cases of progressive disseminated histoplasmosis; however, autopsy data suggest that it occurs in up to 25% of cases.[46] Sites of CNS involvement include the basilar meninges, brain parenchyma with a predilection for the gray-white matter junction, and, rarely, the spinal cord. Isolated involvement

of the thalamus and choroid plexus has also been described.[47] CNS histoplasmosis may occur in 3 forms: meningitis, cerebritis, and vasculitis. The disease may also present as a histoplasmoma, simulating a neoplastic lesion, or as cerebral miliary granulomas.[48]

Histoplasmosis induces a granulomatous reaction that may be weak in immunocompromised patients and children in whom mixed inflammation is evident. Multinucleated giant cells and sheets of foamy histiocytes show intracellular loads of the capsulated yeast form. On GMS stain, the cells show a halo due to the capsule. Granulomas may show extensive central necrosis.

Candidiasis

Human candidiasis is most commonly caused by *Candida albicans*. The rapid multiplication in tissues, production of proteases, adhesions to extracellular matrix proteins, and complement-binding receptors are important virulence factors contributing to its infectivity.[49]

Primary candidiasis of the brain and meninges is rare. CNS involvement occurs in disseminated candidiasis. *Candida* causes focal necrosis around the microcirculation, producing microabscesses, mainly in the region supplied by middle cerebral artery. *Candida* has a predilection for vascular structures causing vasculitis, intraparenchymal hemorrhage, aneurysms, and thrombosis of small vessels with secondary infarction.[50] Histologically, astrocytes, plasma cells, epithelioid cells, and, occasionally, giant cells are evident. The organisms are readily recognized as budding yeasts with narrow base and pseudohyphae in intracellular locations, producing a foamy cytoplasm.

PARASITIC DISEASES

The prevalence of parasitic disease is high in developing countries in Asia, Africa, Central and South America, and Mexico. Although the definite diagnosis of CNS parasitic infection is usually made on histopathology, the clinical diagnosis is generally based on a combination of the ethnicity of the patient, clinical features, serology, and neuroimaging characteristic features. Neuroimaging plays a critical role in diagnosis and management of parasitic disease and provides accurate localization and extent of parasitic load and also the degree of the host's immune response to the parasites. Enzyme-linked immunosorbent assay (ELISA) or indirect hemagglutination of serum or CSF may be useful in the evaluation of patients with nonspecific and inconclusive neuroimaging findings.

Toxoplasmosis

Toxoplasma gondii is an intracellular protozoan that asymptomatically affects a large proportion of the adult population. The latent encysted brady-zoites remain in the tissues and are manifest when there is a decline in immunity, and free tachyzoites are released. Approximately 30% of patients with AIDS develop encephalitis,[51] especially patients with CD4+ cell counts lower than 100/mm[3]. Necrotizing encephalitis is commonly found in the basal ganglia and the corticomedullary junction. Toxoplasma lesions have 3 well-defined zones on pathologic examination: an avascular necrotic center, the intermediate intense inflammatory zone, and the peripheral zone with encysted *Toxoplasma* (**Fig. 9**). The peripheral ring enhancement corresponds with the inflammatory zone, but direct correlation with the central target has not been well documented.[52]

Echinococcosis

Echinococcosis, or hydatid disease, is caused in humans by *Echinococcus granulosus* and *Echinococcus multilocularis*, which are responsible for cystic echinococcosis and alveolar echinococcosis, respectively. The Mediterranean and the Middle East are endemic regions.

For the life cycle to be completed, the hydatid cyst from the intermediate host liver, lung, or brain must be ingested by the definitive host. The definitive host, the dog for the domestic cycle, in turn ingests infected meat harboring hydatid cysts. *E granulosus* infection of the CNS has been estimated at less than 2%, and may be primary, often presenting as solitary parenchymal cysts. Intraventricular and meningeal locations are exceptional. Secondary involvement is caused by the cyst rupture or hydatid fluid dissemination from a distant organ such as the heart. Damage occurs because of cyst formation within the brain, cerebellum, skull, or vertebrae, and, more rarely, in the brain stem or the spinal cord through vertebral or rib infection.[53] On gross evaluation, hydatid cyst shows a smooth, white wall with a lamellated acellular chitin in histologic sections. A lining of membranous germinal layer with hydatid protoscolices, also free floating sand in cyst fluid, is present in viable cysts. The sand represents protoscolices or brood capsules in histology. Eventually the parasite dies and resulting debris, including the hooklets, may remain as hydatid sand. The parenchyma at the periphery is compressed and shows a host-derived capsule with reactive gliosis and fibrosis with variable inflammatory response (**Fig. 10**).

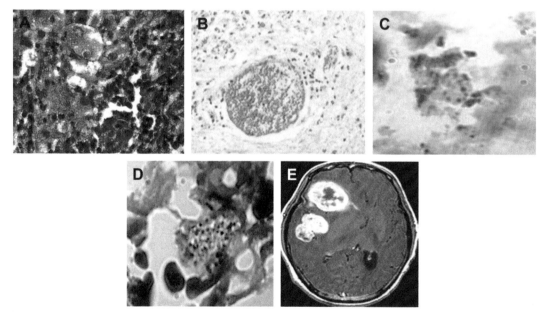

Fig. 9. Toxoplasmosis. (*A*) H&E-stained sections disclosed widespread areas of inflammatory necrosis, circumscribed areas of granulomatous inflammation (400× digital magnification) with (*B*) cysts containing a variable number of microorganisms and *Toxoplasma* free in the damaged tissue (100× digital magnification). (*C*) Squash smear shows oval intracytoplasmic parasites (methylene blue, 400× digital magnification) and (*D*) GMS stain shows clusters of small oval intracytoplasmic parasites (400× digital magnification). (*E*) Axial MR imaging shows multiple enhancing lesions in the right frontotemporal region with mass effect.

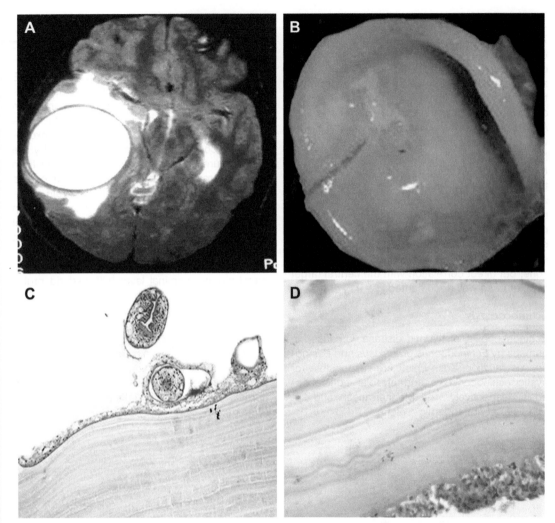

Fig. 10. Hydatid cyst. (*A*) MR image in T2 showing a well-defined round large hypointense lesion with isointense wall and perilesional edema. (*B*) Macrophotograph of the cyst wall showing a translucent white cyst. (*C*) Section showing a viable cyst lined by a germinal layer with brood capsules (H&E, 40× digital magnification). (*D*) Wall showing inflammatory exudate at the periphery of the cyst (H&E, 100× digital magnification).

Amebiasis

Amebic infestations of the brain manifest as secondary brain abscess or primary meningoencephalitis. Secondary amebic abscesses are caused by *Entamoeba histolytica*, which primarily infests the colon directly. The reported incidence of amebic brain abscesses in patients with confirmed amebic liver abscess varies from 0.6% to 8.1%. CNS infection without hepatic involvement is rare.[50] Amebic brain abscesses may be single or multiple, and commonly involve cortical and deep gray matter. The commonest sites of involvement of the brain are the frontal lobe and basal ganglia regions, with the left side being more common than the right by a ratio of 2.3:1.[54] Abscess shows central necrotic and hemorrhagic

anchovy sauce–like pus with inflammation that contains acute and chronic inflammatory cells without granulomas or eosinophils. Trophozoites are evident. Histologic evaluation of this lesion shows a chronic perivascular inflammation with lymphocytes, plasma cells, and macrophages with multinucleated giant cells. The trophozoites are 15 to 40 μm in diameter with a prominent vesicular nucleus and a central nucleolus. The cytoplasm has a blue hue and the nucleus is purple in H&E-stained sections. In PAS, the blue cytoplasm shows flecks of pink. The cysts are surrounded by a double membrane and the cyst wall is also positive with PAS and GMS. Fresh unstained preparations of the aspirated pus or CSF may show characteristic motile trophozoites forming pseudopodia. Subacute or chronic CNS infections caused by *Acanthamoeba* spp, *Balamuthia mandrillaris*, and *Sappinia diploidea*, which occasionally cause cerebral abscess, are termed granulomatous amebic encephalitis. The 2 species are indistinguishable morphologically and may be identified in immunohistochemical evaluation using polyclonal rabbit antisera from the desired species. Cerebral amebiasis is an important and potentially lethal condition in the differential diagnosis of brain abscess, especially when no recognized pathogen is isolated from the pus. Serology is helpful in nonendemic areas only.

Cerebral Malaria

Cerebral malaria is a life-threatening complication of *Plasmodium falciparum* infestation that occurs in approximately 2% of cases.[55] The histologic findings in cerebral malaria include sequestration of infected erythrocyte in brain vessels, mainly cortical and perforating arteries, with perivascular ring hemorrhages and white matter necrosis.[56,57] In some cases, irreversible myelin damage may eventually occur. Recent pathologic and experimental studies have focused on the effect of endothelial activation, nonspecific immune inflammatory response, and subsequent release of cytokines. These factors could lead to vascular engorgement and vasodilatation with cerebral blood flow and edema, which might explain the presence of increased intracranial pressure and brain swelling.[56,57] The hypothesis of brain swelling resulting from vasodilatation and edema may explain the reversal of clinical and MR imaging signs with successful treatment.[58]

NEUROCYSTICERCOSIS

Neurocysticercosis (NCC) is infection of the CNS by the larvae of *Taenia solium*. Pig is the intermediate host, whereas humans are definitive hosts and may accidentally be intermediate hosts as well. Approximately 50 million people are believed to have cysticercosis worldwide. NCC is the most common cause of adult-onset seizures in developing countries. Cysticercosis is endemic in many areas, particularly in several countries in Central and South America, sub-Saharan Africa, India, and Asia.

Cysticercosis occurs by ingestion of eggs by humans; the embryos are released in the small intestine and invade the bowel wall, and they disseminate hematogenously to other tissues and develop into cysticerci in a period of 3 weeks to 2 months. Cysticerci are liquid-filled vesicles consisting of a membranous wall and a nodule containing the invaginated scolex. The scolex has a head with suckers and hooks and a rudimentary body. Humans with cysticercosis are incidental intermediate dead-end hosts.

Four stages of development and regression of NCC have been described on imaging and histopathology and these are grouped as vesicular or cystic, necrotic colloidal, granular nodular, and fibrocalcified stages.[59] In the vesicular or cystic stage, the parasite is viable and composed of well-defined, fluid-filled membrane and scolex, a pathognomonic of NCC. On histologic evaluation, the cysticercus cyst is well separated from the adjacent brain parenchyma, which at this stage shows no evidence of edema or inflammation. The cysticercus comprises a bladder wall with an eccentric single inverted scolex made up of body cavity lined by cuticle with an underlying tall columnar epithelium.[60] Four suckers are present along with a central rostellum with 2 rows of hooklets in the inverted scolex. The bladder wall shows a cuticular and epithelial lining that is thrown into lacelike folds in histologic sections, with underlying loose tissue showing excretory tubules and muscle fibers (**Fig. 11**).

The colloidal stage corresponds to parasite degeneration and the associated inflammatory response in the surrounding parenchyma. The cystic fluid becomes turbid, the surrounding capsule thickens, and an intense inflammatory cell response appears around the cyst. The inflammatory response is predominantly lymphocytic with mostly T cells, mixed with a few B cells. A few eosinophils may also be present. In some cases, a granulomatous reaction may develop. The surrounding parenchyma shows gliosis, fibrosis, and edema.

In the nodular-granular stage, the larva retracts and its fluid content is absorbed. Fibrosis develops with time, progressively occupying the entire lesion. The inflammatory capsule becomes thick and collagenous. The calcified stage is the last stage, in which the fibrous nodule undergoes mineralization and subsequently calcification, which may result from partial dystrophic calcification of the necrotic larva or from the presence of cysticercal calcareous corpuscles.

Parasitic infections like trichinosis, *Toxocara canis*, schistosomiasis, and fasciola may infect the CNS. Isolated cases with MR imaging features have been described and are nonspecific for these conditions.[61]

VIRAL INFECTIONS

Major neurotropic viruses include herpes simplex virus (HSV), varicella-zoster virus (VZV), enteroviruses, and adenoviruses.[62] Viruses gain access

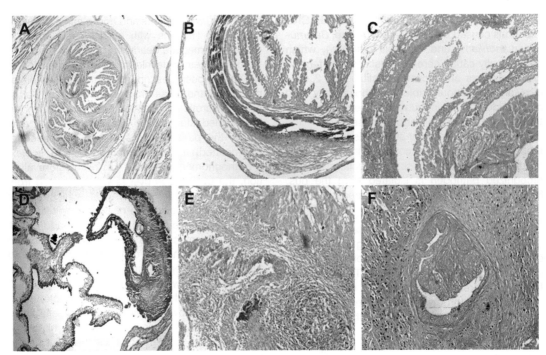

Fig. 11. Stages in the evolution of *Cysticercus cellulosae*. (*A*) Viable cyst. (*B*) Early degeneration with focal calcification. (*C*) Marker inflammation in the surrounding parenchyma. (*D*) Degenerated cyst with edematous bladder wall and partly calcified scolex. (*E*) Granulomatous reaction that may sometimes occur around a degenerating cyst. (*F*) Fibrotic cyst (H&E, 40× digital magnification).

to the CNS through hematogenous dissemination or, less frequently, along the peripheral nerves.[63] Viral infections may cause meningitis or involve gray and white matter, producing either necrotizing or nonnecrotizing panencephalitis.[63,64] Clinical diagnosis is usually based on clinical signs, symptoms, serologic data, and CSF analysis.[65,66] MR imaging, along with advanced techniques such as diffusion imaging and MR spectroscopy, plays an important role in the diagnosis of viral encephalitis. However, the mainstay of diagnosis remains the demonstration of viral DNA or viral serologic markers in the CSF.[67]

HSV

HSV-1 causes viral encephalitis in adults, whereas HSV-2 affects mainly neonates.[68] HSV-1 has a predilection for the limbic system and spreads intracranially, through meningeal branches of the trigeminal nerve, with a tendency to involve the medial temporal and inferior frontal lobes.[69] Temporal lobe abnormality on brain imaging is a strong evidence of herpes simplex encephalitis. Cingulate gyrus and orbitofrontal regions are other commonly involved locations.[70] Histologically, the lesions are characterized by localization,

predominantly to the temporal lobes, where necrotizing, hemorrhagic encephalitis ensues. Necrotic foci show lipid-laden macrophages and perivascular lymphocytic cuffing with pronounced microglial reaction. The lymphocytic response is long-lived and persists even after therapy. Macrophages remain in the necrotic cavities for months to years. However, cells showing the classic cytopathic effects of the virus in the form of intranuclear inclusions in the oligodendroglia, astrocytes, or neurons are not always visible, especially in areas of marked necrosis or when the patient is on antiviral therapy. The diagnosis requires viral cultures or brain tissue or demonstration of HSV DNA by nucleic acid amplification or in situ hybridization. Viral DNA can also be shown by PCR in the CSF.[63,67] A negative PCR obtained during the first 72 hours of disease does not exclude the disease.[68,70]

Japanese Encephalitis

Japanese encephalitis (JE), a *Culex* mosquito–borne flaviviral encephalomyelitis, remains the single most important cause of acute viral encephalitis on a worldwide basis. The largest recent major outbreak of JE occurred in the Uttar Pradesh province of India in 2005.[71]

The JE virus invades the nervous system via the hematogenous route and subsequently spreads along dendritic axons. Early infection is characterized by microglial nodules with polymorphonuclear infiltrate and fat-laden macrophages with perivascular lymphocytic cuffing. As the disease progresses, lesions decrease in cellularity and appear spongy with destruction of axons and myelin. Intense neuronophagia is characteristic of JE infections. Unlike herpes simplex encephalitis, the anterior temporal lobe usually is spared, and insular involvement is rare.[72] The virus infects the neurons, where it multiplies and can be shown by the presence of viral antigens in the neurons and capillary endothelial cells.

Dengue Virus Encephalitis

Dengue virus is transmitted by *Aedes aegypti*.[73] Neurologic involvement occurs in 4% to 5% of dengue infection and may be categorized into (1) patients with direct involvement of brain and spinal cord (encephalitis and myelitis), and (2) secondary involvement (encephalopathy) caused by cerebral edema, cerebral hemorrhage, hyponatremia, hepatic failure, cerebral anoxia, microcapillary hemorrhage, and release of toxic products.[74,75] Rabies is caused by neurotropic RNA viruses in the family Rhabdoviridae, genus *Lyssavirus*.[75] Transmission to humans is mainly through bites of infected rabid dogs, cats, bats, and other wild animals. Other modes of transmission are through inhalation, contact of saliva with an open wound or mucous membrane, and via infected corneal transplants.

The incubation period of rabies is typically 2 to 8 weeks.[76] The virus replicates in the muscle in neuromuscular spindles or motor end plates. Alternatively, the virus may directly affect the sensory nerve endings of the superficial soft tissue. The passage of the virus to the CNS occurs axonally through retrograde axoplasmic flow until the virus reaches the next neuronal cell body.[76] Human rabies manifests in 2 forms: encephalitic and paralytic.[77] In paralytic rabies, the medulla and the spinal cord are mainly involved, whereas in the encephalitic form, the brain stem, cerebrum, and limbic system are involved.[78] Involvement of the basal ganglia and the thalamus is usually seen late in the disease.[78] Both forms of the disease are invariably fatal and most patients die within 10 days of the onset of neurologic symptoms.

The predominant involvement of gray matter of the brain and spinal cord is a hallmark of rabies and is important in differentiating rabies from acute disseminated encephalomyelitis.[79] Cerebral edema is accompanied by a variable amount of perivascular lymphocytic infiltration, microglial proliferation, and neuronophagia. Intraneuronal eosinophilic inclusions (Negri bodies) are diagnostic and are observed best in the Purkinje cells, pyramidal neurons of the cerebral cortex, hippocampus, and large neurons of the cerebellar nuclei. Antimortem diagnosis by a PCR in saliva has been developed recently.[80]

Measles Encephalitis

Measles infection can result in 3 different forms of encephalitis: acute measles encephalitis, subacute sclerosing panencephalitis (SSPE), and measles inclusion body encephalitis.[81] Acute measles encephalitis usually occurs in nonimmunocompromised patients, mostly in children and adolescents but rarely in adults.[81] Diagnosis is usually made from the clinical course and positive immunoglobulin M and immunoglobulin G antibodies to measles in serum and CSF.[82] Pathology shows perivascular inflammation and demyelination. Bilateral striatal necrosis, transient pseudoatrophy, and cerebral vein thrombosis also have been reported.[83,84]

SSPE

SSPE is a rare, postinfectious, progressive form of encephalitis that usually occurs in children and adolescents within a few years after measles infection. The disease is incurable and usually causes death within 2 to 4 years of onset. The diagnosis is based on clinical findings, electroencephalography results, and titers of measles antibodies in the serum and CSF.[85] Early diffuse cerebral swelling may be present in subcortical and periventricular white matter and the basal ganglia region. It can be rapidly progressive and diffuse cortical atrophy is seen in advanced cases.[84] Histologically, the disease is characterized by leptomeningeal, parenchymal, and perivascular inflammation. Reactive gliosis with white matter demyelination accompanies neuronal loss. Intranuclear inclusions are evident in the neurons and oligodendroglia and can be stained using a viral antibody. In later stages, the inclusions may not be evident but viral DNA can be shown by in situ hybridization.[86]

NUTRITIONAL DEFICIENCY DISEASES

Nutritional deficiency is a global problem that is more common and severe in developing countries. Poverty, dietary deficiency, and coexisting infections and infestations contribute to the nutritional deficiency. Protein calorie, minerals, and vitamins, especially of the B complex group, are important in the context of neurologic manifestations. Because of chronic deprivation, there may be multiple deficiencies affecting skin, hair, mucous membrane, bones, and the nervous system. All parts of the nervous system, such as cerebrum, cerebellum, spinal cord, peripheral nerves, and muscles, may be affected in isolation or in various combinations. Neuroimaging may have a role in documentation of the anatomic sites in the CNS (brain and spinal cord). Vitamin B_1 and B_{12} deficiency may show typical imaging features.

Thiamine Deficiency

Thiamine is the precursor of coenzyme thiamine pyrophosphate, which catalyzes the oxidative decarboxylation of pyruvate and α-decarboxylase with production of coenzyme A. The daily requirement of thiamine is 0.3 to 1.6 mg and it is increased with high-carbohydrate diet, pregnancy, lactation, and thyrotoxicosis. Excessive loss of thiamine occurs in diarrhea, hemodialysis, and the diuretic phase of renal failure. Thiamine deficiency results in Wernicke encephalopathy (WE), Korsakoff syndrome (KS), and beriberi. Acute thiamine deficiency is associated with WE, which has marked neuropathologic changes in periventricular nuclei, hypothalamic nuclei, tectal plate, and thalamus. Electron microscopy shows chromatin clumping and swelling of degenerating neurons in diencephalic nuclei in experimental animals.

The chronic stage of WE reveals atrophy of mamillary bodies, cortical thinning, sulcal widening, and ventriculomegaly. Detailed examination reveals loss of brain volume that is obvious in postmortem studies. Multiple subclinical bouts of thiamine or other nutritional deficiencies in alcoholism may contribute to the graded effect of brain regional volume deficits, heterogeneity of clinical syndrome, and the pathologic findings.[87]

Vitamin B_{12} Deficiency

Deficiency of vitamin B_{12} impairs the functions of methionine synthetase and methyl melonyl CoA mutase. Impairment of methyl melonyl CoA mutase results in production of abnormal fatty acids that alter the production of myelin. Methylation of myelin basic protein can stabilize its insertion in the myelin sheath, which may play a role in the pathogenesis of myelin damage.

The most important cause of vitamin B_{12} deficiency is pernicious anemia, which is an autoimmune gastropathy targeting the parietal cells, which produce acid and intrinsic factor. Causes of vitamin B_{12} deficiency are atrophic gastritis caused by *Helicobacter pylori*, gastric resection,

ileal disease, ileal resection, diverticulosis, bacterial overgrowth, pancreatic disease, and tropical sprue. The pathologic changes of vitamin B_{12} deficiency have been reported as subacute combined degeneration of the spinal cord. The main pathologic features are swelling of myelin sheath, followed by demyelination and astrocytic gliosis. These changes start in posterior columns of the lower cervical and upper thoracic spinal cord and spread up and down. Later, the lateral columns are also affected. Optic nerves reveal degeneration of myelinated fibers in the territory of papillomacular bundles. Demyelination has also been seen in cerebral white matter. Axonal degeneration without significant demyelination is seen in the peripheral nerve.[87,88]

The laboratory diagnosis of vitamin B_{12} deficiency is established by low serum vitamin B_{12} level (<211 pg/L), megaloblastic bone marrow, low serum methyl malonic acid, and high homocysteine levels are surrogate markers of vitamin B_{12} deficiency. Blood smear may show macrocytosis, hypersegmented polymorphonuclear cells, and raised mean corpuscular volume. Antiintrinsic factor antibody is specific of pernicious anemia. Antiparietal cell antibody is found in 80% to 90% patients with pernicious anemia, but its specificity is doubtful.

SUMMARY

Tropical diseases of the CNS can be classified into 2 groups: infective and noninfective. Infective CNS diseases, although preventable, remain a major cause of morbidity and mortality in the tropics. A large variety of infectious agents can invade the CNS and cause damage. Specific causal diagnosis of CNS infections continues to be a major challenge and a multimodal diagnostic approach involving neuroimaging, histopathology, and microbial culture may help in resolving the issue. This article describes the pathology of a diverse group of infectious and noninfectious illnesses that affect the CNS in tropical countries. It is important to know the disease burden in a particular tropical region so that triaging of tests, especially for viral pathogens, can be done to rationalize the cost.

REFERENCES

1. Habib AA, Mozaffar T. Brain abscess. Arch Neurol 2001;58:1302–4.
2. Garg M, Gupta RK, Husain M, et al. Brain abscesses: etiologic categorization with in vivo proton MR spectroscopy. Radiology 2004;230:519–27.

3. Prasad KN, Mishra AM, Gupta D, et al. Analysis of microbial etiology and mortality in patients with brain abscess. J Infect 2006;53:221–7.

4. Osenbach RK, Loftus CM. Diagnosis and management of brain abscess. Neurosurg Clin N Am 1992; 3:403–20.

5. Brook I. Brain abscess in children: microbiology and management. J Child Neurol 1995;10:283–8.

6. Roos KL, Tyler KL. Meningitis, encephalitis, brain abscess and empyema. In: Braunwald E, Fauci AS, Kasper DL, et al, editors. Harrison's principle of internal medicine. 16th edition. USA: McGraw-Hill; 2005. p. 2471–89.

7. Whiteman MLH, Bowen BC, Post MJD, et al. Intracranial infection. In: Atlas SW, editor. Magnetic resonance imaging of the brain and spine. 3rd edition. Philadelphia: Lippincott Williams & Wilkins; 2002. p. 1099–177.

8. Luthra G, Parihar A, Nath K, et al. Comparative evaluation of fungal, tubercular, and pyogenic brain abscesses with conventional and diffusion MR imaging and proton MR spectroscopy. AJNR Am J Neuroradiol 2007;28:1332–8.

9. Kao PT, Tseng HK, Liu CP, et al. Brain abscess: clinical analysis of 53 cases. J Microbiol Immunol Infect 2003;36:129–36.

10. Falcone S, Post MJ. Encephalitis, cerebritis, and brain abscess: pathophysiology and imaging findings. Neuroimaging Clin N Am 2000;10:333–5.

11. Zimmerman RD, Weingarten K. Neuroimaging of cerebral abscesses. Neuroimaging Clin N Am 1991;1:1–16.

12. Kielian T. Immunopathogenesis of brain abscess. J Neuroinflammation 2004;1:16.

13. Raviglione MC, Snider DE Jr, Kochi A. Global epidemiology of tuberculosis: morbidity and mortality of a worldwide epidemic. JAMA 1995;273:220–6.

14. Tandon PN, Pathak SN. Tuberculosis of the central nervous system. In: Spillane JD, editor. Tropical neurology. New York: Oxford University Press; 1973. p. 37–62.

15. Shah GV, Desai SB, Malde H, et al. Tuberculosis of sphenoid sinus: CT findings. AJNR 1993;161:681–2.

16. Dastur DK, Manghani DK, Udani PM. Pathology and pathogenic mechanisms in neurotuberculosis. Radiol Clin North Am 1995;33:733–52.

17. Kennedy DH, Fallon RJ. Tubercular meningitis. JAMA 1979;241:264–8.

18. Gupta RK, Gupta S, Singh D, et al. MR imaging and angiography in tubercular meningitis. Neuroradiology 1994;36:87–92.

19. Kioumehr F, Dadsetan MR, Rooholamini AA. Central nervous system tuberculosis: MRI. Neuroradology 1994;36:93–6.

20. Whiteman M, Espinoza L, Post MJD, et al. Central nervous system tuberculosis in HIV-infected patients: clinical and radiographic findings. AJNR Am J Neuroradiol 1995;16:1319–27.

21. Singh I, Haris M, Husain M, et al. Role of endoscopic third ventriculostomy in patients with communicating hydrocephalus: an evaluation by MR ventriculography. Neurosurg Rev 2008;31:319–25.

22. Dastur DK, Lalitha VS, Udani PM, et al. The brain and meninges in tubercular meningitis-gross pathology in 100 cases and pathogenesis. Neurol India 1970;18:86–100.

23. Gupta RK, Jena A, Sharma A, et al. MR imaging of intracranial tuberculomas. J Comput Assist Tomogr 1988;12:280–5.

24. Gajraj A, Grover YK. The impact of CT on the diagnosis of tuberculomas. The International Seminar on Medical Imaging 25th anniversary of the Chinese University of Hong Kong. Hong Kong, June–July, 1988.

25. Jinkins JR, Gupta R, Chang KH, et al. MR imaging of the central nervous system tuberculosis. Radiol Clin North Am 1995;33:771–86.

26. Garcia-Monco JC. Central nervous system tuberculosis. Neurol Clin 1999;17:737–59.

27. Haris M, Gupta RK, Husain M, et al. Assessment of therapeutic response on serial dynamic contrast enhanced MR imaging in brain tuberculomas. Clin Radiol 2008;63:562–74.

28. Whitener DR. Tuberculous brain abscess. Report of a case and review of the literature. Arch Neurol 1978;35:148–55.

29. Brooks WD, Fletcher AP, Wilson RR. Spinal cord complications of tubercular meningitis; a clinical and pathological study. Q J Med 1954;23:275–90.

30. Sharif HS, Aabed MY, Haddad MC. Magnetic resonance imaging and computed tomography of infectious spondylitis. In: Bloem JL, Satoris DJ, editors. MRI and CT of the musculoskeletal system: a text atlas. Baltimore (MD): Williams & Wilkins; 1992. p. 580–602.

31. Oliver K, Isabel W, Matthias M. Neuroimaging of infections. NeuroRx 2005;2:324–32.

32. Miaux Y, Ribaud P, Williams M, et al. MR of cerebral aspergillosis in patients who have had bone marrow transplantation. AJNR Am J Neuroradiol 1995;16:555–62.

33. Ostrow TD, Hudgins PA. Magnetic resonance imaging of intracranial fungal infections. Top Magn Reson Imaging 1994;6:22–31.

34. Tempkin AD, Sobonya RE, Seeger JF, et al. Cerebral aspergillosis: radiologic and pathologic findings. Radiographics 2006;26:1239–42.

35. Awasthi M, Patankar T, Shah P, et al. Cerebral cryptococcosis: atypical appearances on CT. Br J Radiol 2001;74:83–5.

36. Aharon-Peretz J, Kliot D, Finkelstein R, et al. Cryptococcal meningitis mimicking vascular dementia. Neurology 2004;62:2135.

37. Saigal G, Post MJ, Lolayekar S, et al. Unusual presentation of central nervous system cryptococcal

infection in an immunocompetent patient. AJNR Am J Neuroradiol 2005;26:2522–6.

38. Spellberg B, Edwards J, Ibrahim A. Novel perspectives on mucormycosis: pathophysiology, presentation, and management. Clin Microbiol Rev 2005;18:556–69.

39. Horger M, Hebart H, Schimmel H, et al. Disseminated mucormycosis in haematological patients: CT and MRI findings with pathological correlation. Br J Radiol 2006;79:88–95.

40. Terk MR, Underwood DJ, Zee CS, et al. MR imaging in rhinocerebral and intracranial mucormycosis with CT and pathologic correlation. Magn Reson Imaging 1992;10:81–7.

41. Stave GM, Heimberger T, Kerkering TM. Zygomycosis of the basal ganglia in intravenous drug users. Am J Med 1989;86:115–7.

42. Bakleh M, Aksamit AJ, Tleyjeh IM, et al. Successful treatment of cerebral blastomycosis with voriconazole. Clin Infect Dis 2005;40:69–71.

43. Wheat J. Endemic mycoses in AIDS: a clinical review. Clin Microbiol Rev 1995;8:146–59.

44. Cortez KJ, Walsh TJ, Bennett JE. Successful treatment of coccidioidal meningitis with voriconazole. Clin Infect Dis 2003;36:1619–22.

45. Hadley MN, Martin NA, Spetzler RF, et al. Multiple intracranial aneurysms due to *Coccidioides immitis* infection. J Neurosurg 1987;66:453–6.

46. Bradsher RW. Histoplasmosis and blastomycosis. Clin Infect Dis 1996;22:102–11.

47. Tan V, Wilkins P, Badve S, et al. Histoplasmosis of the central nervous system. J Neurol Neurosurg Psychiatry 1992;55:619–22.

48. Gasparetto EL, Carvalho Neto A, Alberton J, et al. Histoplasmoma as isolated central nervous system lesion in an immunocompetent patient. Arq Neuropsiquiatr 2005;63:689–92.

49. Odds FC. Pathogenesis of candida infections. J Am Acad Dermatol 1994;31:2–5.

50. Campbell S. Amoebic brain abscess and meningoencephalitis. Semin Neurol 1993;13:153–60.

51. Porter SB, Sande MA. Toxoplasmosis of the central nervous system in the acquired immunodeficiency syndrome. N Engl J Med 1992;327:1643–8.

52. Post MJ, Chan JC, Hensley GT, et al. Toxoplasma encephalitis in Haitian adults with acquired immunodeficiency syndrome: a clinical-pathological-CT correlation. AJR Am J Roentgenol 1983;140:861–8.

53. Taratuto AL, Venturiello SM. Echinococcosis. Brain Pathol 1997;7:673–9.

54. Lombardo L, Alonso P, Saenz-Arroyo L, et al. Cerebral amoebiasis-report of 17 cases. J Neurosurg 1964;21:704–9.

55. Marsden PD, Bruce-Chwatt LJ. Cerebral malaria. In: Hornabrook RW, editor. Topics on tropical neurology. Philadelphia: FA Davis; 1975. p. 29–44.

56. Janota I, Doshi B. Cerebral malaria in United Kingdom. J Clin Pathol 1979;32:769–72.

57. Turner G. Cerebral malaria. Brain Pathol 1997;7: 569–82.

58. Cordoliani YS, Sarrazin JL, Felten D, et al. MR of cerebral malaria. AJNR Am J Neuroradiol 1998;19: 871–4.

59. Dumas JL, Visy JM, Belin C, et al. Parenchymal neurocysticercosis: follow-up and staging by MRI. Neuroradiology 1997;39:12–8.

60. Del Brutto OH, Rajshekhar V, White AC Jr, et al. Proposed diagnostic criteria for neurocysticercosis. Neurology 2001;24:177–83.

61. Vatsal DK, Kapoor S, Venkatesh V, et al. Ectopic fascioliasis in the dorsal spine: case report. Neurosurgery 2006;59:E706–7 [discussion: E706–7].

62. Hinson VK, Tyor WR. Update on viral encephalitis. Curr Opin Neurol 2001;14:369–74.

63. Rumboldt Z, Thurnher MM, Gupta RK. Central nervous system infections. Semin Roentgenol 2007;42:62–91.

64. Shankar SK, Mahadevan A, Kovoor JME. Neuropathology of viral infections of the central nervous system. Neuroimaging Clin N Am 2008;18:19–39.

65. Uhlmann EJ, Storch GA. Viral encephalitis. Lab Med 2001;32:317–23.

66. Weber W, Henkes H, Felber S, et al. Diagnostic imaging in viral encephalitis. Radiologe 2000;40: 998–1010.

67. Maschke M, Kastrup O, Forsting M, et al. Update on neuroimaging in infectious central nervous system disease. Curr Opin Neurol 2004;17:475–80.

68. Whitley RJ. Herpes simplex encephalitis: adolescents and adults. Antiviral Res 2006;71:141–8.

69. Wong J, Quint DJ. Imaging of central nervous system infections. Semin Roentgenol 1999;34:123–43.

70. Elbers JM, Bitnun A, Richardson SE, et al. A 12 year prospective study of childhood herpes simplex encephalitis: is there a broader spectrum of disease? Pediatrics 2007;119:399–407.

71. Rehle TM. Classification, distribution and importance of arboviruses. Trop Med Parasitol 1989;40:391–5.

72. Pérez-Vélez CM, Anderson MS, Robinson CC, et al. Outbreak of neurologic enterovirus type 71 disease: a diagnostic challenge. Clin Infect Dis 2007; 45:950–7.

73. Bulakbasi N, Kocaoglu M. Central nervous system infections of herpesvirus family. Neuroimaging Clin N Am 2008;18:53–84.

74. Soares CN, Faria LC, Peralta JM, et al. Dengue infection: neurological manifestations and cerebrospinal fluid (CSF) analysis. J Neurol Sci 2006;249: 19–24.

75. Gupta RK, Jain KK, Kumar S. Imaging of nonspecific (nonherpetic) acute viral infections. Neuroimaging Clin N Am 2008;18:41–52.

76. Awasthi M, Parmar H, Patankar T, et al. Imaging findings in rabies encephalitis. AJNR Am J Neuroradiol 2001;22:677–80.

77. Muzaffar J, Venkata Krishnan P, Gupta N, et al. Dengue encephalitis: why we need to identify this entity in a dengue-prone region. Singapore Med J 2006;47:975–7.

78. Bargalló J, Berenguer J, García-Barrionuevo J, et al. The "target sign": is it a specific sign of CNS tuberculoma? Neuroradiology 1996;38:547–50.

79. Desai RV, Jain V, Singh P, et al. Radiculomyelitic rabies: can MR imaging help? AJNR Am J Neuroradiol 2002;23:632–4.

80. Nagaraj T, Vasanth JP, Desai A, et al. Antemortem diagnosis of human rabies using saliva samples from comparison of real time and conventional RT-PCR techniques. J Clin Virol 2006;36:17–23.

81. Jin K, Sato S, Saito R, et al. MRI findings from a case of fulminating adult-onset measles encephalitis. Intern Med 2006;45:783–7.

82. Lee KY, Cho WH, Kim SH, et al. Acute encephalitis associated with measles: MRI features. Neuroradiology 2003;45:100–6.

83. Ruggieri M, Polizzi A, Pavone L, et al. Thalamic syndrome in children with measles infection and selective, reversible thalamic involvement. Pediatrics 1998;101:112–9.

84. Cambonie G, Houdon L, Rivier F, et al. Infantile bilateral striatal necrosis following measles. Brain Dev 2000;22:221–3.

85. Alkan A, Sarac K, Kutlu R, et al. Early- and late-state subacute sclerosing panencephalitis: chemical shift imaging and single-voxel MR spectroscopy. AJNR Am J Neuroradiol 2003;24:501–6.

86. Allen IV, McQuaid S, McMahon J, et al. The significance of measles virus antigen and genome distribution in the CNS in SSPE for mechanisms of viral spread and demyelination. J Neuropathol Exp Neurol 1996;55:471–80.

87. Breslow RA, Guenther PM, Smothers BA. Alcohol drinking patterns and diet quality: the 1999–2000 National Health and Nutrition Examination Survey. Am J Epidemiol 2006;163:359–66.

88. Kunze K, Leitenmaier K. Vitamin B12 deficiency and subacute combined degeneration of the spinal cord (funicular spinal disease). In: Vinken PJ, Bruyn GW, editors. Handbook of Clinical Neurology. In: Vinken PJ, Bruyn GW, Klawans HL, editors. Metabolic and deficiency diseases of the nervous system (part II), vol. 28. Amsterdam: Elsevier; 1976. p. 141–98.

Viral Infections of the Central Nervous System

Sanjeev Kumar Handique, MD

KEYWORDS

• Virus • Infection • Central nervous system • Neuroimaging

Viral infections of the central nervous system (CNS) in humans are uncommon, not because viruses lack neuroinvasive potential, but because access to the CNS is prevented by various factors such as anatomic barriers and virus-specific and nonspecific host immunity. When they do invade the CNS, viruses have the potential to cause infections of any part of the CNS, namely the meninges, brain, or spinal cord, in combination or in isolation, many which have devastating consequences.

Although viruses with CNS-invading potential belong to all families of viruses, those that cause CNS infections in the tropics are different from those of nontropical regions, because of different geographic environments, different insect and animal vectors, frequently compounded by inadequate health care and sanitation facilities in many tropical countries. Ecologic changes of tropical habitats have led to CNS diseases due to emerging viruses in recent times. In an appropriate clinical setting, imaging can often help in establishing possible viral causes of a CNS disease and at times suggest the specific etiologic virus. Imaging becomes more relevant in epidemic encephalitis, where most often the viral cause can be suggested and differentiated from other causes of intracranial infection. As with all CNS infections, magnetic resonance (MR) imaging, with its superior contrast resolution, is preferred to computed tomography (CT) and should be the imaging modality of choice in viral infections of the CNS. This article discusses common causes of viral infections of CNS in the tropics, especially in relation to Asia and the Indian subcontinent, and how imaging can help in the management of these diseases.

VIRAL MENINGITIS

Acute viral meningitis is usually a self-limited disease leading to complete recovery. Enteroviruses (Coxsackie and echoviruses) account for more than half of all cases.[1] Other viruses that may also cause meningitis include mumps, herpes simplex viruses (HSV), and flaviviruses. Enterovirus meningitis may occur in sporadic or epidemic forms and epidemics have been reported from India.[2] However, the etiologic profile of viral meningitides in the Indian subcontinent is largely unknown because the etiologic diagnosis of aseptic meningitis is rarely attempted due to costs, lack of infrastructure, and the self-limiting nature of the disease. One study from China showed meningeal enhancement in MR imaging in 9 out of 23 patients of viral meningitis, whereas CT showed no abnormalities.[3] However, a normal imaging study does not exclude viral meningitis, because both contrast-enhanced MR imaging and fluid-attenuated inversion-recovery (FLAIR) sequences may fail to show any abnormalities.

VIRAL ENCEPHALITIS

Encephalitis is the term used to refer to an infection of the brain, most commonly caused by viruses. Viral encephalitis most commonly presents as an acute illness with fever and altered sensorium with or without focal neurologic deficits. The term acute viral encephalitis or meningoencephalitis is then used; the latter term is used because most viral infections of the brain are accompanied by involvement of the meninges,

Department of Radiology and Imaging, Institute of Neurological Sciences, Dispur, 781006 Assam, India
E-mail address: sanjeevhandique1@gmail.com

Neuroimag Clin N Am 21 (2011) 777–794
doi:10.1016/j.nic.2011.07.012
1052-5149/11/$ – see front matter © 2011 Elsevier Inc. All rights reserved.

neuroimaging.theclinics.com

causing associated aseptic meningitis. Less commonly, viral encephalitis presents as a slower indolent disease process referred to as slow viral infections. In addition, an encephalitic condition that is caused by alteration of immune function in response to a viral illness (acute disseminated encephalomyelitis [ADEM]) needs to be differentiated from acute viral encephalitis in the light of different management for the former condition. This article is limited to acute encephalitides that commonly occur in Asia and the Indian subcontinent, especially those that are endemic to the region and those that are caused by emerging viruses with distinct threat potential. Slow viral infection caused by measles is also discussed because this is a significant problem in Asia and the Indian subcontinent.

The annual incidence of acute encephalitis in the tropics is similar to that in the West, as recent meta-analytical data have shown. In the tropical and Western settings, the annual incidence of encephalitis is 6.34 and 7.4 per 100,000 respectively.[4]

Pathologically, all encephalitides are accompanied by varying degrees of cell necrosis (neuronophagia) and inflammatory changes accompanied by edema.[5] Both areas of cell necrosis and edema are reflected on imaging, especially MR imaging. Variable degrees of inflammation and edema in different encephalitides lead to variability in the diffusion characteristics of the inflamed tissue. For example, in herpes simplex encephalitis (HSE), restriction of diffusion on MR imaging is more marked than in Japanese encephalitis (JE), because the former is a more necrotizing inflammatory disease than the latter.[6] The presence of virus-specific receptors in the cells of the CNS determines susceptibility of the cell to an invading virus. For example, poliovirus invades the anterior horn cells, binding to the CD155 receptor protein. This property lends some specificity to imaging of viral encephalitides. Late sequelae of encephalitis include focal or diffuse atrophy, shrinkage of white matter, and healing of encephalitic and edematous areas by glial reaction.[5] These delayed changes can also be seen on imaging, with residual gliotic lesions of encephalitis tending to be located in the initial areas of involvement. Thus, JE residua may be detected in the thalami, substantia nigra, or basal ganglia.

JE

JE is the most important arboviral encephalitis in the world in terms of incidence, mortality, and morbidity, with more than 50,000 new cases and about 15,000 deaths occurring annually.[7] JE is a mosquito-borne flaviviral encephalitis and is transmitted to man by culicine mosquitoes. It is a zoonosis and the basic cycles of transmission involve the mosquito, pig, and ardeid water birds, with man acting as an incidental dead-end host. Water birds such as herons, egrets, and other ardeid birds are the most important hosts for maintenance of JE virus (JEV), whereas pigs are the most important reservoir and amplifier of the disease. Man-to-man transmission does not occur because viremia in man is low and transient. The geographic area of JE prevalence has been increasing in the past 70 years. Since the first epidemic in Japan in the 1930s, the disease has now become prevalent across several tropical and temperate regions in countries in southern, southeastern, and eastern Asia, the Pacific rim, and recently in the Torres Straits of northern Australia and the Australian mainland. In developed Asian countries such as Japan, Taiwan, and South Korea, JE incidence has dropped considerably as a result of concerted immunization efforts, vector control, improved agricultural practices and animal husbandry, and overall improvement in sanitation. In India, JE is a major public health problem with approximately 2000 to 7000 new cases occurring annually across several Indian states involving almost the entire country.[8,9] Currently, there are more than 10,000 cases being reported annually from China.[10] JE is mostly a disease of children and young adults in endemic areas. In northern Thailand, the annual incidence of JE is estimated to be 40 per 100,000 for ages 5 to 25 years, declining to almost 0 after the age of 35 years.[11,12] When epidemics first occur in new locations such as north and northeastern India, Nepal, and Sri Lanka, adults are also affected. Nonimmune travelers to endemic areas may be particularly susceptible to the disease.[8,13] There are 2 recognized epidemiologic patterns of JE. In the northern areas such as northern Vietnam, northern Thailand, Korea, Japan, Taiwan, China, Nepal, and northern and northeastern India, large epidemics occur during the summer months. In southern areas such as southern Vietnam, southern Thailand, Indonesia, Malaysia, Philippines, Sri Lanka, and southern India, JE tends to be endemic, with peak cases appearing after the start of the rainy season.[14] This variation seems to be related to the temperature rather than the amount of rainfall or different strains of the virus.[15]

After the JEV gains entry through the bite of the mosquito, the virus multiplies locally and in regional lymph nodes. After a period of brief viremia, the virus enters the CNS through the vascular route. Subsequent spread of the virus possibly occurs along the dendrites and axonal processes. The pathologic changes of the brain in fatal cases of JE include vascular congestion, cerebral edema, and brain swelling. Histologically, the leptomeninges show variable degrees of mononuclear inflammation extending along the Virchow-Robin spaces into the brain parenchyma, with formation of perivascular cuffs. Two types of lesions are characteristic microscopically within the brain. The first type of lesion is the cell-rich gliomesenchymal nodule. These lesions are formed by aggregates of microglial cells and lymphocytes around degenerating neurons. They are invariably seen in the medulla. They are also seen in the thalamus, substantia nigra, pontine, and reticular nuclei of brainstem, cerebral cortex, dentate nuclei, and Purkinje cells of the cerebellum. They have also been described in the Ammon's horn of the hippocampus. The second type of lesion is the cell-poor necrolytic lesion seen in the cerebral cortex, thalami, corpus striatum, midbrain, and pons. They are uncommon in the medulla oblongata.[16-18]

JEV infections are mostly asymptomatic and the ratio of clinically apparent to asymptomatic infections may vary from 1:25 to 1:1000.[19] The incubation period of JEV varies from 5 to 15 days.[8] The course of the disease is divided into 3 stages: (1) a prodromal phase preceding CNS features, (2) an encephalitic phase of CNS symptoms, and (3) a late stage in which there is recovery or residual neurologic deficit. Some atypical presentations such as febrile seizures, aseptic meningitis, and acute flaccid paralysis have been described.

The laboratory diagnosis of JE is established by showing (1) a fourfold increase in serum antibody titer, (2) virus isolation, or (3) specific immunoglobulin M (IgM) antibody detection by enzyme immunoassay capture in cerebrospinal fluid (CSF) or serum (Mac-ELISA). The first 2 methods take time and the Mac-ELISA method has the advantage of providing the diagnosis with a single test. However, this test may be positive in CSF in only 50% of patients in the first week of the disease, although it is invariably positive beyond the first week.[17]

The imaging findings of JE reflect the pathologic changes of the brain. The typical imaging findings are lesions in the thalami, substantia nigra, basal ganglia, and hippocampi (Fig. 1). Less commonly, lesions can also be found in the cerebral cortex, midbrain, pons, medulla, cerebellum, and white matter.[20-22] MR imaging has been reported to be more sensitive than CT scan by several investigators and is the imaging investigation of choice. Thalamic lesions are the characteristic finding of JE and are seen in more than 87% to 94% of patients with JE with abnormal MR imaging.[20,23] These can be bilateral or unilateral and are characteristically asymmetric with focal brain swelling in acute lesions (see Figs. 1–3). They appear hyperintense on T2-weighted and FLAIR MR images and slightly hypointense to gray matter on T1-weighted images. On CT, they may appear subtle and slightly hypodense with associated focal brain swelling. JE lesions typically do not enhance after intravenous contrast. Some investigators have reported hemorrhagic lesions, but, in our experience, hemorrhagic changes are rare.[20] In a large series of 62 patients, 89% of the thalamic lesions were bilateral.[23] In a retrospective study of a cohort of patients with CNS infections in a JE-endemic area in southern Vietnam, the presence of thalamic lesions on MR imaging had a sensitivity of 23%, specificity of 100%, positive predictive value of 100%, and a negative predictive value of 42.1% for diagnosis of JE.[24] However, this study used low-field MR imaging (0.06 T), which may explain the low sensitivity found in the study. Our own figures of sensitivity and specificity of thalamic lesions on 1.5-T MR imaging for JE are 93.7% and 54.5% respectively in patients with meningoencephalitic syndrome. In the first week of the disease, the sensitivity and specificity are 90.9% and 50% respectively, which are comparable with Mac-ELISA tests (Handique SK, Deora P, unpublished data, 2011). The presence of thalamic lesions on MR imaging in a JE-endemic area can therefore be a rapid, sensitive, and fairly specific test for separating the patients with JE from those without JE, especially during the summer months when the number of cases of meningoencephalitis increases. Substantia nigra and basal ganglia lesions are the next most common lesions of JE and these too are asymmetric and accompanied by focal brain swelling in acute lesions (see Figs. 1–4). Cortical lesions are most commonly found in the hippocampi, although any part of the cerebral cortex may be involved. We found 17.7% hippocampal involvement in a large series of patients with JE. Hippocampal lesions have a characteristic appearance with predominant involvement of the body and tail with occasional involvement of the head and the amygdalae. Insular involvement is rare (see Fig. 1B, C). The characteristic appearance and associated involvement of the thalami, substantia nigra, and the basal ganglia allow easy differentiation from HSE.[21]

Diffusion-weighted (DW) MR imaging has been reported to help in the early diagnosis and characterize the duration of JE. In a study of 14 patients with JE, lesions appeared either hyperintense on DW imaging, when they were more than or equal to the number of lesions seen on T2-weighted images, or they were hypointense on DW images when more lesions were seen on T2-weighted images. This study found that 9 out of 14 patients showed more lesions on DW images compared

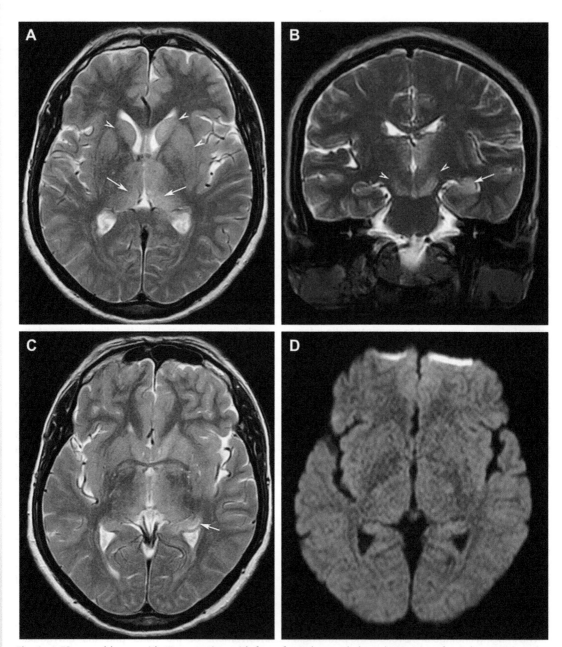

Fig. 1. A 52-year-old man with JE presenting with fever for 7 days and altered sensorium for 2 days. MR imaging was done on day 7 of onset of disease. (*A*) Axial T2-weighted scan showing asymmetric lesions in the thalami (*arrows*) and basal ganglia (*arrowheads*) bilaterally. Note subtle local brain swelling. (*B*) Coronal T2-weighted scan showing bilateral lesions in the substantia nigra (*arrowheads*) and left-sided lesion in the body of the hippocampus (*arrow*). (*C*) Axial T2-weighted scan slightly caudal to (*A*) showing extension of the left hippocampal lesion to the tail (*arrow*). (*D*) Diffusion-weighted (DW) image (b = 1000) does not show any altered diffusion.

with conventional T2-weighted images. Patients with longer disease duration showed significantly raised apparent diffusion coefficient (ADC) values.[25] Others have found different results, however. In a study of 45 patients with JE (n = 38) and HSE (n = 7), patients with acute JE showed significantly less conspicuity of the lesions on DW images than on T2-weighted or FLAIR images. FLAIR images were found to be the best sequence for lesion detection of acute JE. In contrast, patients with acute HSE showed significantly more lesion conspicuity on DW images in comparison with T2-weighted or FLAIR images.[6] Our experience has been similar. Our patients with acute JE

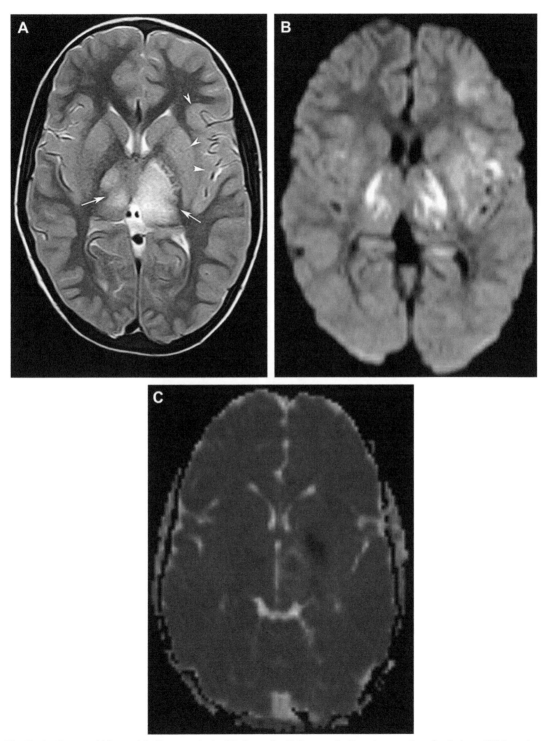

Fig. 2. An 8-year-old boy with JE presented with fever for 5 days and altered sensorium for 2 days. MR imaging was done on day 6 of onset of illness. (*A*) T2-weighted MR imaging shows bilateral asymmetric thalamic lesions (*arrows*) with focal brain swelling. Note subtle lesions in the left putamen and insula (*arrowheads*). (*B*) Diffusion-weighted image and (*C*) apparent diffusion coefficient (ADC) map show restricted diffusion in the left basal ganglia and thalami. Subtle hyperintensities are also noted in the left insula and frontal cortex in (*B*).

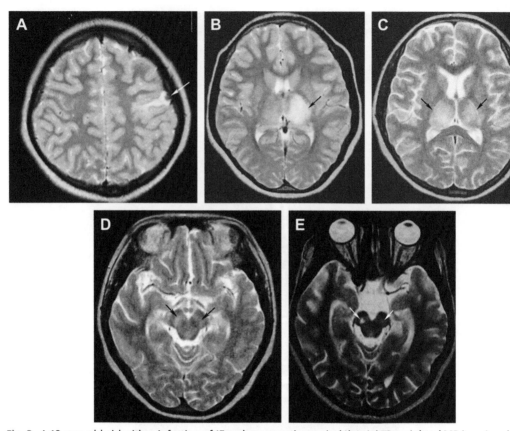

Fig. 3. A 12-year-old girl with coinfection of JE and neurocysticercosis. (*A*) Axial T2-weighted MR imaging done on day 5 after onset of symptoms shows a left frontal cysticercus with T2-hyperintense perifocal edema (*arrow*). This lesion showed ring enhancement with edema on contrast-enhanced CT (not shown). (*B*) Axial T2-weighted MR imaging was done on the same day as (*A*) and shows a left thalamic lesion with mass effect (*arrow*). The substantia nigra was not involved at this stage (not shown). (*C, D*) Axial T2-weighted images done on day 13 show involvement of both thalami (*arrows* in *C*) and substantia nigra (*arrows* in *D*). (*E*) Axial T2-weighted image after 45 days of onset shows residual lesion in substantia nigra (*arrows*). Residual lesions were also seen in both thalami at this stage (not shown). (*From* Handique SK, Das RR, Saharia B et al. Co-infection of Japanese encephalitis with neurocysticercosis: an imaging study. Am J Neuroradiol 2008;29:172; with permission from American Society of Neuroradiology.)

tend to show more lesion conspicuity on conventional scans than on DW images. Often, acute JE lesions also show increased ADC values as well, with lesions appearing isointense on DW images and hyperintense on ADC map images. Less neuronal necrosis in acute JE in comparison with acute HSE and the presence of interstitial edema may explain these findings.[6] DW imaging findings in acute JE are therefore variable, and this needs to be kept in mind while evaluating these patients (see **Figs. 1, 2** and **4**). Increased ADC values are not always seen in chronic JE lesions and must therefore be interpreted with caution (see **Fig. 4**). Other signs of chronic JE lesions such as better definition on T1-weighted and T2-weighted images resembling gliotic lesions and lack of mass effect with associated atrophy should be looked for.

JE rarely presents as a biphasic illness with early relapse of the disease within days or weeks of the first phase of the disease. The clinical manifestations of the second phase may be different from the first phase, but usually conform to the known features of the disease. MR imaging shows fresh areas of brain involvement in the second phase in addition to JE lesions seen in the first phase. We saw 1 such patient in a series of 62 patients with JE. Another study reported 6 patients in a series of 62 patients with JE.[25,26]

Coinfection of JE with neurocysticercosis (NCC) has been reported from India and China.[16,27,28] These diseases have several common epidemiologic and sociodemographic factors, including pig rearing, poor socioeconomic status and hygienic conditions, and malnutrition. More than a casual relationship between the 2 conditions has been suggested by several investigators, with coinfections being advocated as a prognosticator of poor outcome in JE.[16,27] However, others have not

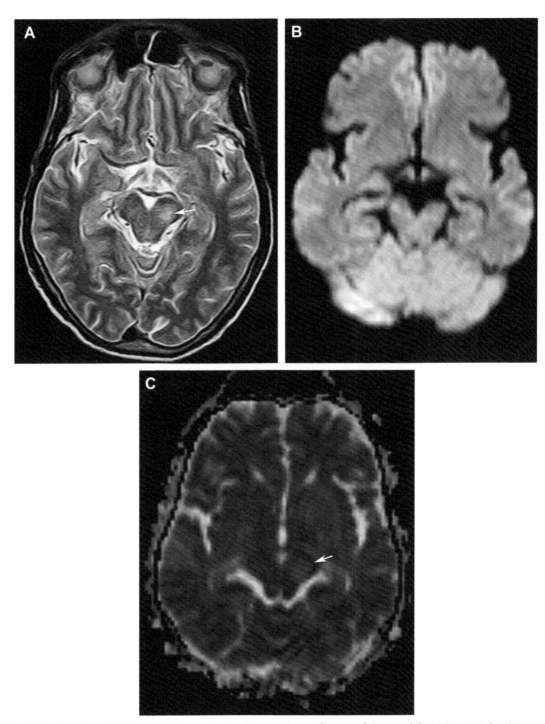

Fig. 4. MR imaging of a 50-year-old man with JE done on day 9 of onset of disease. (*A*) Axial T2-weighted image shows a hyperintense lesion in the left substantia nigra (*arrow*). (*B*) DW image and (*C*) ADC map show facilitated diffusion within this lesion (*arrow* in *C*).

found a significant relationship between the 2 infections.[29] In a prospective study of 62 patients in our hospital, we observed a significantly high association of NCC with JE (19.3%) compared with the prevalence of NCC in controls (1.04%). Lesions of JE were significantly asymmetric with lateralization of the lesions to the side having maximum NCC or a cyst with edema (see **Fig. 4**). More florid JE lesions were seen in coinfections and this was reflected in the significantly higher number of abnormal CT scans in coinfections in contrast to abnormal CT scans in the group. Coinfections were significantly more common in children. We also found evidence of altered immune status in patients with coinfections, with these patients showing significantly lowered JEV IgM levels.[23] Other imaging studies reported similar imaging findings in coinfections.[30] NCC seems to have a synergistic effect on JE and probably facilitates the entry of the JEV into the brain because of the altered immune response.

JE has no specific treatment and the treatment is symptomatic and supportive. Because effective vaccines exist, vaccination of the population at risk is the method of choice for its prevention. Improved farming practices and sanitation, vector control, and reduction of man-mosquito contact are measures that have been effective in the control of the disease.[9]

West Nile Encephalitis

West Nile virus (WNV) is a flavivirus that is closely related to other flaviviruses, such as JEV and dengue virus, and is transmitted to humans by mosquitoes from various species of birds that possibly act as both carriers and amplifiers of the disease. Various species of culicine mosquitoes have been identified to transmit the disease to man. Several birds that act as vertebrate reservoirs have been identified in WNV-prevalent areas.[31,32] Since its first isolation in the West Nile district in Uganda in 1937, WNV has become widely distributed today throughout Africa, the Middle East, Europe, Asia, Canada, Central America, Mexico, the United States, and the Caribbean. It is endemic throughout Africa and the Middle East, whereas large outbreaks have occurred in several countries.[33] In India, WNV was first reported in 1952.[34] Presently it is widely prevalent in India in several states in the southern, eastern, and western parts of the country including Tamil Nadu, Karnataka, Andhra Pradesh, Maharashtra, Gujarat, Madhya Pradesh, Orissa, Rajasthan, and Assam.[31,35] The disease usually presents as a mild febrile illness in this country. Sporadic cases of encephalitis have been reported in children. Despite the abundance of mosquito vectors and neuroinvasive strains of the virus in the country, no major epidemic has been reported to the scale of JE outbreaks. The reason for this is not clear, but may be because of the cross-protection provided by the presence of other flaviviruses in India.[36]

After gaining entry into the blood stream, WNV from a mosquito bite replicates in the reticuloendothelial system. After a second phase of short-lived viremia, the CNS may be invaded, possibly through the hematogenous route, although other routes are possible, such as through the olfactory bulb, choroid plexus epithelial cells, infected immune cells, or retrograde axonal transport through infected peripheral neurons.[37] Because of the rarity of encephalitis, little is known about the neuropathologic findings. Fatal cases show both meningoencephalitis and encephalitis. There is inflammatory change with formation of microglial nodules and neuronophagia with perivascular cuffs in the brain involving the gray and white matter. Brainstem involvement was typical, with involvement of the temporal lobes and basal ganglia. The anterior horns of the spinal cord are involved in patients presenting with spinal cord symptoms. Cranial nerve root involvement is also seen.[38,39]

Seroprevalence studies suggest that most WNV infections are asymptomatic. A small proportion (20%–30%) of infected patients develops a mild febrile syndrome called WNV fever. A smaller subgroup (1 in 150) can develop neuroinvasive disease that may manifest as aseptic meningitis, encephalitis, acute flaccid paralysis, or Guillain-Barré syndrome.[37] Definitive diagnosis of the disease is by showing the WNV-specific antibodies in the serum of CSF.[33]

CT scan does not show any abnormalities in most cases of WNV infection.[40] MR imaging may show abnormalities in more than one-third to more than one-half of the patients.[40–42] Deep gray matter and brainstem involvement was found in 50% of cases in one study of 16 patients by MR imaging. The anatomic areas involved included the basal ganglia, thalami, mesial temporal lobe, midbrain, pons, and cerebellum. Thalamic involvement was seen in 3 (18.75%), a smaller proportion than JE. White matter involvement was seen in 2 patients.[42] Others have reported a higher proportion of white matter disease, with 1 study reporting white matter involvement in as many as 50% (Fig. 5).[41] White matter abnormalities may mimic nonspecific demyelinating lesions and appear hyperintense on T2-weighted and FLAIR images. They show no mass effect or contrast enhancement and usually resolve on follow-up.[40] Some may only be apparent on DW imaging, showing isolated restricted diffusion.[41] Meningeal involvement is seen on contrast-enhanced MR imaging or as sulcal FLAIR hyperintensities (see Fig. 5).[41,42] In patients presenting with acute flaccid paralysis, discreet spinal cord lesions are seen. These lesions may be nonspecific or at times show involvement of the anterior horns. Nerve root enhancement has also been reported.[40–42] DW imaging has been reported to be helpful in lesion detection. In one study, diffusion abnormalities were noted in 50% of the patients.[41] Both gray

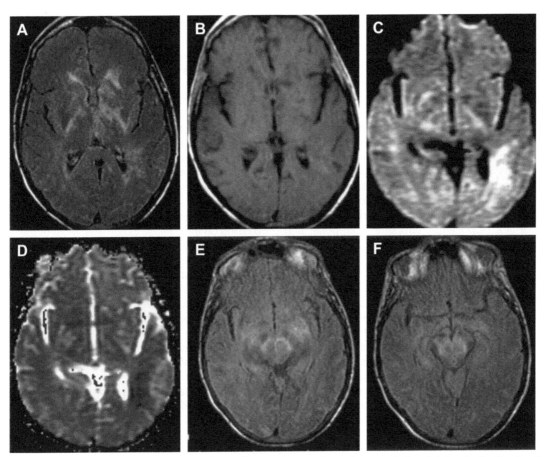

Fig. 5. WNV encephalitis. (*A*) Contrast-enhanced FLAIR image shows increased signal intensity in the basal ganglia and posterior limb of internal capsule bilaterally, left thalamus, and left periventricular white matter, as well as the temporoparietal and occipital sulci. (*B*) Contrast-enhanced T1-weighted image shows no corresponding enhancement. DW image (*C*) and ADC map (*D*) show restricted diffusion in the left periventricular white matter, right basal ganglia, and bilateral posterior limb of internal capsule. (*E* and *F*) Contiguous FLAIR images show increased signal intensity in the midbrain and medial temporal lobes bilaterally, as well as in the right temporal lobe peripherally. Hyperintensity is again shown in the sulci, signifying WNV meningoencephalitis. (*From* Ali M, Safriel Y, Sohi J et al. West Nile virus infection: MR imaging findings in the nervous system. Am J Neuroradiol 2005;26:292; with permission from American Society of Neuroradiology.)

and white matter lesions may show restriction of diffusion. The reason for some lesions showing restricted diffusion is not clear. However, patients with lesions showing isolated restricted diffusion with no corresponding signal abnormality on FLAIR or T2-weighted imaging and patients with normal MR imaging scans have a better outcome than patients with abnormal signal intensity on FLAIR and T2-weighted images. This finding suggests that these areas of isolated restricted diffusion may not be representative of irreversible cell damage or death.[41] Imaging findings of WNV encephalitis have not been reported from Asia or the Indian subcontinent.

There is no definitive treatment of the disease. Treatment is mainly symptomatic and supportive.

No preventive vaccine exists. Disease control therefore is mainly through vector control.[31]

Dengue Encephalitis

Dengue is the most common arboviral disease to infect man and is endemic in more than 100 countries. Approximately 2.5 billion people are at risk for infection. Estimated infections worldwide are 50 million to 100 million, out of which 25,000 die every year.[43] In India, it is reported in more than 18 states of the country.[9] It is caused by a flavivirus transmitted to man by the bite of the infected female *Aedes* mosquito. The infections may be:

a. Asymptomatic; or cause
b. Classic dengue fever or break-bone fever

c. Dengue hemorrhagic fever
d. Dengue shock syndrome
e. Other rarer manifestations like encephalopathy, hepatitis, or myocarditis.

The dengue virus is not generally neuroinvasive, but there is increasing evidence that it may cause encephalitis by direct invasion of the CNS. Isolation of the virus from the CSF, lymphocytic pleocytosis, and demonstration of virus-specific IgM in the CSF by some studies provide this evidence.[44,45] In a series of 9 patients with dengue encephalitis examined by MR imaging in India, abnormality was seen in 1 with lesions in the globus pallidus.[45] Other reports have described lesions in the thalami (like JE), hippocampi, temporal lobe, pons, and spinal cord.[46]

Enterovirus Encephalitis

Enteroviruses (EV) include polio, Coxsackie, echo, and newer enteroviruses that are occasionally neuroinvasive in humans. Although poliovirus has the capability to cause infections of the spinal cord, echo and Coxsackie viruses usually cause aseptic meningitis. Newer EVs occasionally cause neurologic disease that includes aseptic meningitis, encephalitis, acute flaccid paralysis, or other CNS disorders.[47,48] EV71 is an emerging virus that has shown expansion of its geographic range. It causes hand, foot, and mouth disease in children and, in the recent past, several outbreaks have been reported in southeast Asia and Pacific regions. Up to 30% of these patients may show CNS symptoms, although association with neurologic disease is variable.[47] EV71, 76, and 89 encephalitis outbreaks have been reported from north India, whereas EV75 has been reported from the south.[48–50] EV71 was the most common cause of viral encephalitis in children in a study from north India, causing 35.1% of all viral encephalitis.[50] EVs are transmitted through the fecal-oral route, although respiratory-oral spread and spread by fomites is also possible. Invasion of the CNS is through the hematogenous route after viremia occurs. MR imaging findings of EV71 from Taiwan have been reported. Brainstem was the most common site of involvement. The posterior medulla was involved in 75%, posterior pons in 75%, midbrain in 50%, dentate nuclei of cerebellum in 45%, thalamus in 10%, putamina in 5%, and cervical spinal cord in 15% (see **Fig. 6**).[51] In a study from north India, brainstem lesions were the most common and were seen in the midbrain and pons (43% each). Lesions were also noted in the thalamus (43%), cerebellum (28%), cerebral cortex, basal ganglia, and substantia nigra (14% each).[50]

Nipah Virus Encephalitis

Nipah virus encephalitis (NVE) is caused by an emerging zoonotic virus first identified in Malaysia and Singapore in 1998. The Nipah virus (NV) is closely related to the Hendra virus. Both are members of the genus Henipavirus, a new class of virus in the Paramyxoviridae family. It is a neurotropic virus that causes severe encephalitis in humans, with case fatality varying from 40% to 75%. In Malaysia and Singapore, the virus was transmitted to man from infected pigs. The natural hosts of the virus are fruit bats of the Pteropotidae family. Farm animals such as pigs or horses possibly get infected from bat urine or saliva, passing on the disease to humans. Most of the infected in Malaysia were pig farm workers, possibly having contracted the disease from respiratory droplets, throat or respiratory secretions, or from handling infected tissue. Subsequently several NVE outbreaks have occurred in the sub-Himalayan region of the state of West Bengal in India and the adjoining areas of west central Bangladesh since 2001. In Bangladesh and India, infections most likely resulted from consumption of fruit or fruit products such as raw date palm juice contaminated by bat urine or saliva. Unlike in Malaysia and Singapore, man-to-man transmission has been documented in Bangladesh and India with the probable source of infection through handling excretions and secretions of infected patients. In North Bengal, transmission of the virus was reported in a health care setting, with 75% of cases occurring in staff and visitors to hospitals treating the patients.[52,53] Pathologically, an unusual feature is vasculitis with thrombosis and parenchymal necrosis besides other features of encephalitis such as neuronophagia, microglial nodules, and perivascular cuffing.[53] The incubation period varies from 4 to 45 days. Patients present with influenzalike symptoms followed by acute encephalitic syndrome. Survivors may completely recover; however, a small number may show a delayed relapse of encephalitis.[52] In a study from Malaysia, CT scans of patients with NVE were usually normal, but almost all MR imaging scans were abnormal. The most common findings in the acute phase were focal subcortical and deep white matter lesions, and to some extent in the gray matter, that were hyperintense on T2-weighted and FLAIR images, usually without mass effect or edema.[54] In another study from Singapore, patients with acute NVE showed small T2-hyperintense and FLAIR-hyperintense lesions less than 1 cm, mostly in the white matter. Restricted diffusion was observed in some of the larger lesions. Lesions were also seen in the cortex,

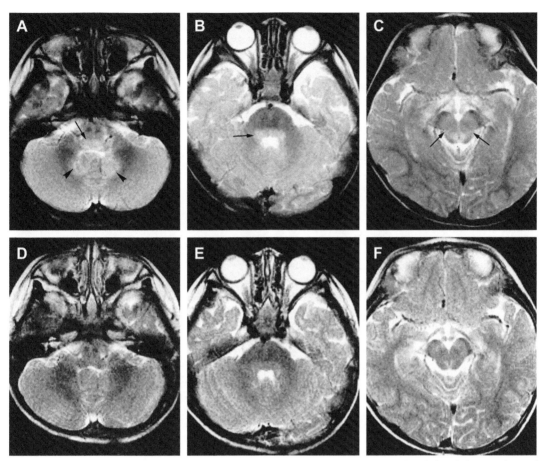

Fig. 6. A 4-year-old boy with acute enterovirus (EV) 71 encephalitis. Patient presented with hand, foot, and mouth disease on June 10, 1998. Two days later, patient developed somnolence, tachycardia, and tachypnea. T2-weighted images show (*A*) hyperintense lesions in the posterior portion of the medulla oblongata (*arrow*) and the bilateral dentate nuclei (*arrowheads*) of the cerebellum; (*B*) hyperintense lesions in the posterior portion of the pons (*arrow*); (*C*) hyperintense lesions in the most central portion of the midbrain (*arrows*); (*D–F*) patient completely recovered without any sequelae. Follow-up MR imaging on July 29, 1998. The hyperintense lesions in the medulla, pons, midbrain, and dentate nuclei had disappeared. (The mild, high signal intensity of the posterior portion of the pons is normal in infants, possibly because of its undermyelinated status.) (*From* Shen WC, Chiu HH, Chow KC et al. MR imaging findings of enteroviral encephalomyelitis: an outbreak in Taiwan. Am J Neuroradiol 1999;20:1891; with permission from American Society of Neuroradiology.)

pons, and cerebral peduncle. Some lesions showed contrast enhancement. These lesions possibly represented microinfarcts from vasculitis-induced thrombosis. Patients who were scanned 1 month after infection showed fresh, tiny foci of T1-hyperintense signal in the cerebral cortex primarily, with lesions also occurring in the white matter, pons, cerebellum, putamen, and thalamus. Only a few of these lesions showed susceptibility on gradient echo sequences. The pathologic correlates of these lesions are unclear but may represent laminar cortical necrosis. Most of the lesions resolved on follow-up in survivors (**Fig. 7**).[55] Imaging findings from India and Bangladesh have not been reported.

No specific treatment or vaccines for NVE exist and treatment is mainly supportive.

Rabies

Rabies (or hydrophobia) is a zoonotic encephalomyelitis and is one of the oldest and most feared diseases known to man, with almost 100% fatality. The rabies virus is a single-stranded RNA virus of the genus Lyssavirus and family Rhabdoviridae. In the Indian subcontinent and other Asian countries, only genotype 1 out of 7 known genotypes is prevalent. It has a worldwide prevalence, although many countries that are geographically isolated, such as Australia and the United

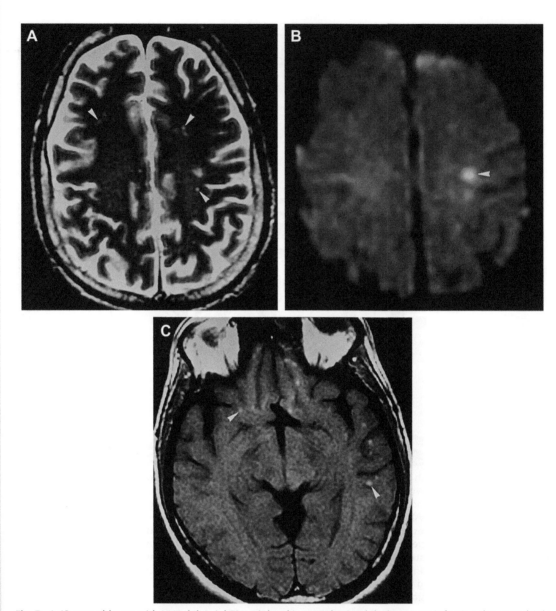

Fig. 7. A 42-year-old man with NVE. (*A*) Axial T2-weighted image obtained during acute infection shows multiple white matter foci of high signal intensity (*arrowheads*) within the cerebral white matter. (*B*) Axial DW image shows only the largest lesion (*arrowhead*) to be hyperintense. Calculated ADC is 0.442 × 10⁻³ mm²/s/s. (*C*) Axial T1-weighted image obtained at 1 month shows multiple punctate hyperintensities (*arrowheads* show some) in the cerebral cortex. These lesions completely disappeared 6 months after the outbreak (not shown). (*From* Lim CC, Lee KE, Lee WL, et al. Nipah virus encephalitis: serial MR study of an emerging disease. Radiology 2002; 222:221; with permission from The Radiological Society of North America.)

Kingdom, are free of the disease. In India, rabies occurs in all parts of the country with the exception of the islands of Andaman and Nicobar, and Lakshadweep. The estimated annual human mortality in the Indian subcontinent is approximately 30,000, but the figure may be 10 times more than that reported. More than 90% of human rabies in India is caused by bites of infected animals, mainly dogs. After inoculation, the virus ascends by retrograde axoplasmic spread to the spinal cord and then to the brain. The initial areas of involvement include the hypothalamus, hippocampus, and the limbic system, with eventual involvement of the entire brain. Despite widespread replication of the virus in the CNS, pathologic changes are minimal, probably because of neuronal apoptosis rather than necrosis and functional derangement of neurotransmitters playing a role in the pathogenesis.[9,56]

After a variable incubation period that may last for days to several years, patients present clinically with the more common classic encephalitic or furious rabies, or the less common paralytic or dumb rabies. Both forms ultimately lead to coma and death. Although the diagnosis of the furious form can be made from the typical clinical symptoms and signs that include the classic hydrophobia (from which rabies gets its other name) and aerophobia, the dumb form can present a diagnostic dilemma because these patients present with ascending paralysis and may lack the classic symptoms of rabies.[56]

There is a lack of imaging literature of rabies, possibly because of difficulty in imaging these patients. CT may show diffuse or focal areas of hypoattenuation in the basal ganglia, hippocampus, periventricular white matter, and brainstem.[57,58] In a study of 5 patients with both furious and paralytic types of rabies, MR imaging showed nonenhancing, ill-defined, subtle T2-hyperintense lesions in the brainstem, hippocampi, hypothalami, deep and subcortical white matter, and deep and cortical gray matter in noncomatose patients. Gadolinium contrast-enhancing lesions were noted in the hypothalami, brainstem nuclei, spinal cord gray matter, and intradural cervical nerve roots only when the patients became comatose. There was no difference in the lesion pattern between furious and paralytic rabies. Differential functional impairment rather than a direct process of virus infection in certain regions of the CNS has been suggested as a possible explanation.[59]

Measles
Measles is an acute, highly infectious disease of childhood and is characterized by fever, upper respiratory symptoms, and the development of a characteristic rash. It is caused by an RNA paramyxovirus and transmission occurs by respiratory droplet infection. Measles is endemic in virtually all parts of the world, but is rare in the developed world because of effective vaccination. An estimated 30 million children are infected worldwide with measles and about 1 million die. In India, the number of measles cases has decreased from about 0.2 million cases in 1987 to about 50,000 cases in 2005.[9] CNS infections by the measles virus can result in acute measles encephalitis (AME), subacute measles encephalitis (SME), or subacute sclerosing panencephalitis (SSPE). SME is a recently recognized condition that occurs in the immunocompromised host and is caused by wild-type measles virus. SSPE is a slow virus infection of the brain caused by measles and characteristically manifests after several years from the initial infection.[60] CNS complications are rare and approximately 1 in 1000 cases results in acute encephalitis.[9] In a study of 155 patients with viral encephalitis from north India, 7% of acute encephalitis was caused by measles virus.[50] SSPE is even rarer and the frequency of occurrence is approximately 1 to 4 cases in 1 million in developed countries, with a possible incidence of up to 21 cases in 1 million in developing countries like India.[61] With the introduction of a mass immunization program for measles in India in 1986, the incidence of SSPE is decreasing in this country.[62] No reports of SME are available from the Indian subcontinent.

AME is caused by direct invasion of the brain by the measles virus and symptoms usually develop within 8 days of onset of measles during the period of measles exanthema. CSF analysis reveals mild pleocytosis, usually mononuclear, mildly increased protein level, and normal glucose level. Detection of specific viral genome in the CSF suggests direct viral invasion of the CNS. Some investigators have not been able to show specific viral RNA in the brain of infected patients, leading to the belief that AME may be caused by autoimmune mechanisms. AME has a mortality of approximately 10% to 20%.[60] MR imaging studies in AME from Korea have shown T2-hyperintense lesions in patients diffusely involving the cortex, corpus striatum, and white matter, with areas of petechial hemorrhage. DW imaging showed restricted diffusion and contrast-enhanced imaging showed cortical and leptomeningeal enhancement.[63,64]

SSPE is a slow virus infection that is a result of persistent measles virus in the CNS. Most patients with SSPE have a history of primary measles infection at an early age. Onset of disease occurs 6 to 8 years after the initial measles attack. Because the incubation period is less than a decade, the disease commonly occurs in childhood but young adults may be affected. Boys are most commonly affected (male/female = 3:1), although measles shows no sex predilection. A close temporal relationship with other viruses, such as Epstein-Barr virus or parainfluenza type 1 virus, has also been suggested as a risk factor for SSPE.[65]

The exact pathogenesis of SSPE is unknown. Measles virus probably gains entry into the brain by infection of the endothelial cells or by circulating inflammatory cells. Despite the long latency period, there is evidence that the measles virus gains entry into the brain soon after the acute infection and subsequently spreads throughout the brain.[65] In the early stages, there is variable inflammation of the meninges, cortical and deep gray matter, and white matter. There is neuronophagia, gliosis, proliferation of astrocytes, perivascular cuffing, lymphocytic and plasma cell infiltration, demyelination, and inclusion bodies in the neurons and glial cells. In the late stages, there is scanty inflammation with severe neuronal loss in the cortex and deep gray matter with thinning of white matter and severe gliosis. Inclusion bodies are scarce.[66] Clinically, the disease starts as minor behavioral and intellectual changes in a previously healthy child. There is development of motor dysfunction and characteristic myoclonic jerks. Within months to years, there is deterioration of sensorium followed by coma.[65] Four stages of the disease have been described, comprising stage I, which includes patients with mild behavioral changes, progressing to stage IV, which includes patients in the vegetative state with loss of cerebral cortical function.[67] Diagnosis is established by clinical presentation, abnormal electroencephalogram findings, increased measles antibodies in serum and CSF, and brain biopsy.[65]

Imaging with CT and MR in SSPE shows white matter changes that appear hyperintense on T2-weighted MR imaging and hypoattenuated on CT scans. These changes are more apparent on MR imaging. In the early stages, white matter changes are asymmetric and more commonly seen in the parietooccipital than in the frontal region. Gray matter changes may also be observed that are more apparent on MR imaging and appear hyperintense on T2-weighted and hypointense on T1-weighted scans. Involvement of the brainstem, cerebral and cerebellar peduncles, and cerebellum may also be seen. The progression of MR imaging findings seems to follow a pattern with focal white matter changes appearing first followed by atrophic changes. In advanced stages, atrophy is more severe and diffuse white matter involvement with thinning of corpus callosum is noted.[68–70] However, despite lesions on conventional MR imaging following a set pattern, MR imaging changes do not correlate well with clinical stages of the disease.[68] DW imaging shows facilitated diffusion within the lesions of SSPE with raised ADC values.[70]

Although conventional MR imaging findings and clinical stages of SSPE are not well correlated, newer MR techniques such as DW imaging, MR spectroscopy, and diffusion tensor imaging (DTI) and diffusion tensor tractography (DTT) have been reported to be of more help in detecting early disease and helping in clinical staging. One study found a significant difference in the ADC values between patients with clinical stage II and stage III of the disease with highest ADC values in stage III disease.[71] Both single and multivoxel MR spectroscopy have been reported to detect early disease

and differentiate between stage II and stage III disease. In one study, children with stage II disease showed no abnormalities on conventional MR imaging, but showed increased choline and myoinositol (MI) levels with normal N-acetyl aspartate (NAA) levels in the frontal subcortical white matter and parietooccipital white matter in comparison with controls. Higher choline levels were observed in the parietooccipital region than in the frontal regions, reflecting the early pathologic changes seen in the former area. However, decreased NAA, increased choline and MI, and increased lactate and lipid peaks were seen in stage III SSPE in relation to controls. These findings probably reflect inflammation in stage II, and demyelination, gliosis, cellular necrosis, and anaerobic metabolism in stage III.[72] DTI has also been reported to detect changes in the early stage of SSPE with normal conventional MR imaging. In a study of 21 patients with stage II SSPE from India, DTI revealed abnormal fractional anisotropy (FA) values in both normal-appearing and abnormal-appearing white matter on T2-weighted images compared with controls. Mean diffusivity (MD) values were significantly increased in the frontal and parietooccipital periventricular white matter (Fig. 8) of patients with both normal-appearing and abnormal-appearing white matter on T2-weighted images.[73] In another study from India by the same group of investigators, tract-specific FA values in some of the major white matter tracts were shown to correlate inversely with clinical grades II to IV.[74]

SME or immunosuppressive measles encephalitis is an infrequent complication of measles in immunosuppressed children, 70% of the cases occurring in acute lymphocytic leukemia. Unlike SSPE, which shows a latency of several years, it has a latency period of few weeks to 7 months. It presents with partial seizure or epilepsia partialis continua, altered sensorium, and variable neurologic deficits. Overall mortality is 85%, with 76% of all patients dying from SME itself. CT is not helpful in imaging these patients. Intravenous ribavirin therapy is effective when administered early.[75] On MR imaging, cortical lesions have been reported in the parietooccipital, frontal, and temporal regions, and in the deep gray matter involving the basal ganglia. Long-term survivors may show cerebral atrophy.[76,77]

Other viruses

Chikungunya is an emerging viral infection that can cause a denguelike illness and, rarely, neurologic manifestations. It is caused by a togavirus and is transmitted to man by the Aedes mosquito. It was first detected in 1952 in Africa and first

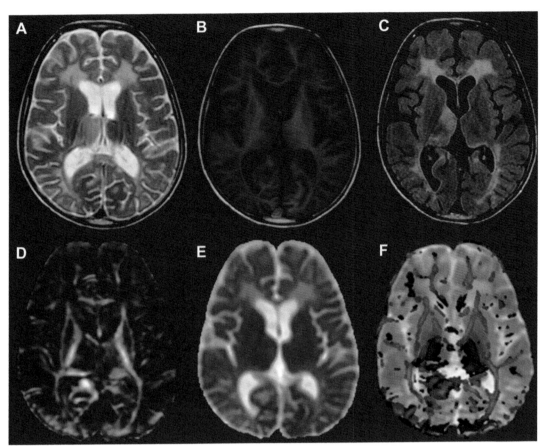

Fig. 8. Subacute sclerosing encephalitis. An 8-year-old boy presented with myoclonic seizures for the last 6 months. He gave a history of measleslike rash at 2 years of age. T2-weighted axial MR imaging (*A*) shows a hyperintense lesion involving the periventricular frontal, occipital, right thalamus, and splenium, which are iso-intense to hypointense on T1 (*B*) and more clearly seen on FLAIR (*C*) images. DTI shows reduction of FA (*D*) and increased MD (*E*) in these regions, more clearly depicted on a color-coded FA map fused with an MD map (*F*). Note the mild ventricular dilatation with generalized atrophy.

reported in India from 1963 to 1973. The virus then disappeared, only to reappear in 2005, and since then it has been reported from 12 Indian states. There were an estimated 1500,000 cases in India in 2006. Neurologic manifestations are rare and include meningoencephalitis, myelopathy, and neuropathy.[78] The imaging features of chikungunya have been described from India. MR imaging was either normal or showed multiple punctuate white matter lesions that were more apparent on DW images than on T2-weighted or T1-weighted images. Although these lesions resembled those of NVE, the prominence on DW images and lack of brainstem or cortical lesions differentiated chikungunya from NVE. Occasional contrast enhancement of these lesions was seen. Nerve root enhancement involving the ventral cauda equina roots has been reported in patients with neuropathy.[78,79]

Chandipura virus (CHP) is a rhabdovirus transmitted to humans by sandflies and mosquitoes.

The virus was first isolated in 1965 and was not considered to have epidemic potential until large outbreaks of acute encephalitis caused by the virus were reported from south India in 2003 and west India in 2004 with high case fatality. Earlier believed to be exclusively Asian, CHP is today prevalent in India, Sri Lanka, and western Africa. Patients showed signs of brainstem encephalitis in a study from south India. CT and MR imaging in these studies has been found to be normal.[80,81]

SUMMARY

Viral infections of the CNS in the tropical countries of Asia and the Indian subcontinent are different from those of the Western and developed world, with the prevalence of several endemic and epidemic viral infections and the added specter of several other emerging viruses that loom as distinct threats. Imaging can help in the management of

CNS viral infections by establishing a working diagnosis in the emergency room, often differentiating viral encephalitis from conditions with clinically similar presentation, such as ADEM, tubercular meningitis, and bacterial meningitis. A working diagnosis of HSE can also be established and early therapy for this condition can be commenced. Many epidemic, endemic, and especially emerging viral encephalitides that plague the tropics and the Indian subcontinent have distinct imaging features that may help in identifying the causative virus.

ACKNOWLEDGMENTS

I would like to acknowledge the work of my colleagues Baijayanta Saharia, Diganta Dutta, Hareswar Meitei, Payal Deorah, and Swagata Baruah in the Japanese encephalitis studies. I would also like to thank the management of GNRC Hospitals Ltd and Mr Rathin Sharma for their help and support.

REFERENCES

1. Kumar R. Aseptic meningitis: diagnosis and management. Indian J Pediatr 2005;72(1):57–63.
2. Sathish N, Scott JX, Shaji RV, et al. An outbreak of echovirus meningitis in children. Indian Pediatr 2004;41(4):384–8.
3. Wang RJ, Wang DX, Wang JW, et al. Analysis of 62 adult patients with viral meningitis. Zhonghua Shi Yan He Lin Chuang Bing Du Xue Za Zhi 2009; 23(3):218–20 [in Chinese].
4. Jmor F, Emsley HC, Fischer M, et al. The incidence of acute encephalitis syndrome in Western industrialised and tropical countries. Virol J 2008;5:134.
5. Booss J, Esiri MM. Pathological features of encephalitis in humans. In: Booss J, Esiri MM, editors. Viral encephalitis in humans. Washington, DC: ASM Press; 2003. p. 3–19.
6. Sawlani V. Diffusion-weighted imaging and apparent diffusion coefficient evaluation of herpes simplex encephalitis and Japanese encephalitis. J Neurol Sci 2009;287:221–6.
7. Solomon T. Viral encephalitis in southeast Asia. Neurol Infect Epidemiol 1997;2:191–9.
8. Misra UK, Kalita J. Overview: Japanese encephalitis. Prog Neurobiol 2010;91:108–20.
9. Park K. Epidemiology of communicable diseases. In: Park K, editor. Textbook of preventive and social medicine. Jabalpur: Banarsidas Bhanot; 2007. p. 123–300.
10. Vaughn DW, Hoke CH. The epidemiology of Japanese encephalitis: prospects for prevention. Epidemiol 1992;14:197–221.
11. Hoke CH, Nisalak A, Sangawhipa N, et al. Protection against Japanese encephalitis by inactivated vaccines. N Engl J Med 1988;319:608–14.
12. Grossman RA, Edelman R, Chiewanich P, et al. Study of Japanese encephalitis virus in Chiangmai Valley, Thailand. II Human clinical infections. Am J Epidemiol 1973;98:121–32.
13. Solomon T, Dung NM, Kneen R, et al. Japanese encephalitis. J Neurol Neurosurg Psychiatry 2000; 68:405–15.
14. Umenai T, Krzysko R, Bektimorov TA, et al. Japanese encephalitis: current worldwide status. Bull World Health Organ 1985;63:625–31.
15. Huong VT, Ha DQ, Deubel V. Genetic study of Japanese encephalitis viruses from Vietnam. Am J Trop Med Hyg 1993;49:538–44.
16. Shankar SK, Vasudev Rao T, Mruthyunjayanna BP, et al. Autopsy study of brains during an epidemic of Japanese encephalitis in Karnataka. Indian J Med Res 1983;78:431–40.
17. Gourie-Devi M, Ravi V, Shankar SK. Japanese encephalitis. An overview. In: Rose C, editor. Recent advances in tropical neurology. Amsterdam: Elsevier Science; 1995. p. 217–35.
18. Zimmerman HM. The pathology of Japanese B encephalitis. Am J Pathol 1946;22:965–91.
19. Solomon T, Winter PM. Neurovirulence and host factors in flavivirus encephalitis evidence from clinical epidemiology. Arch Virol Suppl 2004;18:161–70.
20. Kalita J, Misra UK. Comparison of CT scan and MRI findings in the diagnosis of Japanese encephalitis. J Neurol Sci 2000;174:3–8.
21. Handique SK, Das RR, Barman K, et al. Temporal lobe involvement in Japanese encephalitis–problems in differential diagnosis. Am J Neuroradiol 2006;27: 1027–31.
22. Shoji H, Kida H, Hino H, et al. Magnetic resonance imaging findings in Japanese encephalitis. White matter lesions. J Neuroimaging 1994;4:206–11.
23. Handique SK, Das RR, Saharia B, et al. Co-infection of Japanese encephalitis with neurocysticercosis: an imaging study. Am J Neuroradiol 2008;29:170–5.
24. Dung NM, Turtle L, Chong WK, et al. An evaluation of the usefulness of neuroimaging for the diagnosis of Japanese encephalitis. J Neurol 2009;256:2052–60.
25. Handique SK, Barkataky N. MR imaging in biphasic Japanese encephalitis. Am J Neuroradiol 2008; 29:E3.
26. Pradhan S, Gupta RK, Singh MB, et al. Biphasic illness pattern due to early relapse in Japanese-B virus encephalitis. J Neurol Sci 2001;183:13–8.
27. Desai A, Shankar SK, Jayakumar PN, et al. Co-existence of cerebral cysticercosis with Japanese encephalitis: a prognostic modulator. Epidemiol Infect 1997;118:165–71.
28. Liu YF, Teng CL, Liu K. Cerebral cysticercosis as a factor aggravating Japanese encephalitis. Chin Med J 1957;75:1010–6.
29. Azad R, Gupta RK, Kumar S, et al. Is neurocysticercosis a risk factor in coexistent intracranial disease?

An MRI based study. J Neurol Neurosurg Psychiatry 2003;74:359–61.

30. Singh P, Kalra N, Ratho RK, et al. Co-existent neurocysticercosis and Japanese B encephalitis: MR imaging co-relation. Am J Neuroradiol 2001;22:1131–6.

31. Paramasivan R, Mishra AC, Mourya DT. West Nile virus: the Indian scenario. Indian J Med Res 2003; 118:101–8.

32. Rodrigues FM, Guttikar SN, Pinto BD. Prevalence of antibodies to Japanese encephalitis and West Nile viruses among wild birds in the Krishna-Godavari delta, Andhra Pradesh, India. Trans R Soc Trop Med Hyg 1981;75:258–62.

33. Pattan SR, Dighe NS, Bhawar SB, et al. West Nile fever: an overview. J Biomed Sci Res 2009;1:33–48.

34. Banker DD. Preliminary observations on antibody patterns against certain viruses among inhabitants of Bombay city. Indian J Med Sci 1952;6:733–46.

35. Khan SA, Dutta P, Choudhury P, et al. Co-infection of arboviruses presenting as acute encephalitis syndrome. J Clin Virol 2011;51:5–7.

36. Gajanana A. West Nile virus epidemics: lessons for India. ICMR Bulletin 2002;32(7).

37. Samuel MA, Diamond MS. Pathogenesis of West Nile virus infection: a balance between virulence, innate and adaptive immunity, and viral evasion. J Virol 2006;80:9349–60.

38. Sampson BA, Ambrosi C, Charlot C, et al. The pathology of human West Nile virus infection. Hum Pathol 2000;31:527–31.

39. Kelly TW, Prayson RA, Ruiz AI, et al. The neuropathology of West Nile virus meningoencephalitis: a report of 2 cases and review of the literature. Am J Clin Pathol 2003;119:749–53.

40. Zak IT, Altinok D, Merline JR, et al. West Nile virus infection. AJR 2005;184:957–61.

41. Ali M, Safriel Y, Sohi J, et al. West Nile virus infection: MR imaging findings in the nervous system. Am J Neuroradiol 2005;26:289–97.

42. Petropoulou KA, Gordon SM, Prayson RA, et al. West Nile virus meningoencephalitis: MR imaging findings. Am J Neuroradiol 2005;26:1986–95.

43. World Health Organization. Dengue haemorrhagic fever; diagnosis, treatment, prevention and control. Geneva (Switzerland): WHO; 1997.

44. Solomon T, Dung NM, Vaughn DW, et al. Neurological manifestations of dengue infection. Lancet 2000;355:1053–9.

45. Misra UK, Kalita J, Syam UK, et al. Neurological manifestations of dengue virus infections. J Neurol Sci 2006;244:117–22.

46. Varatharaj A. Encephalitis in the clinical spectrum of dengue infection. Neurol India 2010;58:585–91.

47. Tyler KL. Emerging viral infections of the central nervous system: part 1. Arch Neurol 2009;66:939–48.

48. Lewthwaite P, Perera D, Ooi MH, et al. Enterovirus 75 encephalitis in children, southern India. Emerg

Infect Dis 2010. Available at: http://www.cdc.gov/EID/content/16/11/1780.htm. DOI: 10.3201/eid1611.100672. Accessed August 7, 2011.

49. Sapkal GN, Bondre VP, Fulmali PV, et al. Enteroviruses in patients with acute encephalitis, Uttar Pradesh, India. Emerg Infect Dis 2009;15:295–8.

50. Karmarkar SA, Aneja S, Khare S, et al. A study of acute febrile encephalopathy with special reference to viral etiology. Indian J Pediatr 2008;75:801–5.

51. Shen WC, Chiu HH, Chow KC, et al. MR Imaging findings of enteroviral encephalomyelitis: an outbreak in Taiwan. Am J Neuroradiol 1999;20:1889–95.

52. Nipah virus factsheet (revised in July 2009). Wkly Epidemiol Rec 2010;85:64–7.

53. Tyler KL. Emerging viral infections of the central nervous system: part 2. Arch Neurol 2009;66:1065–74.

54. Goh KJ, Tan CT, Chew NK, et al. Clinical features of Nipah virus encephalitis among pig farmers in Malaysia. N Engl J Med 2000;342:1229–35.

55. Lim CC, Lee KE, Lee WL, et al. Nipah virus encephalitis: serial MR study of an emerging disease. Radiology 2002;222:219–26.

56. Madhusudana SN, Sukumaran SM. Antemortem diagnosis and prevention of human rabies. Ann Indian Acad Neurol 2008;11:3–12.

57. Sing TM, Soo MY. Imaging findings in rabies. Australas Radiol 1996;40:338–41.

58. Awasthi M, Parmar H, Patankar T, et al. Imaging findings in rabies encephalitis. Am J Neuroradiol 2001; 22:677–80.

59. Laothamatas J, Hemachuda T, Mitrabhakdi PW, et al. MR imaging in human rabies. Am J Neuroradiol 2003;24:1102–9.

60. Hosoya M. Measles encephalitis: direct viral invasion or autoimmune-mediated inflammation? Intern Med 2006;45:841–2.

61. Sarkar N, Gulati S, Dar L, et al. Diagnostic dilemmas in fulminant subacute sclerosing panencephalitis (SSPE). Indian J Pediatr 2004;71:365–7.

62. Mishra B, Kakkar N, Ratho RK, et al. Changing trend of SSPE over a period of 10 years. Indian J Public Health 2005;49:235–7.

63. Lee KY, Cho WH, Kim SH, et al. Acute encephalitis associated with measles: MRI features. Neuroradiology 2003;45:100–6.

64. Kim SJ, Kim JS, Lee DY. Neurologic outcome of acute measles encephalitis according to the MRI patterns. Pediatr Neurol 2003;28:281–4.

65. Garg RK. Subacute sclerosing panencephalitis. Postgrad Med J 2002;78:63–70.

66. Esiri MM, Kennedy PG. Virus diseases. In: Adams JH, Duchen LW, editors. Greenfield's neuropathology. 5th edition. London: Edward Arnold; 1992. p. 335–99.

67. Jabbour JT, Garcia JH, Lemni H, et al. Subacute sclerosing panencephalitis presenting as simple partial seizures. J Child Neurol 1990;5:146–9.

68. Brismar J, Gascon GG, von Steyern KV, et al. Subacute sclerosing panencephalitis: evaluation with CT and MR. AJNR Am J Neuroradiol 1996;17: 761–72.

69. Tuncay R, Akman-Demir G, Gokygit A, et al. MRI in subacute sclerosing panencephalitis. Neuroradiology 1996;38:636–40.

70. Sener RN. Subacute sclerosing panencephalitis findings at MR imaging, diffusion MR imaging, and proton MR spectroscopy. Am J Neuroradiol 2004; 25:892–4.

71. Alkan A, Korkmaz L, Sigirci A, et al. Subacute sclerosing panencephalitis: relationship between clinical stage and diffusion-weighted imaging findings. J Magn Reson Imaging 2006;23:267–72.

72. Alkan A, Sarac K, Kutlu R, et al. Early- and late-subacute sclerosing pan encephalitis: chemical shift imaging and single-voxel MR spectroscopy. Am J Neuroradiol 2003;24:501–6.

73. Trivedi R, Gupta RK, Agarawal A, et al. Assessment of white matter damage in subacute sclerosing panencephalitis using quantitative diffusion tensor MR imaging. Am J Neuroradiol 2006;27:1712–6.

74. Trivedi R, Anuradha H, Agarwal A, et al. Correlation of quantitative diffusion tensor tractography with clinical grades of subacute sclerosing panencephalitis. Am J Neuroradiol 2011;32:714–20.

75. Mustafa MM, Weitman SD, Winick NJ, et al. Subacute measles encephalitis in young immuno-compromised host: a review of two cases diagnosed by polymerase chain reaction and treated with ribavirin and review of the literature. Clin Infect Dis 1993; 16:654–60.

76. Poon TP, Tchertkoff V, Win H. Subacute measles encephalitis with AIDS diagnosed by fine needle aspiration biopsy. A case report. Acta Cytol 1998; 42:729–33.

77. Chong HT, Ramli N, Wong KT, et al. Subacute measles encephalitis: a case of long term survival with follow-up MR brain scans. Neurology Asia 2007;12:121–5.

78. Wadia RS. A neurotropic virus (chikungunya) and a neuropathic amino acid (homocysteine). Ann Indian Acad Neurol 2007;10:198–213.

79. Ganesan K, Diwan A, Shankar SK, et al. Chikungunya encephalomyeloradiculitis: report of 2 cases with neuroimaging and 1 case with autopsy findings. Am J Neuroradiol 2008;29:1636–7.

80. John TJ. Chandipura virus – what we know & do not know. Indian J Med Res 2010;132:125–7.

81. Rao NS, Wairagkar NS, Mohan MV, et al. 5. Brain stem encephalitis associated with Chandipura virus in Andhra Pradesh outbreak. J Trop Pediatr 2008;54: 25–30.

Central Nervous System Tuberculosis

Rakesh K. Gupta, MD*, Sunil Kumar, MD

KEYWORDS

- CNS tuberculosis • Tuberculoma • TB meningitis
- TB spondylitis

Key Points: CNS TUBERCULOSIS

- Central nervous system (CNS) tuberculosis is a major cause of sickness and death, especially in developing countries, and is increasing in developed countries because of the emergence of acquired immunodeficiency syndrome (AIDS).

- Isolation of *Mycobacterium tuberculosis* for the definitive diagnosis is possible only in a few patients. Culture has a low yield and needs 6 to 8 weeks.

- In tuberculous meningitis (TBM), precontrast magnetization transfer (MT) T1 imaging shows abnormal meninges with low MT ratio and is characteristic of the disease.

- Tuberculomas have solid and/or liquid caseation on noncontrast MT T1 images, a bright rim around T2 hypointensity is a characteristic feature of tuberculoma; the T2 hypointense rim appears bright in tuberculous abscess.

- When liquefaction of the caseation occurs within tuberculoma as well as abscess, it shows restriction on diffusion-weighted (DW) imaging with low apparent diffusion coefficient (ADC).

- Advanced imaging methods such as perfusion imaging and diffusion tensor imaging (DTI) may be of value in objective assessment of therapy in tuberculoma.

Approximately one-third of the world's population is currently infected with tuberculous bacillus, of which approximately 5% to 10% become sick or infectious at some time during their life. People with human immunodeficiency virus (HIV) are more likely to develop tuberculosis (TB). The World Health Organization (WHO) estimates that there were 9.4 million new cases in 2009, including 1.1 million cases among people with HIV.[1] Approximately 1.7 million people died of TB, including 380,000 people with HIV.[1] Most cases were in the south-east Asian, African, and western Pacific regions (35%, 30%, and 13%, respectively). In 2009, the estimated per capita TB incidence was stable or decreasing in all 6 WHO regions. However, the slow decline in incidence rates per capita is offset by population growth. Consequently, the number of new cases arising each year is still increasing globally in the WHO regions of Africa, the eastern Mediterranean, and southeast Asia.

Neurotuberculosis constitutes 1% of all tuberculosis and 10% to 15% of the extrapulmonary tuberculosis cases, most (>40%) of which are children.[2] Central nervous system (CNS) tuberculosis also accounts for 1.5% to 3.2% of all tuberculosis-related deaths.[3] CNS tuberculosis remains common and, despite the availability of effective antituberculous therapy, continues to cause significant morbidity and mortality. TBM constitutes 70% to 80% of all patients with neurotuberculosis.[4] CNS tuberculosis is a prominent

---

The authors have nothing to disclose.
Department of Radiodiagnosis, Sanjay Gandhi Postgraduate Institute of Medical Sciences, Rae Bareli Road, Lucknow 226014, Uttar Pradesh, India
* Corresponding author.
E-mail address: rakeshree1@gmail.com

Neuroimag Clin N Am 21 (2011) 795–814
doi:10.1016/j.nic.2011.07.004
1052-5149/11/$ – see front matter © 2011 Elsevier Inc. All rights reserved.

cause of sickness and death in developing countries.[5] In developed countries, there has been an increase in the number of CNS TB cases, possibly related to the pandemic of AIDS.[6] M tuberculosis is responsible for almost all cases of tubercular infection in CNS.[5] Tubercular bacilli initiate a granulomatous inflammatory reaction involving different tissue types of the CNS such as meninges, brain, spinal cord, and covering bones. The CNS manifestation is in a variety of forms, such as TBM and its complications, focal cerebritis, tuberculoma, and tubercular abscess. Spinal cord infection is less common and causes either arachnoiditis and/or intramedullary tuberculomas.

Early diagnosis and treatment of CNS tuberculosis is necessary to reduce the morbidity and mortality. Noninvasive imaging modalities such as computed tomography (CT) and magnetic resonance (MR) imaging are routinely used in the diagnosis of CNS TB; however, MR imaging is preferred because it offers greater inherent sensitivity and specificity than CT. This article reviews the various forms of CNS tuberculosis, including its complications and imaging features.

PATHOPHYSIOLOGY
TBM

Tuberculosis is most often a primary infection in children and a postprimary infection in adults. CNS tuberculosis transpires hematogenously from a distant active site such as lung, bone, lymph nodes, or gastrointestinal or genitourinary tract. In the brain, the bacilli lodge in the cortical and subcortical regions and/or meninges, which are richly vascularized.[7] Rarely, there is a direct spread from adjacent infected paranasal sinuses or mastoid air cells.[8] Infection typically begins in a subpial or subependymal cortical location called the Rich focus. The site of this focus determines the type of CNS involvement.[9] Initially, a nonspecific inflammatory reaction, tuberculous cerebritis, develops. Once sensitized, the inflammatory response results in a granuloma. This granuloma may erode into the subarachnoid space and cerebrospinal fluid (CSF), causing basal leptomeningitis. Subsequently, this leads to communicating hydrocephalus, and occasionally obstructive hydrocephalus caused by obstruction of the foramina of Luschka and Magendie. Vasculitis involving the lenticulostriate and thalamoperforating arteries may occur. The adventitial layer of these vessels develop changes similar to those of the adjacent tuberculous exudates followed by the intima, which may eventually be involved or be eroded by a fibrinoid-hyaline degeneration. In later stages, the lumen of the vessel may become completely occluded by reactive subendothelial cellular proliferation and cause small infarcts in the deep gray matter nuclei and deep white matter.[7,10]

Tuberculoma

The initial lesion, a tubercle, consists of a central area of incipient or frank necrosis surrounded by inflammatory cells, lymphocytes, epithelioid and Langerhans giant cells, with an encircling rich vascular zone.[11] These lesions begin as a conglomerate of microgranulomata that join to form a noncaseating tuberculoma.[12] Following the initial infection, most such lesions resolve and reactivation or further evolution of these lesions manifests as caseation within the center of this tuberculoma. Rarely, the lesion may continue to grow by successive addition of layers of granulation tissue and form growth rings.[13]

Subsequently, central caseous necrosis develops in most cases, which is initially solid surrounded by a capsule comprising collagenous tissue, epithelioid cells, multinucleated giant cells, and mononuclear inflammatory cells. The central core of solid caseation consists of a cheesy material high in lipid contents, with macrophage infiltration, regional fibrosis/gliosis, macrophage by-products (free radicals), and perilesional cellular infiltrates. A few bacilli may be present in the center. The caseation then usually liquefies, beginning from the center. The capsule consists of granulation tissue and compressed glial tissue.[10] If abscess formation occurs, this shows central cavitation with chronic inflammatory reaction with fibrosis in the wall and the aspirate from the pus stains positive for acid-fast bacilli. All these lesions are usually accompanied by perilesional edema with some proliferation of astrocytes in the surrounding brain parenchyma.[9]

Spine

M tuberculosis infection in the spine can involve any compartment in the spinal region: vertebrae, intervertebral disk, spinal cord, and its meninges. Meningeal involvement causes spinal meningitis and spinal arachnoiditis.[14] The pathophysiology of spinal meningitis is the same as described earlier in TBM: during primary infection a submeningeal tubercle forms that ruptures into the subarachnoid space.[14] It causes granulomatous inflammation, areas of caseation, and tubercles, with development of fibrous tissue in chronic or treated cases.

CLINICAL FEATURES

Children and older persons are more vulnerable to develop CNS tuberculosis because their immune systems are less robust. TBM is also common in immune-suppressed patients (those with HIV or diabetes, and patients taking steroids or cytotoxic drugs). The onset of TBM is insidious and may be characterized by persistent low-grade fever, malaise, headache, and confusion. Typical clinical features of TBM include fever with nausea, vomiting, headache, neck stiffness, and photophobia.[15] Cranial nerve palsies, especially of third, fourth, and sixth nerves, may also be present. The intracranial tuberculomas manifest with features of a space-occupying lesion of the brain and the patients can present with features of increased intracranial tension, focal or generalized seizures, and focal neurologic deficit. Isolation of *M tuberculosis* for the definitive diagnosis from the tissue on smear or culture is possible only in a few patients. Culture takes 6 to 8 weeks for the result and has a low yield. Thus the index of suspicion is mostly indirect; that is, concomitant tubercular involvement elsewhere (only 10% of cases may show disease elsewhere in the body), malaise, low-grade fever, loss of weight, positive tuberculin test, increased sedimentation rate, history of contact,[16] and so forth.

CSF analysis in TBM normally shows a lymphocytic pleocytosis, increased CSF protein level, and decreased CSF sugar concentration.[17] CSF culture for acid-fast bacilli and CSF polymerase chain reaction (PCR) examination are confirmatory tests for the diagnosis of TBM. The sensitivity of CSF culture for detection of acid-fast bacilli has been reported to be approximately[18] 50%. CSF PCR examination is a new technique, and is more sensitive than the combination of microscopic examination and culture for *M tuberculosis*.[19]

IMAGING

Imaging features of tubercular infections of the CNS, which may involve the meninges, brain, spinal cord, bones covering the brain and spinal cord, are as follows.

Imaging Protocol

The MR imaging protocol for CNS tuberculosis includes T2, T1, fluid-attenuating inversion recovery (FLAIR), magnetization transfer (MT) T1, susceptibility-weighted, DW imaging, and postcontrast T1-weighted images. In addition, inclusion of ^{1}H MR spectroscopy for lesions more than 2 cm is helpful. The closest differential diagnosis of brain tuberculomas is neurocysticercosis (NCC) in the regions endemic for NCC. If lesions around 2 cm appear hyperintense on T2-weighted imaging and showing ring enhancement on postcontrast T1-weighted imaging, isotropic fast imaging excitation

with steady state acquisition (FIESTA) should also be performed to show the scolex within a cyst, which is pathognomonic of NCC.

Cranial Tuberculosis

TBM

TBM is still a common problem in some parts of the world. The meninges are involved either by hematogenous seeding or by local spread from adjoining infected areas.

During the early stages of disease, conventional noncontrast MR imaging studies usually show little or no evidence of any meningeal abnormality. MT T1 imaging is considered superior to conventional spin-echo sequences for imaging the abnormal meninges, which are seen as hyperintense on precontrast T1-weighted MT images.[20] As the disease progresses, mild shortening of T1 and T2 relaxation times may be seen compared with normal CSF. Postcontrast T1-weighted images show abnormal meningeal enhancement (**Figs. 1–3**). The common sites are interpeduncular fossa, pontine cistern, perimesencephalic cistern, suprasellar cistern, and sylvian fissures, with occasional involvement of sulci over the convexities (see **Fig. 1**).[21–23]

MT ratio (MTR) quantification helps in identifying the cause of chronic meningitis; low MTR suggests TBM.[20,24] Ex vivo MR spectroscopy of the CSF shows lactate, acetate, and sugar signals along with cyclopropyl rings (-0.5 to $+0.5$ ppm) and phenolic glycolipids (7.1 and 7.4 ppm), which are not seen in pyogenic meningitis.[25] The combination of ex vivo MR spectroscopy with MT MR imaging may be helpful in diagnosing TBM.

The secondary complications of TBM may develop as the disease progresses or even while the patient is on treatment. The sequelae associated with TBM are as follows.

Hydrocephalus Hydrocephalus develops commonly as a result of blockage of the basal cisterns by the inflammatory exudates (communicating type) (see **Fig. 2**), or occasionally due to mass effect of a focal parenchymal lesion or entrapment of the ventricle by granulomatous ependymitis[26] (obstructive type). Periventricular hyperintensity on T2-weighted or FLAIR images usually suggests seepage of the CSF fluid across the white matter. Atrophy of brain parenchyma may be a late sequela of chronic hydrocephalus. The choroid plexus may serve as an entry point for the pathogens into the CNS. Its involvement, choroid plexitis, presents as prominent contrast enhancement of the choroid plexus and is usually associated with ependymitis, ventriculitis, and meningitis.

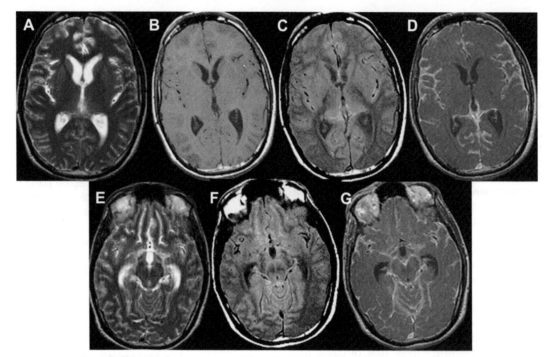

Fig. 1. TBM without hydrocephalus in a young patient. T2 (*A, E*) and T1 (*B*) images at the level of the frontal horn and at the level of the quadrigeminal cistern are unremarkable. MT T1 images at the corresponding levels show bright meninges (*C, F*) that enhance diffusely on postcontrast T1 images (*D*) and (*G*).

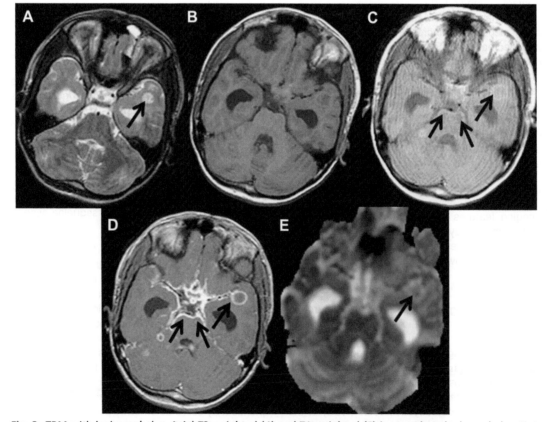

Fig. 2. TBM with hydrocephalus. Axial T2-weighted (*A*) and T1-weighted (*B*) images show hydrocephalus. Note the hyperintense lesion in the left anterior temporal lobe (*arrow*), which is hypointense on the T1-weighted image. Precontrast MT T1 image (*C*) shows hyperintensity around the pons as well as tuberculomas (*small arrow*) that show enhancement on postcontrast T1-weighted images (*D*). ADC map shows low ADC in the left anterior temporal lobe tuberculoma (*E*). The CSF findings and CSF PCR were consistent with TBM.

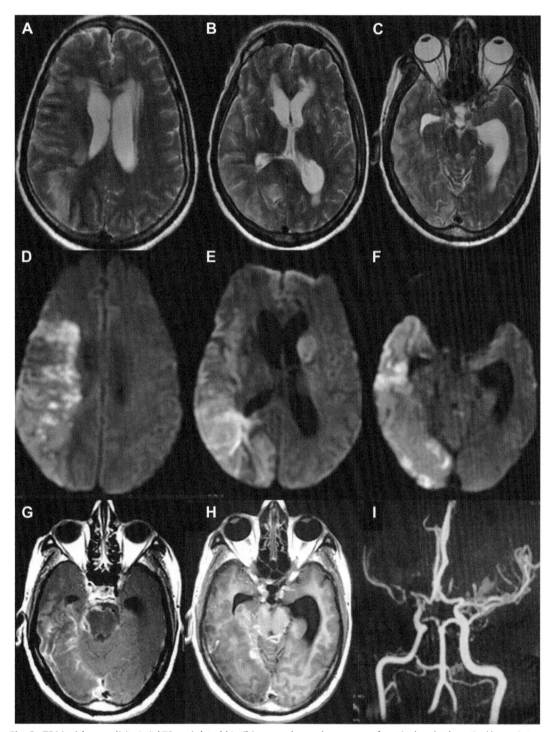

Fig. 3. TBM with vasculitis. Axial T2-weighted (*A–C*) images show a large area of cortical and subcortical hyperintensity in the right frontal-parietal and occipital regions, left basal ganglia, and in the periventricular region with mild ventricular dilatation. DW images (*D–F*) show a large area of restricted diffusion in the right middle cerebral artery and posterior cerebral artery territory and left basal ganglia. Axial MT T1 (*G*) image shows basal exudates and abnormal meninges, which appear bright. Postcontrast T1 (*H*) image shows abnormal meningeal enhancement in the MT T1 bright regions (*G*). MR angiogram (*I*) of the circle of Willis shows segmental narrowing involving the supraclinoid portion of the right internal carotid artery, middle cerebral artery, and right posterior cerebral artery.

Vasculitis Vasculitis is another common complication seen at autopsy in cranial TBM involving small and medium-sized vessels and causing ischemic cerebral infarction.[26] Most of the infarcts are in the basal ganglia and internal capsule regions because of the involvement of the lenticulostriate arteries; however, involvement of the large vascular territory such as the middle cerebral artery may also be encountered.[10,21,27] MR angiography may help in the detection of vascular involvement (see **Fig. 3**). Intracerebral inflammatory aneurysms may also be seen in CNS tuberculosis.[28] MR angiography can reveal this rare vascular complication.[25] DW imaging helps in early detection of infarcts.[27] Vascular complications are usually seen following initiation of specific therapy, possibly due to the healing and fibrosis of meninges resulting in the occlusion of embedded vasculature.

Focal or diffuse pachymeningitis CNS TB may involve the dura mater, causing pachymeningitis, which may occur either in isolation or with pial or parenchymal disease. Pachymeningitis may present as focal or diffuse involvement of the dura mater and occur secondary to hematogenous spread.[29,30] Thickened dura mater may be evident on precontrast studies but is detected usually as abnormal enhancement on postcontrast images. However, the appearance of focal and diffuse pachymeningitis on MR imaging is nonspecific and may be seen in a large number of inflammatory and noninflammatory conditions.

Cranial nerve neuropathy Clinical involvement of the cranial nerves is seen in 17.4% to 40% of patients with TBM caused by vascular compromise resulting in ischemia of the nerve or caused by entrapment of the nerves by the exudates.[25]

Intracranial tuberculoma
Brain tuberculoma is a space-occupying mass of granulomatous tissue that is encountered more frequently in developing countries and is responsible for high morbidity and mortality.[5] The incidence of tuberculoma is higher in the developing world (15%–50% of all intracranial lesions), compared with developed countries where the incidence is about 0.2% of all biopsied brain lesions.[13] Early recognition and treatment of this condition on imaging plays an important role in patient management. Intracranial tuberculomas may be solitary or multiple and variable in size. These tuberculomas are found across all age groups; however, a predilection for children has been reported.[13] The common sites include cerebral hemispheres, basal ganglia, cerebellum, and brainstem. Rarely, ventricular system and meninges are also involved.[13,31]

Extra-axial tuberculomas may also occur, which may cause widening of the basal foramen or adjacent bone destruction.[32] Tuberculoma in the hypophyseal region is rare and it is frequently associated with thickening of the pituitary stalk.[33]

MR features From the appearance on T2-weighted imaging, the intra-axial tuberculomas may be classified as:

1. T2 hyperintense lesion
2. T2 hypointense lesion
3. T2 hyperintense center with peripheral hypointense rim
4. Lesion with mixed/heterogeneous signal intensity.

T2 hyperintense lesion Noncaseating tuberculomas, typically less than 1.5 cm in diameter, appear hyperintense on T2-weighted images, isointense to hypointense on T1, hyperintense on MT T1, and FLAIR, and show nodular or ring enhancement on postcontrast studies. On DW imaging, these lesions may show hyperintensity with low ADC.[20,25] These tuberculomas may be part of miliary tuberculosis or TBM (**Fig. 4**). This appearance may resemble metastases, lymphomas, demyelinating plaques, and other infective granulomas. The presence of a bright rim on noncontrast MT T1 along with low MTR may help in its differentiation from other lesions.

T2 hypointense lesion Tuberculomas with solid caseation are usually isointense to hypointense on both T2-weighted and T1-weighted images. These lesions are surrounded by a rim of variable thickness that may appear hyperintense on T1-weighted and T2-weighted images. On DW images, there is no restriction seen in the solid caseation of the tuberculoma with a high ADC. On noncontrast MT T1 images, this rim shows hyperintensity, a characteristic feature seen in tuberculomas, and the solid caseation remains hypointense (**Figs. 5–7**). The rim comprises inflammatory cells, some of which may contain fragmented portions of the lipid-rich cell wall of *M tuberculosis*. Lipids are known to have no MT effect; the rim has a lower MT ratio than the core and appears bright on MT. Biochemically, the core contains necrotic tissue and macromolecules that are responsible for the higher MT ratio compared with the rim.[34] The rim shows enhancement on postcontrast T1 images, whereas solid caseation does not enhance. The solid caseation contains cheesy material high in lipid contents, with macrophage infiltration, regional fibrosis/gliosis,

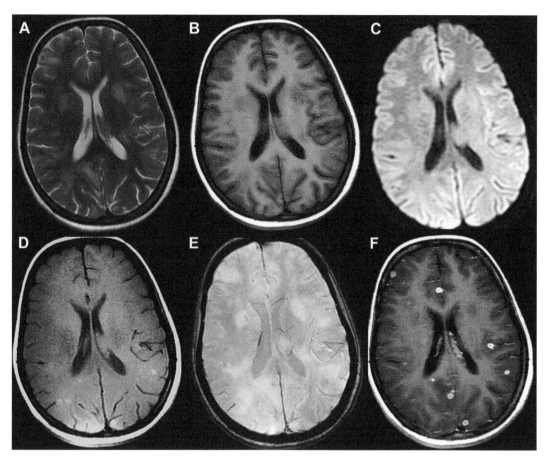

Fig. 4. Miliary tuberculomas. Multiple areas of focal hyperintensity are seen on T2-weighted axial image (A). These areas are seen as slight hypointensities on a T1-weighted image (B). DW image (C) does not reveal any abnormality. MT T1 (D) shows multiple small lesions with bright rims in the regions of hyperintensity noted on T2 (A). Susceptibility-weighted imaging (E) does not show any blooming that would indicate calcification or bleeding. Contrast-enhanced T1-weighted image (F) confirms the presence of multiple small lesions with rim enhancement in the areas of MT T1 (D) and T2 hyperintensities (A). Chest skiagram of the patient showed miliary tuberculosis.

and macrophage by-products (free radicals), components that are possibly responsible for the hypointensity seen on T2-weighted images.[25] These MT T1 visible constituents of tuberculoma closely match the histologic appearances.[34] The MT ratio of the core has been shown to be much lower than similar-appearing cysticerci lesions.[20] In vivo MR spectroscopy of these tuberculomas reveals the presence of lipid peaks.[35] The presence of serine at 3.7 to 3.9 ppm on ex vivo/in vitro MR spectroscopy of the tuberculoma sample suggest the presence of *M tuberculosis* because serine is found in abundance in the wall of this bacterium.[25] T2 hypointensity is seen in some lymphomas, glioblastoma, metastases from colonic carcinoma or melanoma, fungal granulomas, or cysticerci lesions. Hemorrhage, hemorrhagic tumor, occult cerebrovascular malformation, and calcification may also appear as

T2 hypointense lesions. Susceptibility-weighted sequences such as SWAN may differentiate hemorrhage and calcification from other T2 hypo-intense lesions.

T2 hyperintense center with peripheral hypointense rim When liquefaction of the caseation occurs within a tuberculoma, it appears as a T2 hyperintense lesion with peripheral hypointense rim. On T1-weighted and MT T1-weighted images, the centers of these lesions are hypointense. Tuberculomas with liquid caseation show restriction on DW images (see **Figs. 2, 5,** and **8**). There is rim enhancement on postcontrast studies. The MTR remains significantly lower in tuberculoma compared with other conditions such as NCC. This appearance of a T2 hyperintense center with peripheral hypointense rim may also be seen in other conditions such as pyogenic or tubercular

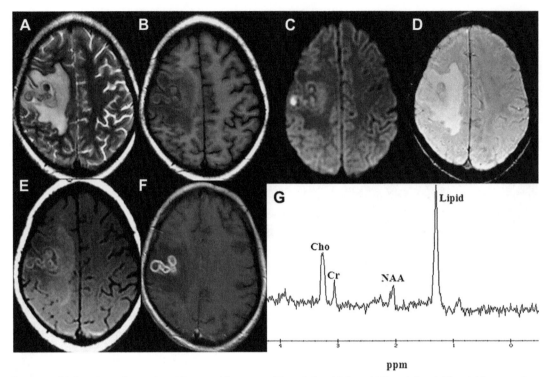

Fig. 5. Multiple tuberculomas in a 32-year-old woman. T2-weighted (*A*) and T1-weighted (*B*) axial images show multiple lesions with mixed intensity on T2-weighted as well as T1-weighted images in the right frontal region with perilesional edema. DW image (*C*) shows bright intensity in one of the lesions, suggesting liquefied caseation with restricted diffusion. SWAN image (*D*) does not reveal any blooming, eliminating the possibility of calcification or hemorrhage. MT T1-weighted (*E*) and contrast-enhanced T1-weighted images (*F*) show rim of hyperintensity around the lesions (*E*) that enhances on contrast. ¹H MR spectroscopy (*G*) reveals the prominent lipid peak with slightly increased choline and reduced *N*-acetyl aspartate (NAA) and creatine. Minimal increase in choline is seen from the cellular component of the tuberculoma; reduced NAA and creatine are caused by the partial volume effect and lipids represent the caseation. The patient had pulmonary tuberculosis and was on treatment. She responded to antituberculous therapy and lesions regressed in a period of 18 months.

abscesses, degenerating NCC, toxoplasmosis, and metastases. In NCC, the scolex appears as an eccentrically placed hypointense nodule on T2-weighted imaging that differentiates it from tuberculoma. The susceptibility-weighted and isotropic T2-weighted imaging techniques are helpful in differentiating these lesions from neurocysticercosis. MR spectroscopy may differentiate this stage of tuberculomas from pyogenic abscesses by showing cytosolic amino acids resonances in the latter.

Lesion with mixed/heterogeneous signal intensity At times, tubercular lesions show mixed intensity on spin-echo imaging with a rim of variable thickness that may appear minimally hyperintense on T1 and show variegated enhancement (**Fig. 9**). Similar-appearing lesions include lymphomas, glioblastoma, metastases, fungal granulomas, and toxoplasmosis. ¹H MR spectroscopy may be nonspecific in its differentiation. This type of

tubercular lesions show large choline and lipid resonances with variable creatine resonance and correlate with predominantly cellular infiltrate along with small areas of solid caseation on histopathology.[36] It is suggested that the presence of choline is caused by the contribution from the cellular component in this type of tuberculoma.[36] On MT images, the rim shows hyperintensity, whereas the caseous regions are heterogeneously hypointense.

Miliary tuberculosis Miliary brain tuberculosis is a result of hematogenous spread of infection in which multiple, small miliary tubercles of less than 2 mm are seen. It is usually associated with TBM. These lesions may not be visible on conventional spin-echo MR images or show only tiny foci of hyperintensity on T2-weighted images. The spin-echo invisible lesions are clearly visible on MT T1-weighted imaging. T1-weighted images after gadolinium administration show numerous small, homogeneous enhancing lesions

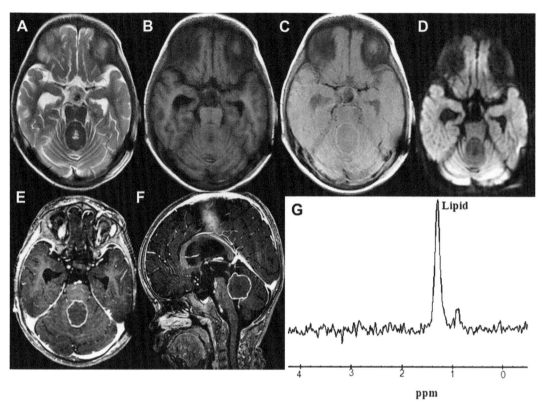

Fig. 6. Vermian tuberculoma in a 17-year-old boy. T2-weighted axial image (A) shows a hypointense mass with small central hyperintensity in the vermis that appears isointense with central hypointensity on the T1-weighted image (B) with obstructive hydrocephalus. The rim of the lesion is hyperintense on the MT T1 image (C). No diffusion restriction is noted on the DW image (D). Postcontrast BRAVO axial (E), and sagittal (F) images show rim enhancement. ^{1}H MR spectroscopy (G) shows prominent lipid peaks. Histology confirmed it as tuberculoma.

(see **Fig. 4**). MT T1 imaging helps in defining the true disease load in these patients.[20]

Role of advanced imaging In a recent study, Gupta and colleagues performed dynamic contrast enhancement MR (DCE-MR) imaging in 13 patients with brain tuberculoma and showed that the regional cerebral blood volume (rCBV) of the cellular portion significantly correlated with the cellular fraction volume, microvascular density (MVD), and vascular endothelial growth factor (VEGF) of the excised tuberculomas. MVD also correlated significantly with VEGF. Correlation between rCBV, MVD, and VEGF confirms that rCBV is a measure of angiogenesis in the cellular fraction of the brain tuberculoma.[37,38] In another recent DCE-MR imaging study in brain tuberculoma, the investigators reported a significant positive correlation between physiologic indices (K^{trans} and v$_e$) and matrix metalloproteinase-9 (MMP-9) expression (a marker of blood-brain barrier disruption) in excised tuberculoma. However, a weak correlation between physiologic indices and

VEGF expression in excised tuberculoma suggests a limited role of VEGF in opening of the blood-brain barrier. Correlation between K^{trans} and MMP-9 suggests that K^{trans} can be used as a surrogate marker of blood-brain barrier disruption. These parameters may be useful in assessment of therapeutic response in tuberculomas.

Diffusion tensor MR imaging (DTI) has been widely used for the detection of white matter abnormality in various clinical conditions.[39–41] A recent serial DTI study showed strong negative correlation of MMP-9 expression in excised tuberculoma with fractional anisotropy (FA), linear anisotropy (CL), and planar anisotropy (CP), and significant direct correlation with spherical anisotropy (CS). The investigators also reported significant increase in FA, CL, and CP along with significantly decreased CS with time in patients who were serially followed up with antitubercular therapy[42] (ATT). These methods may be of value in objective assessment of therapy in tuberculoma and guide the clinician in modulation of treatment.

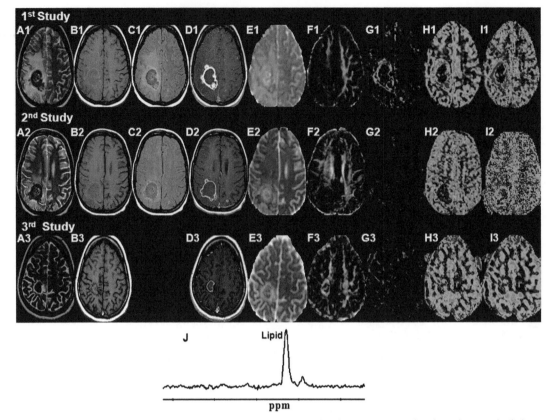

Fig. 7. Right parieto-occipital tuberculoma showing regression with therapy. T2-weighted axial image (*A1*) shows a hypointense lesion with areas of small hyperintensity and perifocal edema that gradually regressed after 6 months (*A2*) and 14 months (*A3*) of therapy. Note the corresponding changes on T1 (*B1–3*), MT T1 (*C1–2*), postcontrast T1-weighted images (*D1–3*). ADC maps (*E1–3*) show gradual regression in the lesion, whereas FA maps show increase in FA (*F1–3*) in the periphery, suggesting disappearance of edema and increase in fibrosis around the lesion. T1 contrast perfusion maps such as K^{trans} (*G1–3*), corrected CBV (*H1–3*) and CBF (*I1–3*) show gradual normalization suggesting healing of the lesion. Note the persistence of rim enhancement (*D3*) in the absence of any significant K^{trans} (*G3*), suggesting the presence of false disease activity. Single-voxel ^1H MR spectroscopy done on the first study shows only the presence of lipids (*J*).

Tuberculous brain abscess

Tuberculous brain abscesses constitute approximately 4% to 7% of the total CNS TB in developing countries. These abscesses are diagnosed from macroscopic evidence of abscess formation along with histologic demonstration of vascular granulation tissue in the wall containing both acute and chronic inflammatory cells, and isolation of *M tuberculosis*.[43]

On MR imaging, these appear as large, solitary, and frequently multiloculated ring-enhancing lesions with surrounding edema and mass effect.[44] DW imaging in tuberculous abscesses shows restricted diffusion with low ADC values.[45–48] High lipid-containing *M tuberculosis* bacilli are probably responsible for significantly lower MTR values from the rim of tuberculous abscesses (19.89 ± 1.55) compared with pyogenic abscesses (24.81 ± 0.03).[49]

In vivo ^1H MR spectroscopy in tuberculous abscesses shows only lactate and lipid signals (at 0.9 and 1.3 ppm), without any evidence of cytosolic amino acids. This pattern may be useful but is not characteristic because a similar pattern may also be seen in staphylococcal abscess. Quantitative MT T1 imaging may be needed to help in its differentiation (**Fig. 10**).

Spinal Tuberculosis

Intraspinal TB

The MR features of spinal meningitis are usually visible on contrast-enhanced images in which at times a thin, diffuse meningeal enhancement may be noted. In arachnoiditis, imaging features include CSF loculation and obliteration of the spinal subarachnoid space with loss of outline of the spinal cord and clumping of the nerve roots

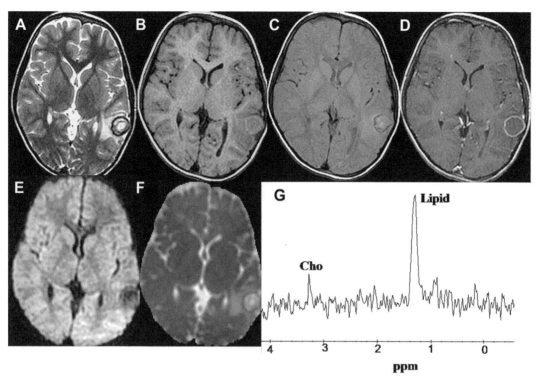

Fig. 8. A large tuberculoma in the left temporal region. T2-weighted axial image (A) shows central hyperintensity with a peripheral hypointense rim and perifocal edema. The lesion appears hypointense in the center with peripheral isointensity on the T1-weighted (B) image. MT T1 image (C) shows a hyperintense rim beyond the T2 hypointensity, suggesting a cellular rim of the tuberculoma that enhances on the postcontrast T1-weighted image (D). The lesion does not show restriction of diffusion on the DW image (E) with high ADC (F). ¹H MR spectroscopy (G) shows prominent lipid resonance at 1.3 ppm with small resonance of choline. Histology confirmed it as tuberculoma.

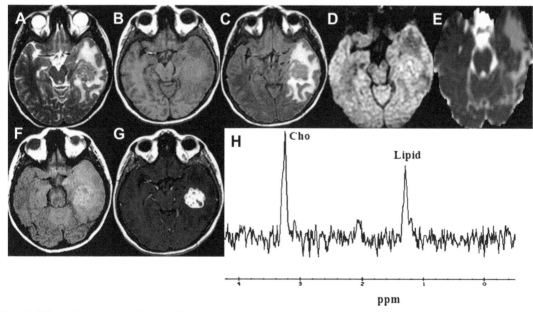

Fig. 9. Tuberculoma presenting as a heterogeneous mass in the left temporal lobe in a 40-year-old man. A mass lesion with mixed signal intensity appears with surrounding edema on T2-weighted (A), T1-weighted (B), and FLAIR (C) images. Small areas of hyperintensity are seen within this mass on DW images (D), which have low signal on the ADC map (E). MT T1 image shows multiple small hyperintense rings around these hyperintense DW imaging lesions (F), which enhance on the postcontrast T1-weighted image (G). ¹H MR spectroscopy (H) of this lesion reveals a large lipid with increase in choline. Histology confirmed it as tuberculoma.

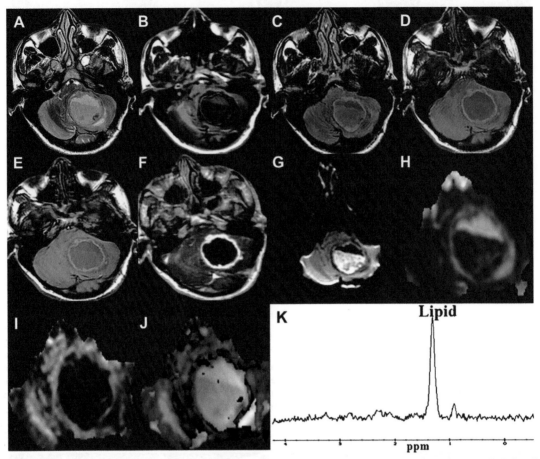

Fig. 10. Tubercular abscess in the left cerebellar hemisphere. Axial T2-weighted image (*A*) shows a well-defined, round, heterogeneously hyperintense lesion with peripheral hypointense rim. On the T1-weighted image (*B*), the lesion is heterogeneously hypointense centrally with a peripheral isointense rim. Axial FLAIR (*C*) image shows minimal perilesional edema. On the MT T1 images, with MT pulse off (*D*) and pulse on (*E*), the T2 hypointense rim appears hyperintense. Axial postcontrast T1-weighted (*F*) image shows thick nodular rim enhancement. The DW image (*G*) shows restriction in the dependent part of the cavity with corresponding low ADC (*H*) suggesting cellular debris. FA map (*I*) and color-coded FA map (*J*) show high FA in the wall as well as in parts of the cavity of the lesion. ¹H MR spectroscopy (*K*) shows dominant lipid resonances. Histology from the wall was consistent with tuberculous abscess. Pus culture was positive for *M tuberculosis*.

in the lumbar region. Contrast studies may show nodular, thick, linear dural enhancement, often completely filling the subarachnoid space on postcontrast MR images.[50–52] In chronic stages of disease, there may not be any enhancement even though unenhanced images show signs of arachnoiditis.[50,51] The spinal cord may be involved secondarily and show infarction, syringomyelia, myelitis, and tuberculoma formation. Syringomyelia is seen as cord cavitation with CSF-like intensity that does not show any enhancement on postcontrast images.[50,51]

Myelitis

Tuberculous myelitis is usually associated with tuberculous intracranial involvement of the meninges or brain parenchyma, or with tuberculous arachnoiditis of the spine (**Fig. 11**). Intramedullary tuberculomas are uncommon and have similar imaging features to brain tuberculomas.[53,54] MR imaging features of spinal tubercular abscess, another rare condition, are similar to cerebral tubercular abscess. As the treatment begins, there is reduction in the T2 hyperintensity in the spinal cord and enhancement becomes more clearly defined on postcontrast T1-weighted images.[55] The surrounding edema continues to be extensive. These findings suggest the beginning of intramedullary abscess formation with imaging features seen in brain abscesses.[55] The abnormalities visible on T2-weighted images subside in weeks, whereas contrast enhancement may persist for months.[55]

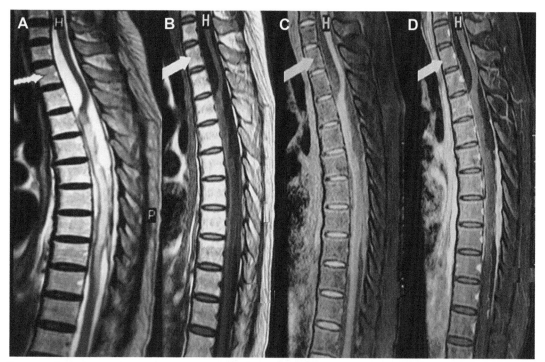

Fig. 11. Tubercular myelitis with arachnoiditis. Midsagittal T2, T1, and fat-suppressed precontrast and postcontrast T1-weighted images (*A–D*) of the dorsal spine show nonenhancing CSF-like signal intensity collection anterior (*arrow*) (C6–D2 level) and posterior (D3–D5 level) to the spinal cord. The underlying upper dorsal cord is kinked. The spinal cord from D3 to D9 shows diffuse central hyperintensity (*A*). The midsagittal fat-saturated postcontrast T1-weighted (*D*) image shows thick continuous meningeal enhancement posteriorly from D5 to D8 with diffuse leptomeningeal enhancement. White arrow denotes the second dorsal vertebra.

Dural and subdural disorders

Tuberculous pus formation may occur between the dura and the leptomeninges and appear as a loculation. This appears hyperintense on T2-weighted images and isointense to hypointense on T1-weighted images. However, the dural granulomas appear hypointense to isointense on T2-weighted images and isointense on T1-weighted images. Peripheral enhancement can be seen on postcontrast images.[51]

Epidural tuberculous abscesses may be seen in isolation or in association with arachnoiditis, myelitis, spondylitis, and intramedullary and dural tuberculomas.[51,55] These lesions appear to be isointense to the spinal cord on T1-weighted images and show mixed intensity on T2-weighted images (**Fig. 12**). Uniform enhancement is seen if the TB inflammatory process is phlegmonous in nature on postcontrast images, which converts to peripheral enhancement if epidural abscess formation or caseation develops.[51,55]

Tuberculous spondylitis

Tuberculous spondylitis is a frequent occurrence in developing countries and is an important cause of spine-related morbidity. Early diagnosis and prompt treatment are required to avoid permanent damage or deformity in the spine.

Tuberculous spondylitis commonly involves vertebral bodies; however, disease in other structures, such as posterior osseous elements, epidural space, paraspinal soft tissue, and intervertebral disks, is also seen.[56] The most commonly involved sites in tuberculous spondylitis are dorsal and lumbar spine, especially the thoracolumbar junction. Usually more than 1 vertebral body is affected, but solitary vertebral lesions can also occur.

MR has the unique ability to detect marrow abnormalities before any bony destruction; hence it has assumed the role of primary imaging modality. The involved vertebrae are hyperintense on T2-weighted images and hypointense on T1-weighted images.[56,57] As the disease progresses, diskovertebral involvement may be visible. Features such as vertebral intraosseous abscesses (**Figs. 13–15**), paraspinal abscesses, diskitis, skip lesions, and spinal canal encroachment can all be seen. Reduction in disk height and morphologic alteration of the paraspinal soft tissue is a late occurrence. Enhanced MR studies are valuable for characterizing tuberculous spondylitis by

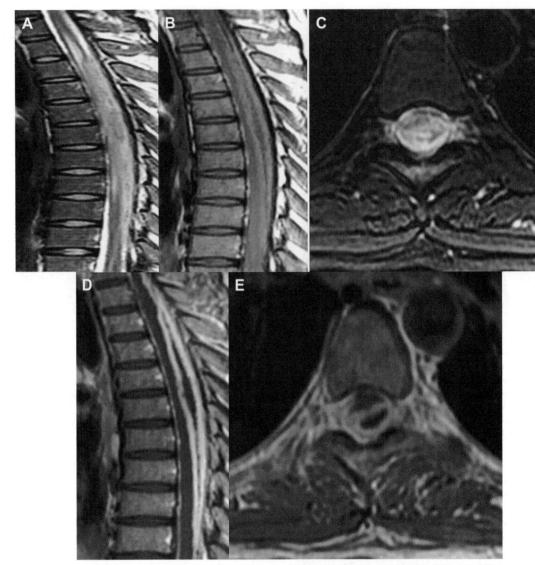

Fig. 12. Posterior epidural tuberculous abscess in an HIV-positive patient. Sagittal T2-weighted image (*A*) shows a curvilinear area of increased signal intensity in the posterior subarachnoid space of the mid-dorsal spinal canal. The corresponding area is hypointense on the T1-weighted image (*B*). The underlying spinal cord is compressed and shows increased signal intensity with almost complete obliteration of the subarachnoid space (*A–C*) caused by mass effect. Sagittal (*D*) and axial (*E*) postcontrast T1-weighted images show thick peripheral wall enhancement with a central nonenhancing area of liquefaction suggesting epidural abscess. No abnormal enhancement is noted in the adjacent vertebral bodies and intervertebral disks.

showing rim enhancement around intraosseous and paraspinal soft tissue abscesses (see **Figs. 13–15**) and, rarely, in lesions with solid caseation.[57] Therapeutic response is assessed by showing progressive increase in signal intensity on T1-weighted images (**Fig. 16**) in the affected vertebrae caused by fatty marrow deposition that indicates healing.[56]

Demonstration of bone fragments in the intra-spinal and/or extraspinal soft tissue is considered characteristic of tuberculous spondylitis.[56] This is

caused by the lack of proteolytic enzymes that lyse the bone in the tuberculous inflammatory exudate. These fragments are best shown on CT; however, T2*-weighted images can also show these by accentuating the diamagnetic suscepti-bility properties of the calcium salt present in the bone fragments. The presence of bone fragment is characteristic of tuberculous spondylitis even in the absence of abscess formation.[57]

As in brain, diffusion imaging is useful for demonstrating restriction of diffusion in spinal

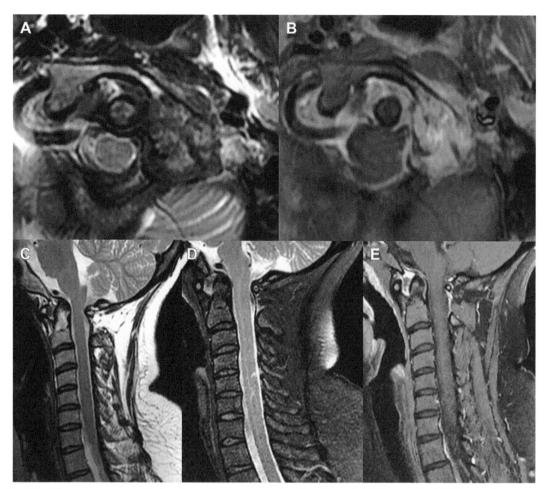

Fig. 13. Tuberculous spondylitis involving the craniovertebral junction. Axial T2-weighted (*A*) image shows area of heterogeneous signal intensity in the occipital condyle and lateral mass of atlas on the left side. Axial (*B*) and midsagittal (*E*) fat-suppressed postcontrast T1-weighted image shows moderate heterogeneous contrast enhancement of the altered area. (*C–D*) Extension of the enhancing soft tissue between the anterior arch of atlas and dens on T2 images resulting in atlantoaxial dislocation (AAD) of 4.3 mm with mild basilar invagination causing mild narrowing of the foramen magnum. No abnormal cord signal intensity or enhancement is seen.

infections.[58] Tubercular abscesses in soft tissues as well as within the vertebrae also behave in a similar manner and show restriction of diffusion (see **Fig. 15**) with low ADC.

TUBERCULOSIS IN HIV/AIDS

Tuberculosis has seen a resurgence in the past 2 decades because of the increasing numbers of patients with AIDS.[59] A total of 5% to 9% of patients with AIDS develop tuberculosis, and, of these, 2% to 18% have CNS involvement.[23,60,61] CNS tuberculosis may be the initial clinical manifestation of AIDS and may result from reactivation of a previous infection or from a primary, newly acquired infection.[59] The predominant mechanism of disease spread is hematogenous.

Pathologic Features

The most common intracranial manifestation of tuberculosis is basal meningitis; however, tuberculomas, tuberculous abscess, and cerebral infarction are also seen. HIV infection may alter the pathologic features of TBM. Fewer basal exudates and greater numbers of acid-fast bacilli occur in the brain parenchyma and meninges in patients with HIV infection.[62]

Imaging Features

Imaging features depend on the site of infection. In TBM, hydrocephalus and meningeal enhancement are seen.[60] The hydrocephalus results primarily from obstruction of the basal

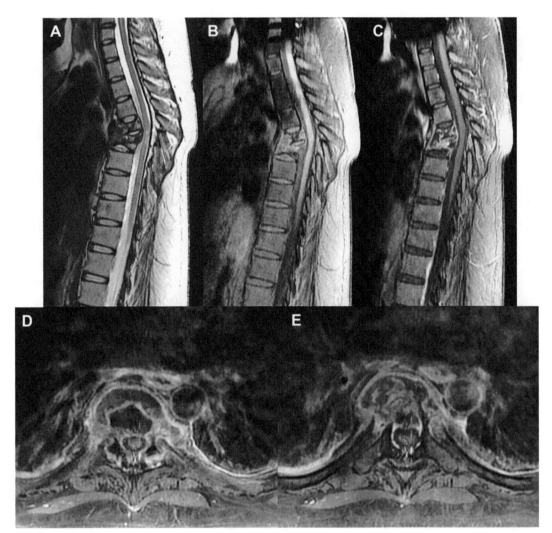

Fig. 14. Tuberculous spondylitis of the dorsal spine. Midsagittal T2-weighted (*A*) and fat-saturated T1-weighted (*B*) images show contiguous involvement with an area of altered signal intensity in D2 and D3 vertebral bodies and the intervening disk, resulting in wedge collapse and kyphotic deformity. Hyperintense signal intensity that indicates edema is noted in the underlying cord caused by mass effect. Fat-suppressed postcontrast T1-weighted (*C*) image shows moderate heterogeneous enhancement of the altered signal area within the vertebral bodies. Axial postcontrast T1-weighted (*D, E*) images show a thick-walled abscess in the prevertebral and paravertebral region. Bilateral minimal pleural effusion is also noted.

cistern by inflammatory exudates. In addition, cerebral abscesses and tuberculomas may be seen.[60]

Tuberculomas occurred in 24% of patients in a study by Whiteman and colleagues.[23] The appearance of tuberculomas in AIDS is similar to those seen in patients who do not have HIV and was described earlier. On postcontrast images, noncaseating tuberculomas show nodular homogeneous enhancement. Caseating tuberculomas have ring enhancement. Tuberculous abscesses are more common in HIV-infected patients. Among patients with CNS

tuberculosis, 4% to 8% of those without HIV infection developed abscesses, compared with 20% in the group of patients with HIV.[23] Abscesses tend to be larger than tuberculomas, frequently greater than 3 cm. Abscesses are also more frequently solitary unlike tuberculomas. The imaging features of tubercular abscesses are described in an earlier section.[9]

Cerebral infarction complicates CNS tuberculosis and was seen in 36% of the patients in the study by Whiteman and colleagues.[23] Imaging features are similar to those described in patients without HIV.

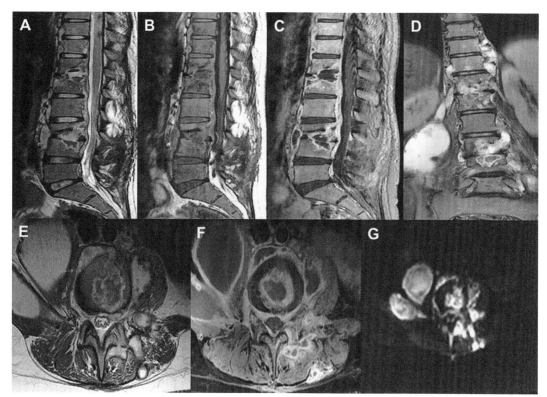

Fig. 15. Tuberculous spondylitis of lumbar spine. Midsagittal T2-weighted (*A*) and T1-weighted (*B*) images show areas of abnormal signal intensity which are hyperintense on T2-weighted, and hypointense on T1-weighted, images in D12, L1, L3, and L4 vertebral bodies and intervertebral disks at D12/L1 and L3/4 levels, with partial wedge collapse of L3 vertebra. Fat-suppressed postcontrast sagittal T1-weighted (*C*) image shows heterogenous enhancement of the altered signal area with central areas of liquefaction. Coronal T2-weighted (*D*) image shows craniocaudal extent of the right paravertebral abscess. Axial T2-weighted (*E*) and axial fat-suppressed postcontrast T1-weighted (*F*) images show hyperintense prevertebral, bilateral psoas muscles, and left paraspinal collection with peripheral enhancement. DW (*G*) image shows restriction inside the collection.

ASSESSMENT OF THERAPEUTIC RESPONSE

Once the diagnosis is made on imaging and other laboratory investigations, the patients are given antitubercular treatment[63,64] (ATT). MR imaging is the modality of choice for following these patients. Serial imaging in responding patients usually shows a decrease in lesion size after 3 to 4 months and its disappearance by 12 months.[64] Rarely, a paradoxic progression of intracranial tuberculomas or development of new lesions during the treatment of CNS tuberculosis has also been recognized.[65] Advanced imaging techniques such as perfusion imaging and DTI may be useful in the assessment of response in these patients (see **Fig. 7**). It has been shown that changes in K^{trans} and v_e closely match the therapeutic response in brain tuberculoma even in the presence of a paradoxic increase in the lesion volume.[37]

A reduction in the intensity of the meningeal enhancement is considered a positive response to treatment in patients with TBM. In a recent serial DTI study in TBM, it was shown that the cortical FA values decreased on treatment (0.13 ± 0.02) compared with baseline values (0.15 ± 0.03). The investigators also reported a significant positive correlation between FA and proinflammatory molecules (PMs), thereby suggesting that the DTI metrics may be used as noninvasive surrogate marker of PMs in assessing therapeutic response in patients with TBM.[37]

Calcification of the meninges and parenchymal tuberculoma is seen as sequelae of TBM, and usually appear markedly hypointense on all spin-echo sequences. An isointense or hypointense core with a hyperintense rim on T2-weighted and FLAIR images is the most common imaging appearance.[66]

SUMMARY

CNS tuberculosis is a major cause of sickness and death in developing countries and is being increasingly seen in the developed world because

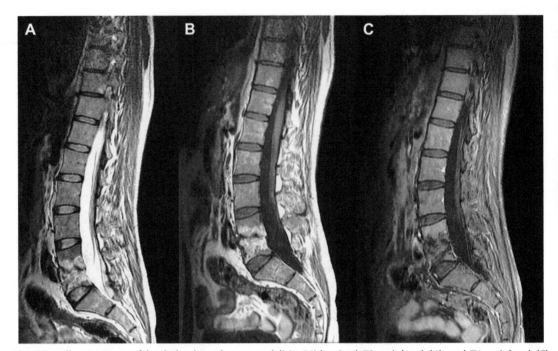

Fig. 16. Follow-up case of healed tuberculous spondylitis. Midsagittal T2-weighted (*A*) and T1-weighted (*B*) images show abnormal hyperintensity in the paradiscal area of L4 and 5 vertebral bodies showing suppression with no obvious enhancement on a sagittal fat-suppressed postcontrast T1-weighted (*C*) image, suggesting fatty replacement. No residual prevertebral or epidural collection is seen. The intervening disk is hypointense and thinned out, suggesting sclerosis.

of the emergence of AIDS. It spreads hematoge-neously and involves meninges, brain paren-chyma, spinal cord, and covering bones. The presenting clinical features vary according to the site of infection, and are usually nonspecific. Isola-tion of *M tuberculosis* for the definitive diagnosis is possible only in a few patients. MR imaging plays an important role in its early recognition. MT-T1 imaging is considered superior to conventional spin-echo sequences for imaging the abnormal meninges and tuberculomas. The MT ratio of tu-berculomas remains significantly lower compared with other conditions such as cysticercosis. Use of ^{1}H MR spectroscopy in combination with other MR imaging techniques may also help in its differenti-ation from similar diseases. Imaging characteris-tics of tuberculomas in HIV remain the same as in patients without HIV. Advanced imaging methods such as perfusion imaging and DTI may be of value in objective assessment of therapy in tuberculoma and guide the clinician in modulation of treatment.

REFERENCES

1. WHO 2010/2011 tuberculosis global facts. Available at: www.who.int/tb/publications/2010/factsheet_tb_2010.pdf. Accessed March 31, 2011.

2. Garg RK. Classic diseases revisited: tuberculosis of the central nervous system. Postgrad Med J 1999; 75:133–40.

3. Rock RB, Olin M, Baker CA, et al. Central nervous system tuberculosis: pathogenesis and clinical aspects. Clin Microbiol Rev 2008;21: 243–61.

4. Thwaites GE, Tran TH. Tuberculous meningitis: many questions, too few answers. Lancet Neurol 2005;4: 160–70.

5. Tandon PN, Pathak SN. Tuberculosis of the central nervous system. In: Spillane JD, editor. Tropical neurology. New York: Oxford University Press; 1973. p. 37–62.

6. Hopewell PC. Overview of clinical tuberculosis. In: Bloom BR, editor. Tuberculosis: pathogenesis, pro-tection, and control. Washington, DC: American Society of Microbiology; 1994. p. 25–46.

7. Dastur DK, Manghani DK, Udani PM. Pathology and pathogenic mechanisms in neurotuberculosis. Ra-diol Clin North Am 1995;33:733–52.

8. Shah GV, Desai SB, Malde H, et al. Tuberculosis of sphenoid sinus: CT findings. AJR Am J Roentgenol 1993;161:681–2.

9. Garcia-Monco JC. Central nervous system tubercu-losis. Neurol Clin 1999;17:737–59.

10. Dastur DK, Lalitha VS, Udani PM, et al. The brain and meninges in tuberculous meningitis-gross

pathology in 100 cases and pathogenesis. Neurol India 1970;18:86–100.

11. Gray F, Alonso JM. Bacterial infections of the central nervous system. In: Graham DI, Lantos PL, editors. Greenfield's neuropathology. 7th edition. London: Arnold (Hodder Headline Group); 2002. p. 151–93.

12. Jinkins JR, Gupta RK, Chang KJ, et al. MR imaging of the central nervous system tuberculosis. Radiol Clin North Am 1995;33:771–86.

13. Gupta RK, Jena A, Sharma A, et al. MR imaging of intracranial tuberculomas. J Comput Assist Tomogr 1988;12:280–5.

14. Brooks WD, Fletcher AP, Wilson RR. Spinal cord complications of tuberculous meningitis; a clinical and pathological study. Q J Med 1954;23:275–90.

15. Leonard JM, Des Prez RM. Tuberculous meningitis. Infect Dis Clin North Am 1990;4:769–87.

16. Dott NM, Levine E. Intracranial tuberculoma. Edin Medical J 1939;46:36–41.

17. Kennedy DH, Fallon RJ. Tuberculous meningitis. JAMA 1979;241:264–8.

18. Zuger A, Lowy FD. Tuberculosis. In: Scheld WM, Whitley RJ, Durack DT, editors. Infection of the central nervous system. 2nd edition. Philadelphia: Lippincott-Raven; 1997. p. 417–43.

19. Bonington A, Strang JI, Klapper PE, et al. Use of Roche AMPLICOR Mycobacterium tuberculosis PCR in early diagnosis of tuberculous meningitis. J Clin Microbiol 1998;36:1251–4.

20. Gupta RK, Kathuria MK, Pradhan S. Magnetization transfer MR imaging in CNS tuberculosis. AJNR Am J Neuroradiol 1999;20:867–75.

21. Gupta RK, Gupta S, Singh D, et al. MR imaging and angiography in tuberculous meningitis. Neuroradiology 1994;36:87–92.

22. Kioumehr F, Dadsetan MR, Rooholamini AA. Central nervous system tuberculosis: MRI. Neuroradiology 1994;36:93–6.

23. Whiteman M, Espinoza L, Post MJD, et al. Central nervous system tuberculosis in HIV-infected patients: clinical and radiographic findings. AJNR Am J Neuroradiol 1995;16:1319–27.

24. Kamra P, Azad R, Prasad KN, et al. Infectious meningitis: prospective evaluation with magnetization transfer MRI. Br J Radiol 2004;77:387–94.

25. Gupta RK. Tuberculosis and other non-tuberculous bacterial granulomatous infections. In: Gupta RK, Lufkin RB, editors. MR imaging and spectroscopy of central nervous system infection. New York: Kluwer Academic/Plenum Publishers; 2001. p. 95–145.

26. Tandon PN, Bhatia R, Bhargava S. Tuberculous meningitis. In: Vinken PJ, Bruyn GW, Klawans HZ, editors, Handbook of clinical neurology, vol. 8. Amsterdam: Elsevier; 1988. p. 196–226.

27. Shukla R, Abbas A, Kumar P, et al. Evaluation of cerebral infarction in tuberculous meningitis by diffusion weighted imaging. J Infect 2008;57:298–306.

28. Kim IY, Jung S, Jung TY, et al. Intracranial tuberculoma with adjacent inflammatory aneurysms. J Clin Neurosci 2008;15(10):1174–6.

29. Brismar T, Hugosson C, Larsson SG, et al. Tuberculosis as a mimicker of brain tumor. Acta Radiol 1996; 37:496–505.

30. Goyal M, Sharma A, Mishra NK, et al. Imaging appearance of pachymeningeal tuberculosis. AJR Am J Roentgenol 1997;169:1421–4.

31. Whelan MA, Steven J. Intracranial tuberculoma. Radiology 1981;138:75–81.

32. Kesavadas C, Somasundaram S, Rao RM, et al. Meckel's cave tuberculoma with unusual infratemporal extension. J Neuroimaging 2007;17:264–8.

33. Salem R, Khochtali I, Jellali MA, et al. Isolated hypophyseal tuberculoma: often mistaken. Neurochirurgie 2009;55:603–6.

34. Gupta RK, Hussian N, Kathuria MK, et al. Magnetization transfer MR imaging correlation with histopathology in intracranial tuberculomas. Clin Radiol 2001;56:656–63.

35. Gupta RK, Roy R, Dev R, et al. Finger printing of Mycobacterium tuberculosis in patients with intracranial tuberculomas by using in vivo, ex vivo, and in vitro magnetic resonance spectroscopy. Magn Reson Med 1996;36:829–33.

36. Venkatesh SK, Gupta RK, Paul L, et al. Spectroscopic increase in signal is not specific marker for differentiation of infective/inflammatory from neoplastic lesions of the brain. J Magn Reson Imaging 2001;14:8–15.

37. Haris M, Gupta RK, Husain M, et al. Assessment of therapeutic response on serial dynamic contrast enhanced MR imaging in brain tuberculomas. Clin Radiol 2008;63:562–74.

38. Gupta RK, Haris M, Husain N, et al. Relative cerebral blood volume is a measure of angiogenesis in brain tuberculoma. J Comput Assist Tomogr 2007; 31:335–41.

39. Hasan KM, Gupta RK, Santos RM, et al. Diffusion tensor fractional anisotropy of the normal-appearing seven segments of the corpus callosum in healthy adults and relapsing remitting multiple sclerosis patients. J Magn Reson Imaging 2005;21: 735–43.

40. Thomalla G, Glauche V, Weiller C, et al. Time course of Wallerian degeneration after ischemic stroke revealed by diffusion tensor imaging. J Neurol Neurosurg Psychiatry 2005;76:266–8.

41. Gupta RK, Saksena S, Agarwal A, et al. Diffusion tensor imaging in late posttraumatic epilepsy. Epilepsia 2005;46:1465–71.

42. Gupta RK, Haris M, Husain N, et al. DTI derived indices correlate with immunohistochemistry obtained matrix metalloproteinase (MMP-9) expression in cellular fraction of brain tuberculoma. J Neurol Sci 2008;275:78–85.

43. Whitener DR. Tuberculous brain abscess. Report of a case and review of the literature. Arch Neurol 1978;35:148–55.

44. Farrar DJ, Flanigan TP, Gordon NM, et al. Tuberculous brain abscess in a patient with HIV infection: case report and review. Am J Med 1997; 102:297–301.

45. Gupta RK, Prakash M, Mishra AM, et al. Role of diffusion weighted imaging in differentiation of intracranial tuberculoma and tuberculous abscess from cysticercus granulomas—a report of more than 100 lesions. Eur J Radiol 2005;55:384–92.

46. Mishra AM, Gupta RK, Saksena S, et al. Biological correlates of diffusivity in brain abscess. Magn Reson Med 2005;54:878–85.

47. Luthra G, Parihar A, Nath K, et al. Comparative evaluation of fungal, tubercular, and pyogenic brain abscesses with conventional and diffusion MR imaging and proton MR spectroscopy. AJNR Am J Neuroradiol 2007;28:1332–8.

48. Reddy JS, Mishra AM, Behari S, et al. Role of diffusion-weighted imaging in the differential diagnosis of intracranial cystic mass lesions: a report of 147 lesions. Surg Neurol 2006;66:246–50.

49. Gupta RK, Vatsal DK, Husain N, et al. Differentiation of tuberculous from pyogenic brain abscesses with in vivo proton MR spectroscopy and magnetization transfer MR imaging. AJNR Am J Neuroradiol 2001;22:1503–9.

50. Kumar A, Montanera W, Willinsky R, et al. MR features of tuberculous arachnoiditis. J Comput Assist Tomogr 1993;17:127–30.

51. Gupta RK, Gupta S, Kumar S, et al. MRI in intraspinal tuberculosis. Neuroradiology 1994;36:39–43.

52. Chang KH, Han MH, Kim IO, et al. Tuberculous arachnoiditis of the spine: findings in myelography, CT, and MR imaging. AJNR Am J Neuroradiol 1989;10:1255–62.

53. Jena A, Banerji AK, Tripathi RP, et al. Demonstration of intramedullary tuberculomas by magnetic resonance imaging: a report of two cases. Br J Radiol 1991;64:555–7.

54. Lu M. Imaging diagnosis of spinal intramedullary tuberculoma: case reports and literature review. J Spinal Cord Med 2010;33(2):159–62.

55. Murphy KJ, Brunberg JA, Quint DJ, et al. Spinal cord infection: myelitis and abscess formation. AJNR Am J Neuroradiol 1998;19:341–8.

56. Sharif HS, Aabed MY, Haddad MC. Magnetic resonance imaging and computed tomography of infectious spondylitis. In: Bloem JL, Satoris DJ, editors. MRI and CT of the musculoskeletal system: a text atlas. Baltimore (MD): Williams & Wilkins; 1992. p. 580–602.

57. Gupta RK, Agarwal P, Rastogi H, et al. Problems in differentiating spinal tuberculosis from neoplasm on MRI. Neuroradiology 1996;38:S97–104.

58. Eastwood JD, Vollmer RT, Provenzale JM. Diffusion-weighted imaging in a patient with vertebral and epidural abscesses. AJNR Am J Neuroradiol 2002; 23:496–8.

59. Smith AB, Smirniotopoulos JG, Rushing EJ. Central nervous system infections associated with human immunodeficiency virus infection: radiologic- pathologic correlation. Radiographics 2008;28:2033–58.

60. Villoria MF, de la Torre J, Fortea F, et al. Intracranial tuberculosis in AIDS: CT and MRI findings. Neuroradiology 1992;34:11–4.

61. Bishburg E, Sunderam G, Reichman LB, et al. CNS TB with AIDS and its related complex. Ann Intern Med 1986;105:210–3.

62. Katrak SM, Shembalkar PK, Bijwe SR, et al. The clinical, radiological and pathological profile of tuberculous meningitis in patients with and without human immunodeficiency virus infection. J Neurol Sci 2000; 181:118–26.

63. Gupta RK, Jena A, Singh AK, et al. Role of magnetic resonance (MR) in the diagnosis and management of intracranial tuberculomas. Clin Radiol 1990;41: 120–7.

64. Awada A, Daif AK, Pirani M, et al. Evolution of brain tuberculomas under standard antituberculous treatment. J Neurol Sci 1998;156:47–52.

65. Bas NS, Guzey FK, Emel E, et al. Paradoxical intracranial tuberculomas requiring surgical treatment. Pediatr Neurosurg 2005;41:201–5.

66. Ku BD, Yoo SD. Extensive meningeal and parenchymal calcified tuberculoma as long-term residual sequelae of tuberculous meningitis. Neurol India 2009;57:521–2.

Parasitic Diseases of the Central Nervous System

Ahmed Abdel Khalek Abdel Razek, MD[a,*],
Arvemas Watcharakorn, MD[b,c], Mauricio Castillo, MD[b]

KEYWORDS

- Imaging • Parasitic • Infection • Central nervous system
- Cysticercosis • Toxoplasmosis

Parasitic diseases are distributed worldwide, with increased prevalence in areas of poor sanitation. Although these diseases occur much more frequently in developing countries, sporadic cases occur in nonendemic areas because of an increase in international travel and immunosuppression caused by posttransplantation therapy or HIV infection. Parasitic diseases can involve the central nervous system (CNS) with multiple clinical presentations. The most common parasitic infection of the CNS is cysticercosis; other less frequent infections are toxoplasmosis, echinococcosis, and schistosomiasis. Rare parasitic diseases are sparganosis, paragonimiasis, malariasis, amebiasis, toxocariasis, and American and African trypanosomiases. MR imaging is the most helpful tool because it identifies characteristic features of the illness studied. Some advanced techniques, such as diffusion MR, perfusion MR, and MR spectroscopy, provide more clues for differentiation of parasitic diseases of the CNS from simulating lesions. The radiologist plays a vital role in the diagnostic work-up of these infections. By interfacing with clinicians, the radiologist can help direct appropriate testing and treatment, ultimately decreasing the morbidity and mortality associated with these infections.[1–5]

CYSTICERCOSIS

Cysticercosis is the most common parasitic infection of the CNS. It is found worldwide, particularly in Central and South America, India, Africa, East Asia, and Eastern Europe. Cysticercosis is caused by the encysted larvae of the tapeworm *Taenia solium*. It develops after ingestion of eggs from the feces of a tapeworm carrier, which is followed by hematogenous spread to neural, muscular, and ocular tissue. Intracranially, the oncospheres, the primary larval form of *T solium*, develop into a secondary larval form called "cysticerci." There are many types of cerebral cysticercosis. The parenchymal type is the most common type, whereas the subarachnoid (cisternal), intraventricular, and mixed types are also observed.[6–9] Cysticercosis affects males and females equally and manifests predominantly in young adults, with a peak occurrence at 25 to 35 years of age. The clinical presentation is nonspecific. Patients present with epilepsy (50%–70%), headache (43%), symptoms of cerebrospinal fluid (CSF) flow obstruction (33%), and signs of meningeal irritation (<2%). Seizures are a result of perilesional inflammation in degenerating cysts, although infarction, vasculitis, and even calcified granulomas may also act

No funding support.
The authors have nothing to disclose.
[a] Diagnostic Radiology Department, Mansoura Faculty of Medicine, Mansoura, Egypt
[b] Division of Neuroradiology, Department of Radiology, University of North Carolina at Chapel Hill, Chapel Hill, NC, USA
[c] Department of Radiology, Faculty of Medicine, Thammasat University, Pathumthani, Thailand
* Corresponding author.
E-mail address: arazek@mans.edu.eg

Neuroimag Clin N Am 21 (2011) 815–841
doi:10.1016/j.nic.2011.07.005

as predisposing factors. The cysticercus-specific IgG antibody level, in either serum or CSF, has a specificity and sensitivity of 100% and 98%, respectively. The common sites of cysticercosis are the CNS, the eye, and muscle tissue. It commonly involves the brain parenchyma; the ventricles (20%–25%); or the subarachnoid space (2%–3%). The corticomedullary junction is the primary location of the parenchymal form of this parasite. More than one anatomic site is often involved, and one patient can have lesions in different stages of the disease simultaneously.[6–12]

Parenchymal Cysticercosis

Parenchymal cysticercosis is divided into four stages: (1) vesicular, (2) colloidal vesicular, (3) granular nodular, and (4) nodular calcified.

Vesicular stage (active)
This stage consists of a viable larva with a scolex. On imaging, the larva appears as a cyst (4–20 mm) with signal intensity similar to that of CSF on T1- and T2-weighted images. The cyst wall is thin, with little or no enhancement. The scolex appears as a mural nodule of low signal intensity on the T2-weighted image, high signal intensity on T1-weighted and FLAIR images (similar to a hole with a dot or a pea in a pod) that may show some enhancement (Fig. 1).

Colloidal vesicular stage (active)
When the larva degenerates, the fluid becomes turbid, and its capsule thickens. Degenerating cysts may be hyperintense on both T1- and T2-weighted images because of their contents. Ring-like enhancement is seen in two-thirds of cases. Edema and contrast enhancement are also seen in this stage (Fig. 2).

Granular nodular stage (active)
When the larva dies, the cyst begins to collapse, the capsule thickens, the scolex calcifies, and edema develops. It has an imaging appearance similar to the colloidal stage but with thicker, intensely enhanced walls and more surrounding edema (Fig. 3).

Nodular calcified stage (inactive)
The lesion is completely mineralized with no active immune response from the host. A small, calcified lesion measuring 2 to 10 mm is typical. Usually, there are no mass effects or contrast enhancement. However, contrast enhancement or perilesional edema has been identified in some lesions and is likely related to recent seizure activity originating from chronic regions (Fig. 4).[6,9,12–16]

Delayed contrast MR imaging is a sensitive method for detection of lesions in the degenerative phase, which are prone to show enhancement related to the active inflammatory reaction of these stages.[13] By diffusion-weighted imaging (DWI), the cysts have signal intensities similar to or slightly higher than that of CSF, and the scolex is detectable as a hyperintense nodule within the vesicle.[17] MR spectroscopy helps to differentiate cysticercosis from abscesses and cystic metastasis. The presence of succinate alone or increased amounts of both succinate and acetate indicates the presence of degenerating cysticerci and differentiates them from anaerobic or tuberculous abscesses.[18,19] The choline/creatine ratio may be increased, probably because of the presence of inflammatory cells. Perfusion (reduced regional cerebral blood volume [rCBV]) map shows low perfusion of a benign lesion (see Fig. 2).

When the cysticercosis grows larger than 1 to 2 cm in size, it may show surrounding edema, wall enhancement, or mural nodules. With these appearances, it can resemble tumor, so-called "pseudotumoral" form (Fig. 5). This form is rarely seen. It may occur in the cerebral hemisphere but rarely in the cerebellar hemisphere. The main differential diagnosis includes glioma and echinococcus.[20,21] Encephalitic cysticercosis occurs when multiple lesions are simultaneously in the granular stage and there is diffuse brain edema and overwhelming inflammation around the cyst.[9] The disseminated miliary form represents a massive cysticercus infestation of the CNS and is characterized by multiple small cystic formations diffusely spread out in the brain parenchyma.[8]

During the vesicular stage of cysticercosis, the lesions may be difficult to distinguish from echinococcosis (usually a large, solitary cyst in the region of distribution of the middle cerebral artery); sparganosis (seen in patients from Southeast Asia, multiple cystic lesions); cystic metastases; and multiple abscesses. During the colloidal vesicular and granular nodular stages of cysticercosis, both solitary and multiple cysts may be difficult to distinguish from metastases. DWI may be helpful in differentiating abscesses from cysticercosis. Pyogenic abscesses are nearly always bright by DWI, whereas cysticercal cysts are darker.[6–9]

Treatment of cysticercosis depends on the form and the type of disease and the location and number of cysts. Treatment is a combination of cysticidal agents (ie, albendazole and praziquantel) and corticosteroids to control the host inflammatory response, because cysticidal therapy itself initiates a host inflammatory response that may result in more symptoms. Surgical intervention is rarely used because of early diagnosis.[22] Imaging has been used to follow-up on the lesions after treatment (Fig. 6).

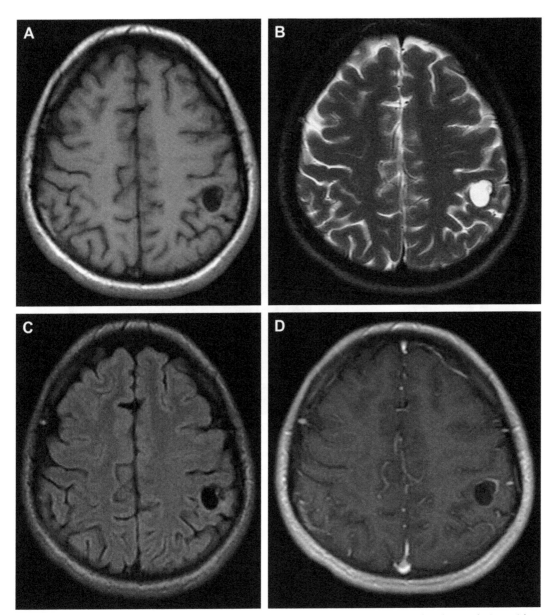

Fig. 1. Vesicular stage of cysticercosis. (*A*) Axial T1-weighted image shows a well-defined cystic lesion with no discernible wall containing a small area of high signal intensity representing the scolex. (*B*) Axial T2-weighted image shows similar findings. Note the absence of surrounding edema. (*C*) Axial FLAIR image more clearly delineates the scolex. (*D*) Axial contrast T1-weighted image shows minimal marginal enhancement.

Intraventricular Cysticercosis

The ventricular system is the second most common site (54%) of cysticercosis. This form of the illness commonly occurs in isolation, but it may be associated with parenchymal disease (24%). The most common site of intraventricular cysticercosis is the fourth ventricle (53%), followed by the third ventricle (27%), the lateral ventricle (11%), and the aqueduct (9%). Cysticercosis reaches the ventricular cavity by way of the choroid plexus, and the intraventricular form has an aggressive clinical course. The parasite may occlude CSF communication, causing acute episodes of ventriculomegaly with sudden death or mass effects. Larval death initiates ependymitis, which produces hydrocephalus or ventricular entrapment.[6,23–25]

Intraventricular lesions are cyst-like and may be difficult to identify on CT. However, intraventricular metrizamide applied through the ventriculoperitoneal shunt may help to delineate the cyst. MR

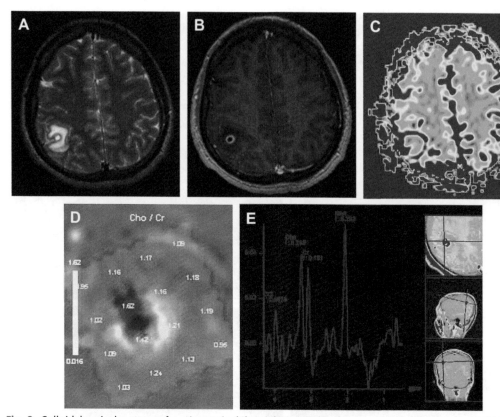

Fig. 2. Colloidal vesicular stage of cysticercosis. (*A*) Axial T2-weighted image shows a well-defined thick-walled cystic lesion with moderate surrounding edema. (*B*) Axial contrast-enhanced T1-weighted image shows marginal enhancement of the lesion. (*C*) Perfusion (rCBV) map shows low perfusion centrally of the lesion at the right parietal lobe but increased perfusion peripherally. (*D, E*) Two-dimensional MR spectroscopy imaging (TE = 144 ms, TR = 4000 ms): maximal choline/creatine ratio is 1.62, probably caused by inflammation and presence of inflammatory cells.

imaging is the imaging method of choice. The cyst contents are generally isointense to CSF on T1- and T2-weighted and FLAIR images. Occasionally, they are slightly brighter than CSF on FLAIR images. On T1-weighted images, they may be isointense to the brain and may show contrast enhancement on postcontrast T1-weighted images (**Fig. 7**). A thin, hypointense rim may be seen, particularly on T2-weighted imaging.[6,7,25] High-resolution highly T2-weighted sequences, such as the constructive interference in the steady state (CISS, FIESTA) technique, allow for better delineation of the cyst and the scolex (**Fig. 8**).[23] Cisternal MR imaging allows for detection of the cyst, which appears as a hypointense lesion surrounded by contrast material. Cysts in the vesicular stage may migrate from one ventricle to another and may be trapped in the aqueduct of Sylvius, leading to acute obstructive hydrocephalus. During the colloidal vesicular and granular nodular stages, the cysts may show enhancement of their walls or the adjacent ependyma. Some cysts may have a scolex. These intraventricular

cysts often lead to obstructive hydrocephalus and ventriculitis because of ependymal inflammatory response or to adhesions caused by prior ventricular infestation. Ependymitis manifests as ependymal and subependymal hyperintensity on T2-weighted images, and contrast enhancement of ventricular wall may be seen.[6,13]

Cisternal (Subarachnoid) Cysticercosis

Cysticercosis may occur in the basal cisterns (3.5%). The cisternal cysticercosis mainly involves the cerebellopontine angle and suprasellar cisterns and may be in the perimesencephalic, magna, and sylvian cisterns. The racemose form presents as large multiloculated cystic lesions with a "bunch-of-grapes" appearance separated by the septa. Racemose cysts can be seen on T1- and T2-weighted sequences, but the cyst contents tend to blend in with the CSF. Usually, minimal to no enhancement of the cyst wall is seen. However, the enhancement of the cisternal cysticercosis is variable and some lesions can

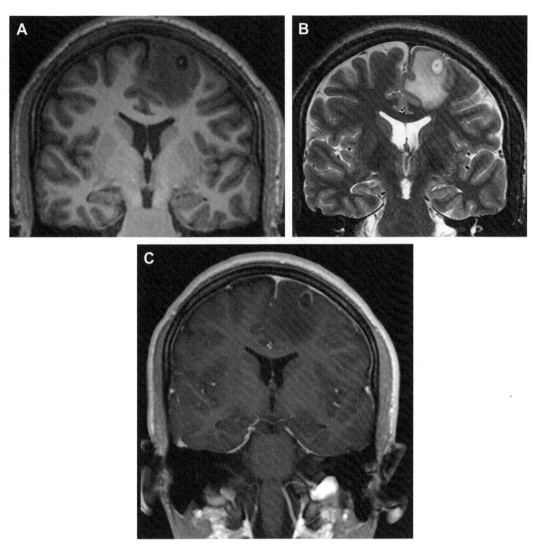

Fig. 3. Granular nodular stage of cysticercosis. (*A*) Coronal T1-weighted image shows a cyst with a hyperintense scolex and marked surrounding edema. (*B*) Coronal T2-weighted image shows high signal intensity with the bullseye of the scolex. (*C*) Coronal contrast-enhanced T1-weighted image shows intense contrast enhancement of the cyst wall.

show intense enhancement (**Fig. 9**). There is associated mass effect, causing local subarachnoid enlargement with a multiloculated appearance. The scolex is rarely seen. Cisternal cysticercosis may appear also as a single bladder measuring 3 to 18 mm with an invaginated scolex. The cyst contents tend to follow the CSF on all pulse sequences and easily can be overlooked (**Fig. 10**). Enlargement of a cisternal space or hydrocephalus may be the only clue to abnormality. High-resolution highly T2-weighted sequences, such as the CISS technique, are sensitive for cisternal cysticercosis.[25–29]

Vasculitis must be suspected when segmental narrowing, a beaded appearance, or an abrupt or tapered area of vascular obstruction is noted after angiography (**Fig. 11**). Arteritis is seen in up to 53% of patients with subarachnoid cysticercosis, including asymptomatic patients, with the middle and posterior cerebral arteries being most commonly affected. Multivessel involvement is noted in 50% of cases, and infarction associated with arteritis is seen in 2% to 12% of cases.[6] Calcification of the middle cerebral artery in young adults has been reported. Arachnoiditis can be either focal (ie, contrast enhancement involves only one cerebral basal cistern) or diffuse (ie, contrast enhancement involves multiple basal cisterns) (**Fig. 12**). It may represent an initial sign of cystic degeneration or be the result of cystic attachment to the ependyma, which elicits a granulomatous response.[6,7,25]

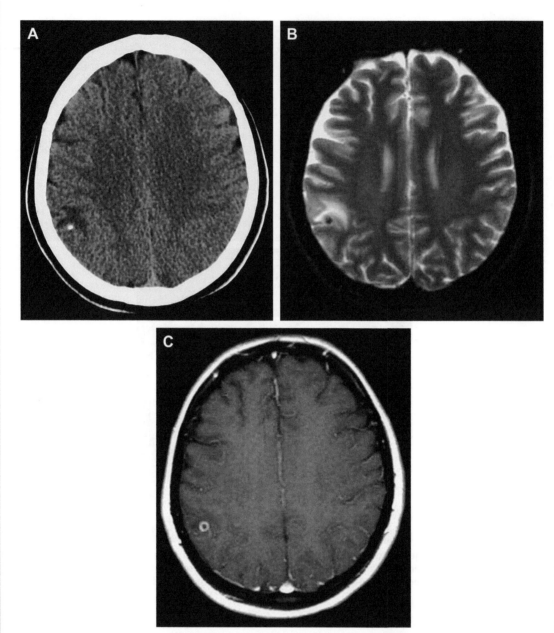

Fig. 4. Nodular calcified stage of cysticercosis. (*A*) Axial CT scan shows a calcified lesion with mild surrounding edema. (*B*) Axial T2-weighted image shows a signal void lesion with surrounding edema. (*C*) Axial contrast-enhanced T1-weighted image shows mild marginal enhancement of the cyst wall.

Spinal Cysticercosis

The spinal form of cysticercosis occurs in 1% to 5% of patients with neurocysticercosis. Two forms of spinal neurocysticercosis are recognized. The leptomeningeal (extramedullary) form is six to eight times more common than the intramedullary form (**Fig. 13**). The leptomeningeal form occurs as a consequence of downward migration of larvae from the cerebral to the spinal subarachnoid space. The intramedullary form is uncommon and occurs through hematogenous or ventriculoependymal migration. The parasite commonly lodges itself in the thoracic spinal cord.[9] Spinal neurocysticercosis reveals signal intensity similar to cerebral parenchymal cysts on all pulse sequences. Differential diagnosis includes neoplastic, inflammatory, demyelinating, vascular, and granulomatous lesions.[30–33]

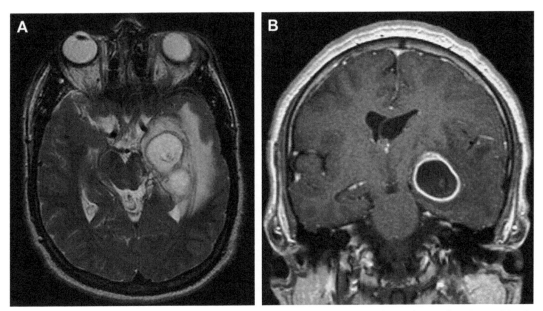

Fig. 5. Pseudotumoral cysticercosis. (A) Axial T2-weighted image shows a cystic lesion larger than 2 cm with a hypointense scolex and surrounding edema. (B) Coronal contrast-enhanced T1-weighted image shows thick marginal enhancement of the lesion and enhancement of the scolex.

TOXOPLASMOSIS

Toxoplasmosis is an opportunistic protozoan infection primarily affecting patients with immune deficiencies. It is more common in Central Europe than in North America. Toxoplasmosis is most commonly seen in patients with HIV and is rarely seen after allogeneic bone marrow transplantation (BMT) (1%–7.6%). Toxoplasma is found in 10% to 34% of all AIDS autopsies. Cerebral toxoplasmosis results from infection by an intracellular protozoan, *Toxoplasma gondii*. In the United

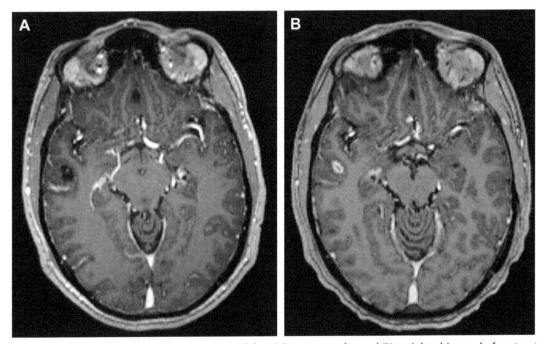

Fig. 6. Cysticercosis before and after treatment. (A) Axial contrast-enhanced T1-weighted image before treatment shows a marginal-enhancing lesion with an enhancing scolex. (B) Axial contrast-enhanced T1-weighted image after treatment shows decreased size of the cyst with collapsed lumen and disappearance of the scolex.

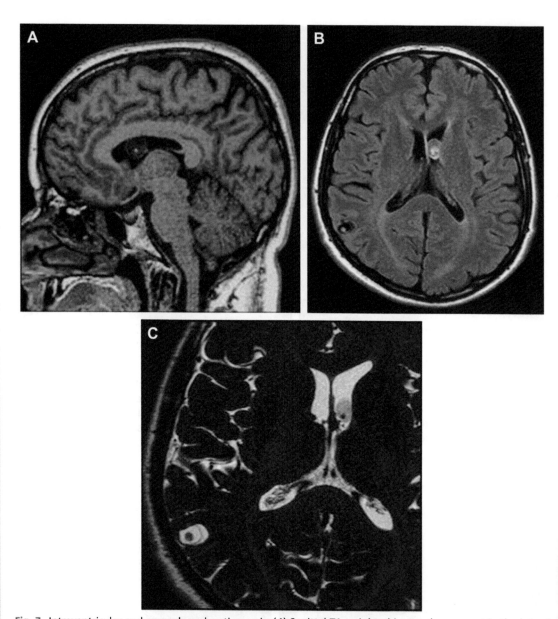

Fig. 7. Intraventricular and parenchymal cysticercosis. (*A*) Sagittal T1-weighted image shows a cyst in the lateral ventricle. The scolex appears as a hyperintense lesion. (*B*) Axial FLAIR image shows a left intraventricular cyst with a hyperintense scolex. There is also a parenchymal cystic lesion with a scolex. (*C*) Axial CISS image better delineates the cyst wall and scolex of the intraventricular and intraparenchymal lesions.

States, 20% to 70% of adults are seropositive for toxoplasma. After the acute infection, the latent form, called "encysted bradyzoites," remains in the tissues until a decline in immunity. Rupture of the cysts releases the free tachyzoite, which causes acute illness.[34–36] Patients may present with symptoms from mass effect, focal neurologic deficits, seizures, or cranial nerve palsies. Polymerase chain reaction testing of peripheral blood samples or CSFs has high sensitivity and specificity for the diagnosis of cerebral toxoplasmosis.

HIV-infected patients become most susceptible to developing active toxoplasmosis when their CD4 counts reach less than 100 cells/µL. The basal ganglia, thalamus, and corticomedullary junction regions are affected most often; however, the brainstem and corpus callosum may also be involved. The lesions are characterized by three zones. The central zone consists of coagulative necrosis with few organisms. The intermediate zone is hypervascular and contains numerous inflammatory cells mixed with tachyzoites and

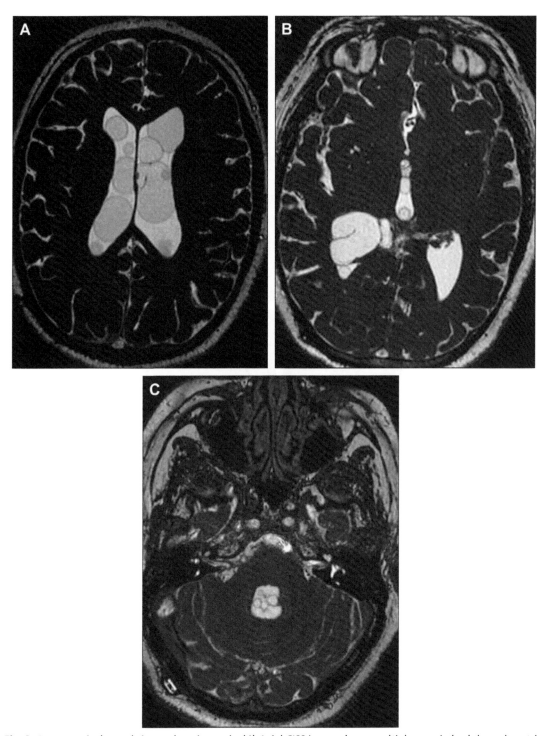

Fig. 8. Intraventricular and cisternal cysticercosis. (A) Axial CISS image shows multiple cysts in both lateral ventricles. (B) Axial CISS image shows multiple intraventricular cysts in the third ventricle. Note the hypointense scolex. Also, there are cysts with entrapment of the right occipital horn. (C) Axial CISS shows multiple cysts in the fourth ventricle with multiple small cysts in the cerebellopontine angle.

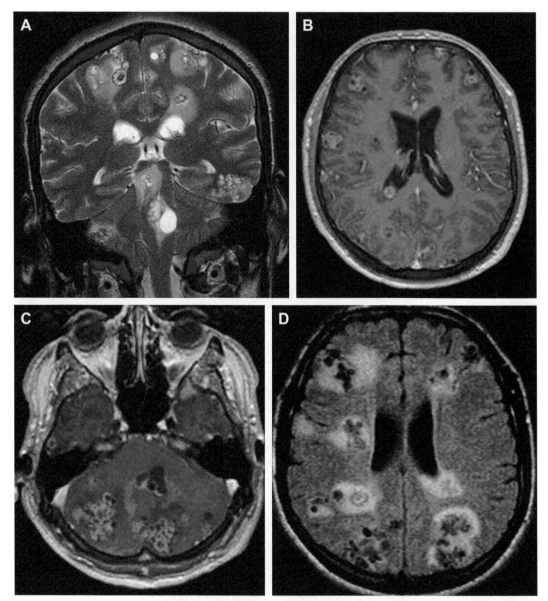

Fig. 9. Cisternal cysticercosis. (*A*) Coronal T2-weighted image shows that multiple cysts are seen scattered in the brain and cortical sulci. (*B, C*) Axial contrast-enhanced T1-weighted images at two levels show that multiple enhancing cysts are seen scattered within the sulci of the supratentorial region and in major horizontal fissure of the cerebellum and fourth ventricle. (*D*) Axial FLAIR image shows the cysts in mixed locations, some with surrounding edema.

encysted organisms. Finally, the peripheral zone is composed of encysted parasite. Surrounding vasogenic edema of the lesions is noted. Toxoplasma lesions do not have a capsule. Lesions from toxoplasmosis are usually multiple (85%) but may be solitary (15%).[35–38]

On nonenhanced CT scans, toxoplasma lesions are hypodense with edema and mass effect. Solid, nodular-enhancing, or ring-enhancing lesions are typically observed on postcontrast studies

(**Fig. 14**).[36] On T2 and FLAIR images, the lesion may show a target sign with central hyperintensity-correlated with necrosis, a hypointense rim correlating with an inflammatory zone, and peripheral hyperintensity correlating with surrounding edema. Contrast T1-weighted images show ring enhancement of the inflammatory zone (**Fig. 15**).[36–38] An eccentric (asymmetric) target sign is characterized by a small nodule along the wall of the enhancing ring. This finding is highly suggestive

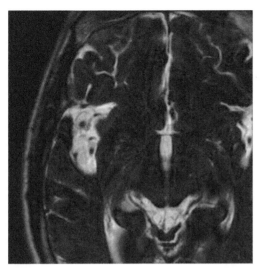

Fig. 10. Cisternal cysticercosis. Axial CISS image shows cisternal cysticercosis with a thin hypointense wall and a hypointense scolex.

of toxoplasmosis; however, it is relatively insensitive and is seen in less than 30% of cases (Fig. 16).[39,40] Toxoplasmosis sometimes involves the corpus callosum with a butterfly appearance simulating multiform glioblastoma.[41] Imaging in the acute phase may demonstrate foci of nodular enhancement, predominantly in the periventricular and subpial regions with slight perilesional edema.[35–37]

Primary toxoplasma encephalitis is often difficult to distinguish from CNS lymphoma. The criteria suggestive of toxoplasmosis are subcortical location, multiplicity, and eccentric target sign. MR spectroscopy in toxoplasmosis reveals elevated lipid and lactate peaks, consistent with an anaerobic acellular environment within an abscess. In contrast, primary CNS lymphoma shows a mild to moderate increase in lactate and lipids, a markedly elevated choline peak, and variably decreased levels of N-acetylaspartate and creatine. Perfusion MR imaging shows reduced rCBV in toxoplasma lesions and increased rCBV in lymphoma. Reduced rCBV in toxoplasmosis is probably attributable to a lack of vasculature within the abscess, whereas the hypervascularity of lymphoma is the reason for its increased rCBV.[42] DWI shows restricted diffusion of lymphoma, whereas toxoplasmosis demonstrates a wide range of diffusion characteristics, which can overlap with those of lymphoma (Fig. 17).[43–45] Toxoplasmosis reveals a lower magnetization transfer ratio than lymphoma. Thallium-201 brain single-photon emission computed tomography is positive for CNS lymphoma in an HIV-seropositive patient, whereas negative results are presumed to be caused by an infectious agent.[46] The results of previous studies have shown that [18F] fluorodeoxyglucose positron emission tomography can accurately differentiate lymphoma from infections. The standardized uptake values for cerebral lesions were much higher in lymphomas than in toxoplasma lesions.[36,37]

After therapy with pyrimethamine sulfadiazine and folic acid, there is a decrease in the number and size of the lesions, with a reduction in edema and mass effect within 10 days. Full resolution of the lesions may take 6 months, and healed foci may calcify or show changes consistent with leukomalacia.[36,37] Paradoxic worsening of the systemic inflammatory clinical response after treatment is associated with a paradoxic increase in the size and number of lesions, and perilesional

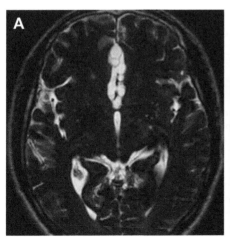
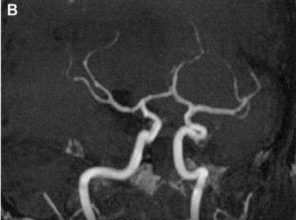

Fig. 11. Cisternal cysticercosis with vasculitis. (A) Axial T2-weighted image shows racemose cisternal cysticercosis in the interhemispheric fissure. (B) MR angiography shows irregularity with segmental narrowing of bilateral anterior cerebral arteries.

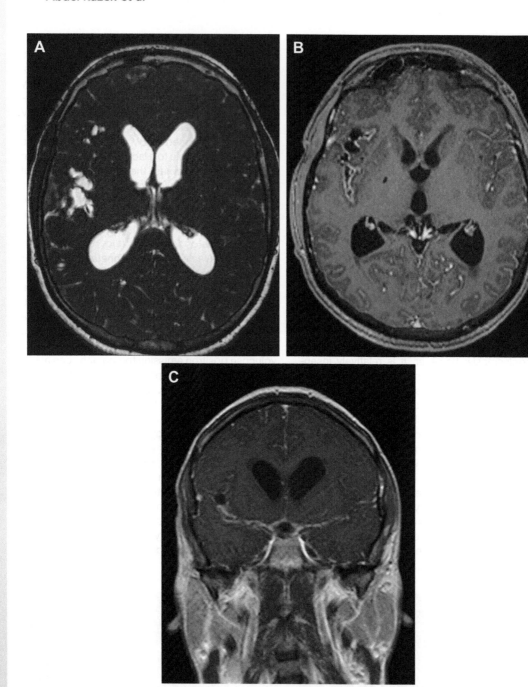

Fig. 12. Cisternal cysticercosis with arachnoiditis. (*A*) Axial CISS image demonstrates multiple cysts in right sylvian cistern. (*B*) Axial contrast-enhanced T1-weighted image shows peripheral enhancement of the cysts in the right sylvian cistern. (*C*) Coronal contrast-enhanced T1-weighted image reveals associated enhancement along the basal cisterns.

edema, and greater enhancement of the lesion is seen in patients with immune reconstitution inflammatory syndrome.[47]

Toxoplasmosis in BMT

Toxoplasmosis encephalitis may manifest differently in AIDS patients versus post-BMT patients.

AIDS is characterized by selective CD4 cell loss, whereas post-BMT patients have a more global loss of immune cells. Post-BMT patients may not mount a sufficient inflammatory response at the blood–brain barrier, allowing for passage of gadolinium and vasogenic edema. MR imaging of toxoplasmosis in patients with BMT shows only subtle, irregular meningeal enhancement, with possible

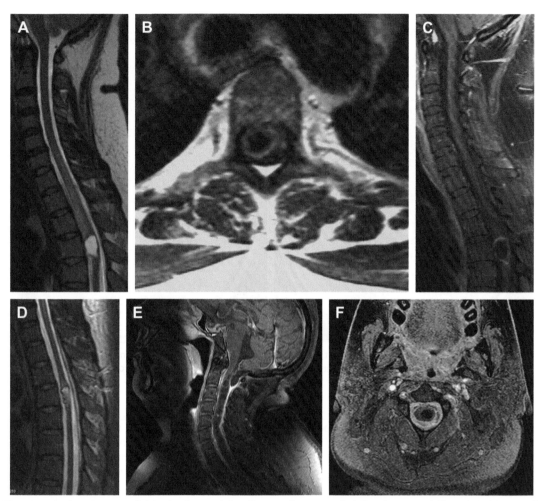

Fig. 13. Spinal cysticercosis. (*A*) Sagittal T2-weighted image shows a well-defined intramedullary cystic lesion with a thin wall at the T3 vertebral level. (*B*) Axial T1-weighted image shows the intramedullary location of the lesion. (*C*) Sagittal contrast-enhanced T1-weighted image shows mild marginal enhancement of the cystic lesion. (*D*) Sagittal T2-weighted follow-up image shows that the intramedullary cystic lesion has decrease in size after treatment for neurocysticercosis. (*E, F*) Sagittal and axial contrast-enhanced T1-weighted images in another patient reveal an intradural extramedullary cystic lesion at craniocervical junction and several intramedullary cystic lesions in cervical spinal cord. Diffuse leptomeningeal enhancement also is noted.

extension to the cortex and white matter–gray matter junction. Most of the parenchymal lesions are nonenhancing because of a more global loss of the immune system. Despite a lack of enhancement, mass effect and edema are usually present. The parenchymal lesions may have undergone hemorrhagic transformation.[48]

Congenital Toxoplasmosis

Toxoplasmosis is a common cause of congenital infection. Clinically significant abnormalities occur when the fetus is infected before 26 weeks of gestational age. Neuroimaging studies reveal hydrocephalus and intracranial calcifications (**Fig. 18**) (most commonly in the cortex and basal

ganglia and more diffuse than those seen in cytomegalovirus). The classic triad of hydrocephalus, multifocal parenchymal calcifications, and chorioretinitis is demonstrated in a minority of cases.[49]

ECHINOCOCCOSIS

CNS infestation occurs in 2% of patients with echinococcosis. The two main types of the disease are cystic echinococcosis (CE) and alveolar echinococcosis, which are caused by *Echinococcus granulosus* and *E multilocularis*, respectively. CE occurs in rural areas and is usually self-limited; it is more frequent, and most cases occur in Australia, New Zealand, the Middle East, and

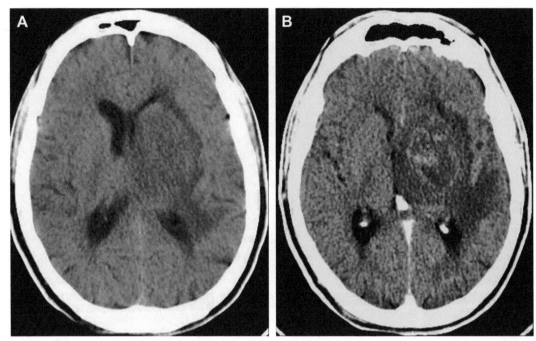

Fig. 14. Toxoplasmosis. (*A*) Axial noncontrast CT scan shows a hypodense lesion with mass effect, and edema in the left thalamic region. (*B*) Axial contrast-enhanced CT scan shows a heterogeneous contrast enhancement of the lesion with surrounding edema.

South America. Alveolar echinococcosis occurs in children with an infiltrative pattern and is less frequent; it often occurs in North America, Central Europe, Russia, and China. Humans are secondarily infected by ingestion of food or water contaminated with eggs of the parasite.[50–53]

CNS CE

Parenchymal CE

CE has three layers: (1) the outer layer (pericyst), which is dense and fibrous; (2) the middle laminated membrane (ectocyst), which is acellular and permits the passage of nutrients; and (3) the inner layer (endocyst), a germinal layer that produces daughter vesicles. The scolices (larval stage) are seen within the daughter vesicles. Daughter vesicles are formed from cysts and may form within main cyst. They are seen in the supratentorial region, often along the territory of the middle cerebral artery. Patients present with symptoms of space-occupying lesions, including headache, seizure, and focal neurologic deficits.[53–56] A serologic test helps to diagnose CE.

The World Health Organization Informal Working Group on Echinococcus classifies CE according to its viability into active fertile (CE1 and CE2); transitional (CE3); and degenerated, inactive, and infertile cysts (CE4 and CE5).[50] The CE1 type is the most common type of CE, which appears as well-defined, smooth, thin-walled, homogeneous CSF-isointense cystic lesions that are spherical or oval and may reach up to 15 cm in size. The hypointense rim on T2-weighted MR images represents the three layers. A thin rim of contrast enhancement limited to the capsule region may be detected. Cerebral edema around the cyst may occur (**Fig. 19**). CE2 cysts appear as unilocular cysts with small, peripherally arranged daughter vesicles. The presence of daughter cysts is considered to be pathognomonic of a hydatid cyst (**Fig. 20**). The CE3 type appears as a primary maternal cyst with multiple large daughter cysts. These daughter cysts may produce wheellike, rosettelike, or honeycomblike structures. The CE4 type appears as a cystic lesion with serpentine bands or floating membranes representing the detached or ruptured membranes. The CE5 is dead cysts characterized by a thick calcified wall in 50% of patients. The degree of calcification varies from partial to complete calcification of the cyst.[56] Peaks from lactate, succinate, acetate, and pyruvate by MR spectroscopy help in diagnosis of cestodal cysts. Pyruvate and succinate are markers of identification and viability for parasitic cysts.[57,58]

Treatment of cerebral hydatid cysts is primarily surgical. The cysts must be removed intact without spillage of the cyst contents to avoid an

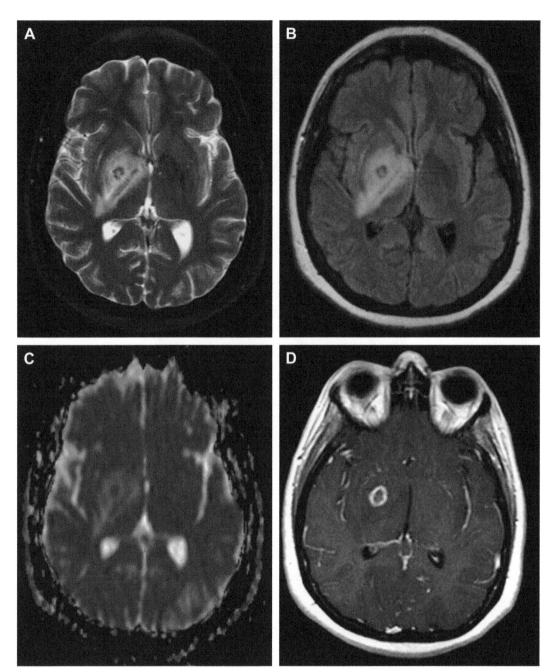

Fig. 15. Target sign of toxoplasmosis. (*A*) Axial T2-weighted image shows right thalamic hypointense lesion with central hyperintensity and surrounding hyperintense edema. (*B*) Axial FLAIR shows similar pattern. (*C*) Apparent diffusion coefficient map shows restricted diffusion of the lesion with free diffusion of surrounding edema. (*D*) Axial contrast-enhanced T1-weighted image shows ring enhancement of the lesion.

anaphylactic reaction or recurrence. Injection with formaline, 20% saline, or medical treatment with anthelmintic agents can reduce the cyst size.[59]

Cisternal and ventricular CE
Subarachnoid spaces are the second most common location of the disease in the CNS, although occurrence in these areas is far less frequent. Epidural and intraventricular cysts have been reported. Cysts are usually singular and may be unilocular or multilocular. They may be seen after surgery.[60,61]

Spinal CE
Spinal involvement accounts for less than 1% of echinococcosis. The thoracic segment of the spine

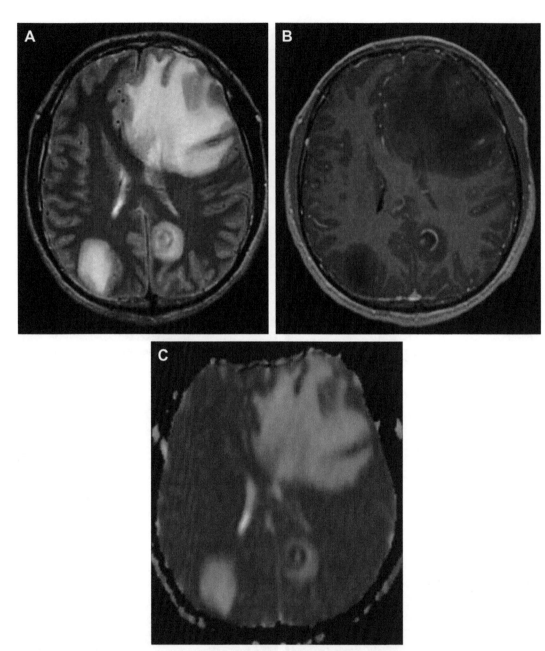

Fig. 16. Eccentric target sign of toxoplasmosis. (*A*) Axial T2-weighted image shows an eccentric target sign in the left occipital lobe associated other lesions with surrounding edema. (*B*) Axial contrast-enhanced T1-weighted image better delineates the eccentric target sign. (*C*) Axial apparent diffusion coefficient map can delineate the target sign of the lesion.

is the most frequently affected (50%), followed by the lumbar (20%), sacral (20%), and cervical segments (10%). The cysts tend to grow along the points of least resistance and cause cortical bony erosion extending to the vertebral canal.[62]

Cerebral Alveolar Echinococcosis

Alveolar echinococcosis features alveolar structures composed of numerous irregular cysts with

a diameter between 1 and 20 mm that are not sharply demarcated from surrounding tissue. Central cystic cavities can result from necrosis of the inner part of the cyst. An irregularly thickened and partially calcified wall is present in most cases. This wall lies in the deep gray matter but may be in the posterior fossae. On CT and MR imaging, the lesions mainly appear as solid or multilocular cystic masses. Calcification and surrounding edema are

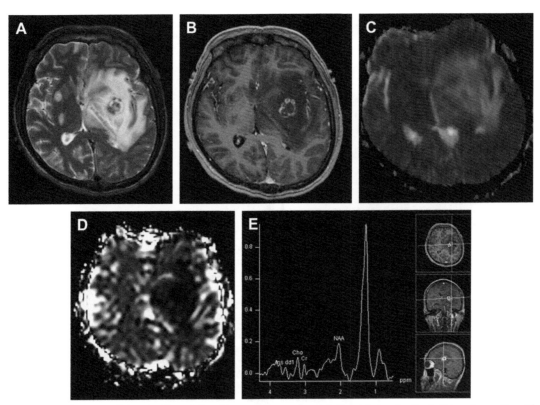

Fig. 17. Toxoplasmosis. (*A*) Axial T2-weighted image shows a well-defined lesion in the left basal ganglia with surrounding edema. There is another lesion at right basal ganglia. (*B*) Axial contrast-enhanced T1-weighted image shows heterogeneous ring enhancement of the lesion in the left basal ganglia. (*C*) Apparent diffusion coefficient map shows restricted diffusion of the lesion with free diffusion in the surrounding edema. (*D*) Perfusion map shows decreased perfusion of the lesion. (*E*) MR spectroscopy shows high lipid peak.

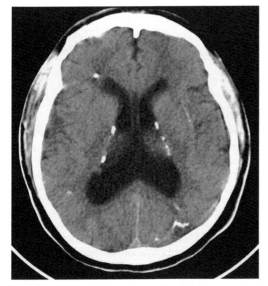

Fig. 18. Congenital toxoplasmosis. Axial noncontrast CT scan shows multiple discrete intraparenchymal and periventricular calcifications.

common findings in these lesions. Peripheral ring-like, heterogeneous, nodular, and cauliflowerlike enhancement patterns have all been reported. Perfusion-weighted imaging reveals low rCBV within the lesions because of gliosis and higher values in the periphery because of surrounding inflammation. This infection may mimic malignancy as a result of invasion of adjacent structures and destructive tissue growth.[63,64]

SCHISTOSOMIASIS (BILHARZIASIS)

Schistosomiasis (bilharziasis) of the CNS is an uncommon entity. *Schistosomia mansoni* and *S haematobium* are almost always associated with spinal infection, and *S japonicum* affects the brain. *S mansoni* is endemic to tropical Africa and parts of the Near East, northeastern South America, and the eastern Caribbean islands. *S hematobium* is found in Africa and the Middle East. *S japonicum* is found in Asia, where it is endemic to southern and eastern China, Taiwan, Japan, and the Philippines.[65] *Schistosoma* species have a complex life cycle. The host

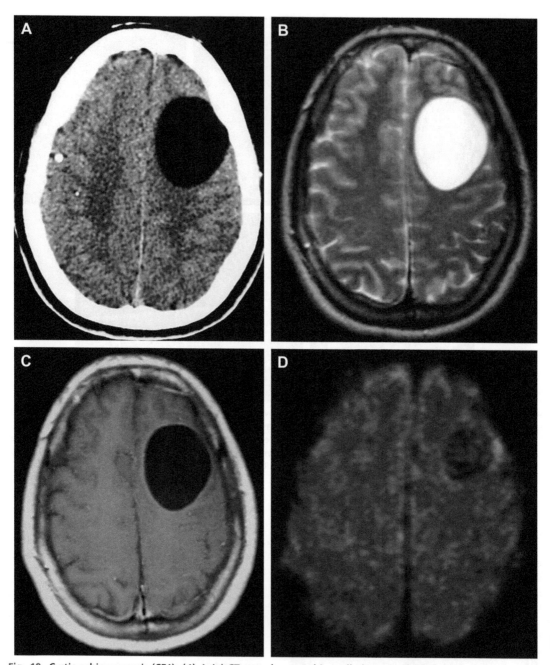

Fig. 19. Cystic echinococcosis (CE1). (*A*) Axial CT scan shows a thin-walled cyst in the left high parietal region. Another small calcified lesion is seen in the right parietal region. (*B*) Axial T2-weighted image shows a large, well-defined, round, unilocular hyperintense cyst with a hypointense rim. (*C*) Postcontrast axial T1-weighted image shows no enhancement along the cyst wall. (*D*) Diffusion MR imaging shows free diffusion within the lesion.

is the freshwater snail that releases *Schistosoma* cercariae into the water. The cercariae infect humans percutaneously and transform into schistosomula. The schistosomulae migrate to the lungs and the liver and then descend to the mesenteric venous system. *S mansoni* and *S japonicum* inhabit the portal veins, whereas *S haematobium* occupies the veins of the bladder.[66–70]

Cerebral Schistosomiasis

The routes for spreading of schistosomiasis to the brain include embolization of eggs through the arterial system, especially if a pulmonary arteriovenous fistula exists; retrograde venous spread by way of Batson's plexus; and anomalous migration of worms through the brain. Patients with cerebral

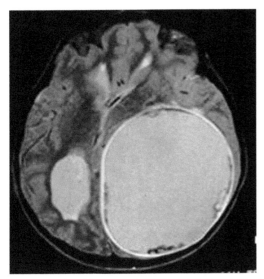

Fig. 20. Cystic echinococcosis (CE2). Axial T2-weighted image of the brain shows multiple small daughter vesicles arranged peripherally within the huge maternal cyst.

schistosomiasis are commonly asymptomatic (90%) and may present with signs of space-occupying lesions, such as headache, seizures, papilledema, and visual and oral disturbances. These lesions may be found in the cerebrum, cerebellum, brainstem, leptomeninges, and choroid plexus. CT usually demonstrates a hyperdense area surrounded by a hypodense halo of edema. MR imaging shows foci of low signal on T1 and high signal on T2, with contrast enhancement. A characteristic MR imaging pattern of lesions is a large mass comprising multiple intensely enhancing nodules, sometimes with areas of linear enhancement.[5,65] Central linear enhancement surrounds multiple enhancing punctate nodules, forming an "arborized" appearance. Although this pattern is highly suggestive, it is not present in all cases. Anthelmintic treatment usually improves the patient's condition within 6 weeks, with complete resolution within 6 months.[65–67]

Spinal Schistosomiasis

Spinal schistosomiasis is seen in young male patients. Its localization in the lower cord and conus region is explained by the free anastomosis between the pelvic veins and the valveless vertebral venous plexus. The pathologic types are myelitis, granulomatous, radicular, and vascular. The most frequent form is myeloradiculopathy. Blood and CSF analysis usually show eosinophilia and intrathecal specific antibodies. MR imaging shows moderate expansion of the distal spinal cord.

Abnormalities are isointense to the cord on T1 and hyperintense in a patchy pattern on T2-weighted images. The enhancement may be intramedullary nodular, peripheral, or linear radicular. Intramedullary nodular enhancement correlates to multiple schistosomiasis microtubercles. Peripheral enhancing lesions correlate to thickened leptomeninges, and linear radicular enhancement correlates with thickened nerve roots (**Fig. 21**).[5,71–86]

AMEBIASIS

Cerebral amebiasis is unusual, and its incidence is reported to be 0.7% to 0.8%. Most patients are between the second and fourth decade of life and most are male. *Entamoeba histolytica* rarely affect the CNS. *Acanthamoeba* and *Naegleria* organisms are responsible for causing granulomatous amebic encephalitis (GAE) and primary amebic meningoencephalitis (PAM), respectively. They have distinctive epidemiology, organisms, patterns of presentation, clinical courses, pathology, and imaging findings.[72–74]

Granulomatous Amebic Encephalitis

GAE is a subacute to chronic infection caused by *Acanthamoeba* and *Leptomyxida* organisms. *Acanthamoeba* species are found in all types of environment. It occurs in debilitated or immunocompromised patients who have AIDS or were subjected to chemotherapy or steroid therapy. The clinical course is characterized by a long duration of focal neurologic symptoms. Pathologically, there is focal edema of the cerebral hemispheres. Multifocal parenchymal lesions of the posterior fossa structures, the diencephalon, and the thalamus are seen. Microscopically, there is evidence of leptomeningitis, which is most prominent adjacent to the parenchymal lesions. There may be necrotizing angiitis. Intralesional hemorrhage caused by necrotizing angiitis is considered to be an important diagnostic feature. The lesions of GAE are thought to represent focal areas of cerebritis or microabscesses.[72,73]

Imaging findings for GAE are either in the form of large solitary masslike lesions, multifocal patterns, or a combination of the two findings. The masslike lesion (pseudotumoral pattern) often demonstrates a linear and superficial gyriform pattern of enhancement, which is a useful indicator of the diagnosis (**Fig. 22**). This pattern possibly represents a combination of enhancement in the inflamed meninges and the underlying cortex. There may be a border zone and microabscesses caused by infiltration of brain substance, with amebae along the pial vessels. The multifocal pattern shows T2 hyperintensity and a heterogeneous or ringlike pattern of

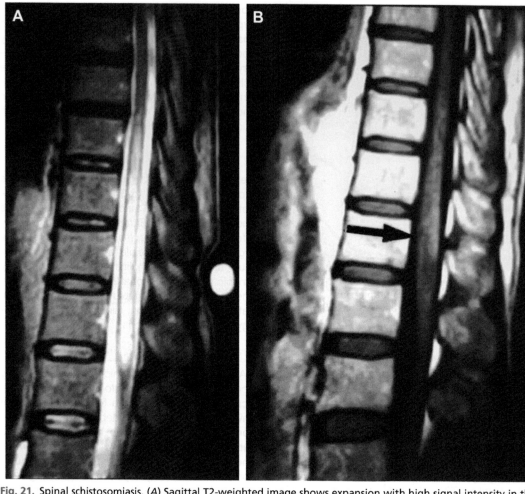

Fig. 21. Spinal schistosomiasis. (*A*) Sagittal T2-weighted image shows expansion with high signal intensity in the lower part of the spinal cord. (*B*) Contrast T1-weighted image shows mild heterogeneous enhancement (*arrow*) along the posterior aspect of the spinal cord lesion.

enhancement, with a predilection for the diencephalon, thalamus, brainstem, and posterior fossa structures. Multiple punctate focal areas of enhancement are seen bilaterally throughout the cerebellar hemispheres, in addition to a few scattered lesions at the corticomedullary junction. Surgical removal of granulomatous mass lesions, combined with chemotherapy, such as amphotericin B or clotrimazole, provides the best chance of survival.[5,72]

Primary Amebic Meningoencephalitis

PAM is caused by *Naegleria fowleri*, with most patients having an acute onset of symptoms with rapid progression and almost fatal meningoencephalitis within 48 to 72 hours. The affected patients are children and young adults who are not immunocompromised. The mode of entry of

organisms is through the olfactory tract during contact with contaminated water or by inhalation of contaminated dust or soil. The pathologic changes seen in PAM are extensive damage to the brain parenchyma, ependyma, and meninges. Congestion of the meningeal vessels, the edematous cortex, with herniation of the uncus and the cerebellum are other features. Microscopically, there is purulent leptomeningeal exudate with hemorrhage and necrosis of the cerebral hemispheres, brainstem, and cerebellum.[72]

The imaging features of PAM are nonspecific, with evidence of brain edema and subsequent basilar meningeal enhancement. Imaging reveals a pattern of brain edema and hydrocephalus, with rapid progression of the disease. There is also evidence of obliteration of the cisterns with enhancing basilar exudates. In addition, there is infarction of the right basal ganglia, possibly

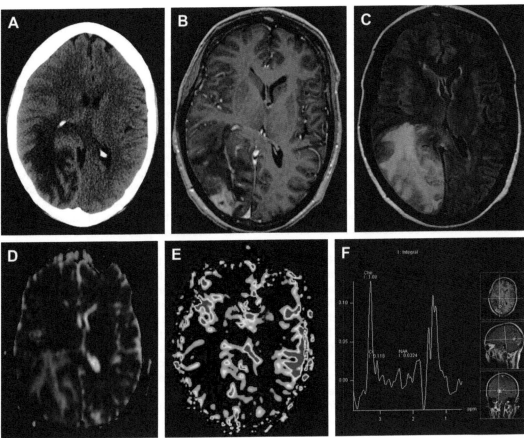

Fig. 22. Granulomatous amebic encephalitis. (*A*) Unenhanced CT shows an ill-defined low-density area involving the right parieto-occipital regions with mass effect. (*B*) Postcontrast MR image shows patchy and linear enhancement of the lesion. (*C*) FLAIR image shows hyperintensity in the lesion. (*D*) No definite areas of restricted diffusion in the lesion are seen on the apparent diffusion coefficient map. (*E*) Perfusion MR imaging (rCBV map) shows decreased perfusion of the lesion. (*F*) MR spectroscopy reveals elevated lactate (inverted peak), mildly elevated choline (Cho) and diminished *N*-acetylaspartate (NAA). Diagnosis was confirmed by biopsy.

caused by obliteration of the perforating vessels by the extensive exudates. Cerebral infarctions have been described in cases of PAM. The mainstays of treatment for PAM are amphotericin B, rifampicin, and miconazole.[72,73]

MALARIASIS

Malaria is caused by different species of the genus *Plasmodium*. Cerebral malaria occurs in 2% of patients infected by *P falciparum*. Human infection occurs by female mosquitoes of the genus *Anopheles*. The disease is seen in children and visitors to endemic areas. The neurologic signs of this illness are nonspecific with a high mortality rate (20%–50%). The parasites first multiply in the liver cells and later in the erythrocytes. There is diffuse petechial hemorrhage caused by occlusion of the cerebral capillaries by infected erythrocytes. Infarction

with surrounding edema is also seen and is caused by cerebral toxicity of cytokines after breakdown of the blood–brain barrier.[3,75–77]

Imaging findings in cerebral malaria include cerebral edema, cortical and subcortical ischemic lesions, and multiple petechial hemorrhages. Detection of hemorrhage and infarction in a single patient has been reported. Imaging reveals cerebral edema with thalamic and cerebellar white-matter hypodensity on CT and focal or diffuse hyperintense lesions on T2 and FLAIR images.[3] DWI is sensitive for detection of areas of ischemic changes and cerebral edema.[77] The susceptibility-weighted sequence is helpful in the detection of small hemorrhages as hypointense lesions. Cerebral malaria may be associated with central pontine myelinolysis and myelinolysis in the upper medulla. Multifocal petechial hemorrhages in the white matter may simulate acute multifocal hemorrhagic encephalopathy caused by sepsis and disseminated intravascular coagulation. Differentiation between these two situations should be made based on clinical data.[75]

SPARGANOSIS

Sparganosis is a parasitic infection caused by migrating larvae of *Spirometra mansoni*. It has a high incidence in Southeast Asia, Japan, China, and Korea. Humans become infected by drinking contaminated water; ingesting the raw or inadequately cooked flesh of snakes, fish, or frogs; or by applying infected flesh as a poultice to an open wound or the eye. The larvae may migrate through the loose connective tissues of the foramina of the skull base to reach the brain. The live worm is thread-shaped (5–18 cm) with serpiginous peristalsis. The degenerated worm is usually surrounded by collagen fibers, inflammatory cells, and gliosis. Cerebral infection has nonspecific signs and symptoms, such as headache, seizure, or neurologic deficits. The course of the disease varies from 8 months to 30 years. Enzyme-linked immunosorbent assay (ELISA) is useful for reaching the correct diagnosis. Most of the lesions are located in the white matter of the parietal, occipital, temporal, or frontal lobe and may be in the basal ganglia, insula, and cerebellum.[78–83]

There are three characteristic findings of cerebral sparganosis. The primary characteristic of cerebral sparganosis is the presence of a tunnel sign caused by a live worm migrating with an undulating motion. The tunnel appears hypointense on T1-weighted images, slightly hyperintense or isointense on T2-weighted images, and column- or fusiform-shaped with a solid or shallow appearance on post-contrast MR images. The enhancing tunnels are caused by reactive inflammatory tissue or by a granuloma entrapping the worm. The second finding is conglomerated ring or bead-shaped enhancement, which represents an inflammatory granuloma. The wall of the ring-shaped granuloma is hypointense on T1-weighted images and slightly hypointense on T2-weighted images. The third finding is various stages of disease in the same image.[80,81] In the acute stage, extensive perifocal edema and mass effect are present, whereas in the chronic stage, cortical atrophy, a dilated ipsilateral ventricle, and punctate calcification are apparent. Diffusion MR imaging shows isosignal intensity lesion. MR spectroscopy reveals increased choline and decreased *N*-acetylaspartate peaks with additional peaks: the doubling peak at 1.3 ppm of lipid or lactate, implying necrosis, and the alanine peak at 1.4 to 1.8 ppm. Perfusion MR imaging shows no definite increased cerebral perfusion.[79]

PARAGONIMIASIS

Paragonimiasis is a parasitic disease endemic to East and Southeast Asia, including Korea, China, and Japan. The disease is caused by *Paragonimus westermani*. Human infections are caused by ingestion of infected undercooked fresh water crabs or crayfish. Brain involvement has been reported in 2% to 27% of cases.[84] The neurologic presentation is nonspecific as a headache and focal neurologic deficits. An ELISA test is sensitive and specific for the diagnosis of paragonimiasis.[85] Toxic substances produced by the parasite are responsible for aseptic inflammation or granulomatous reaction to the parasite or its eggs.[5] The initial intracranial lesions include exudative aseptic inflammation, cerebral hemorrhage, and infarction. The wandering adult *Paragonimus* makes tunnels along the track of migration.[5,86]

On MR imaging, conglomerates of multiple ring-shaped shadows or enhancement of so-called "grape cluster" or "soap bubble" forms in one hemisphere is the most suggestive pattern of this disease. The appearance of a tunnel caused by a wandering adult worm has been reported in one patient. The tunnel sign usually presents as a 4 × 0.8 cm columnar or fusifrom low signals on T1-weighted images and high signals on T2-weighted images. There is hemorrhage of various degrees with surrounding edema that is different from a pure hemorrhage because it results from both hemorrhage and aseptic inflammation. A large calcified area made up of clustered nodules has been reported. DWIs show restricted diffusion of the abscess cavity or a heterogeneous signal from hemorrhage caused by the T2 shine-through effect.[85] On CT, multiple calcifications with round or oval shapes surrounded by low-density areas, cortical atrophy, and ventricular dilation are seen.[84] Early active lesions can be treated by chemotherapy with bithionol or praziquantel.[85]

AMERICAN TRYPANOSOMIASIS (CHAGAS DISEASE)

American trypanosomiasis (Chagas disease) exists only in Latin America and is caused by *Trypanosoma cruzi*, which is transmitted to humans by blood-sucking insects (Triatominae). In the acute phase, patients present symptoms with myocarditis, and clinical signs of CNS involvement rarely occur. The chronic phase is the most prevalent and is characterized by cardiomyopathy and progressive esophageal and colonic dilation (Chagas megacolon and

Chagas megaesophagus). CNS involvement may be a late presentation of the acute phase or caused by reactivation (eg, in the immunosuppressed and AIDS patients). Chagas meningoencephalitis may manifest as the first presentation of AIDS. The definitive diagnosis depends on characterizing the parasite in CSF tests or by histologic analysis of the cerebral parenchyma. In imaging studies, Chagas meningoencephalitis usually manifests as multiple expanding hyperintense lesions on T2-weighted images with nodular or annular enhancement. Involved areas include the corpus callosum, the periventricular white matter, the deep white matter, the subcortical regions, and the cerebellum (**Fig. 23**). Additionally, it may be seen in the spinal cord. It may be impossible to differentiate Chagas meningoencephalitis from toxoplasmosis and CNS lymphoma.[5,87]

AFRICAN TRYPANOSOMIASIS

African trypanosomiasis (sleeping sickness) is an endemic chronic disease found mainly in central and western Africa that is transmitted in the salivary gland of the infected bloodsucking vector *Glossina* or tsetse flies, which are found only in Africa. *Trypanosoma brucei rhodesiense* (more virulent) and *Trypanosoma brucei gambiense* (most common) are the two parasites responsible

for human disease.[5] African trypanosomes invade the brain parenchyma by two routes. One is by early seeding in the choroid plexus and secondary passage into the CSF. The other is direct passage into the cerebral capillaries. Once these vessels are involved, the large extracellular spaces within the white matter allow the parasite to move into the brain tissue. On CT, meningeal enhancement and diffuse hypoattenuated areas affecting the white matter of the centrum semiovale, periventricular regions, and basal ganglia have been reported in the late stages. MR imaging initially reveals meningeal thickening, followed by multiple white-matter T2 hyperintense lesions (which may be symmetric) in the central gray matter, internal capsule, cerebellar peduncles, corpus callosum, and cortex.[5,88]

TOXOCARIASIS

Toxocariasis is a common roundworm in dogs. Human infection with *Taenia canis* rarely affects the CNS. *Toxocara* may be seen on some tropical islands. The highest incidence is seen in Thessaloniki, Greece. Humans become infected after ingesting embryonated eggs from the soil or after exposure to dirty hands, raw vegetables, or larvae from undercooked giblets. The three forms of the disease are (1) visceral larva migrans, (2) occult, and (3) ocular.[89] A patient with visceral larva migrans syndrome has generalized illness, with hypereosinophilia and symptoms arising from larval invasion of different organs. Involvement of the liver, lungs, and eyes is common, but CNS infestation is rare. A patient with CNS infection may present with epilepsy, encephalitis and meningoencephalitis, eosinophilic meningitis, arachnoiditis, meningoradiculitis, optic neuritis, and meningomyelitis.[90,91] The *Toxocara* larvae are metabolically active and produce an array of enzymes and waste products that cause tissue damage and a marked inflammatory reaction, of which eosinophils are a major component. High serum titers of *T canis* antibodies by ELISA, eosinophilia in the blood, or CSF helps with diagnosis of toxocariasis.[89]

Cerebral Parenchymal Toxocariasis

Cerebral toxocariasis mainly manifests as a granulomatous process. MR images show multifocal, circumscribed lesions in the brain with strong contrast enhancement or a combination of circumscribed and diffuse changes in chronic infections. Multiple subcortical, cortical, or white matter lesions that are hypodense on CT, hyperintense on T2-weighted images, and homogeneously enhancing are seen. Associated focal meningeal

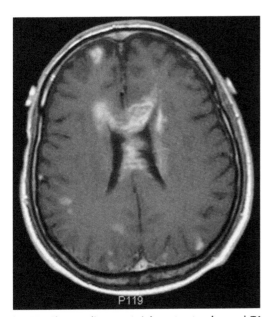

Fig. 23. Chagas disease. Axial contrast-enhanced T1-weighted image shows multiple enhancing lesions in the corpus callosum, periventricular, and deep white matter, and cortical and subcortical regions. Diagnosis was confirmed by biopsy.

enhancement near the lesion may also be observed. There is a marked decrease in the size and number of the lesions after anthelmintic treatment.[89,90]

Spinal Toxocariasis

Spinal cord involvement with solitary or multiple lesions that are hyperintense on T2-weighted images and strongly enhanced on postcontrast T1-weighted images has been reported. The enhancing foci are homogenous and closely confined to the posterior segment of the cord. These features distinguish a parasitic process from pyogenic infections, which commonly lead to central necrosis and peripheral ring enhancement.[90,91]

CEREBRAL TRICHINOSIS

Cerebral trichinosis is characterized by eosinophilic meningoencephalitis; vascular (arteriolar) thrombosis; and small white and gray matter infarctions. By CT, multifocal hypodense small white matter and cortical lesions have been described, along with cortical infarctions with ring enhancement. Diffuse white matter hypodensity of the centrum semiovale may also be present. In one case report, MR imaging showed multiple microinfarctions at the border zones of major vascular territories, in the periventricular white matter, and in the corpus callosum.[92] The lesions appear hyperintense on T2-weighted and FLAIR images with reduced apparent diffusion coefficient and show no contrast enhancement. Most lesions regressed over time (3 weeks and 3 months follow-up). In another case report, focal lesional contrast enhancement and bilateral diffuse T2 hyperintensities in the centrum semiovale have been described.[93]

SUMMARY

The radiologist plays a central role in the diagnosis and management of patients with parasitic infections. CT is helpful in detecting calcified lesions. MR imaging is much more sensitive for accurate localization, characterization of the lesions, delineation of associated parenchymal changes, determining the activity of some lesions, and monitoring the patient after therapy. Combining these techniques with advanced MR imaging, such as diffusion MR, perfusion MR, or MR spectroscopy, helps with differentiation of parasitic infections from abscesses and malignancy. A thorough understanding of the imaging patterns associated with common intracranial parasitic infections allows the radiologist to narrow down the options for differential diagnosis and to facilitate the timely implementation of appropriate therapies. Combining the imaging features of parasitic diseases with their epidemiologic, clinical, and physiopathologic characteristics may help to narrow the diagnosis when imaging features are nonspecific.

REFERENCES

1. Aiken A. Central nervous system infection. Neuroimaging Clin 2010;20:557–80.
2. Foerster B, Thurnher M, Malani P, et al. Intracranial infections: clinical and imaging characteristics. Acta Radiol 2007;48:875–93.
3. Restrepo C, Raut A, Riascos R, et al. Imaging manifestations of tropical parasitic infections. Semin Roentgenol 2007;42:37–48.
4. Chang KH, Cho SY, Hesselink JR, et al. Parasitic diseases of the central nervous system. Neuroimaging Clin N Am 1991;1:159–78.
5. da Rocha A, Junior A, Ferreira N, et al. Granulomatous diseases of the central nervous system. Top Magn Reson Imaging 2005;16:155–87.
6. Kimura-Hayama E, Higuera J, Corona-Cedillo R, et al. Neurocysticercosis: radiologic-pathologic correlation. Radiographics 2010;30:1705–19.
7. Yeaney G, Kolar B, Silberstein H, et al. Solitary neurocysticercosis. Radiology 2010;257:581–5.
8. Amaral L, Ferreira R, Rocha A, et al. Neurocysticercosis evaluation with advanced magnetic resonance techniques and atypical forms. Top Magn Reson Imaging 2005;16:127–44.
9. Castillo M. Imaging of neurocysticercosis. Semin Roentgenol 2004;39:465–73.
10. Zee CS, Go JL, Kim PE, et al. Imaging of neurocysticercosis. Neuroimaging Clin N Am 2000;10:391–407.
11. Rahalkar MD, Shetty DD, Kelkar AB, et al. The many faces of cysticercosis. Clin Radiol 2000;55:668–74.
12. Litt AW, Mohchyt T. Neurocysticercosis. Radiology 1999;211:472–6.
13. Lucato LT, Guedes MS, Sato JR, et al. The role of conventional MR imaging sequences in the evaluation of neurocysticercosis: impact on characterization of the scolex and lesion burden. AJNR Am J Neuroradiol 2007;28:1501–4.
14. Lalitha P, Reddy B. Unusual extensive T1 hyperintense signals on MR imaging in neurocysticercosis. AJNR Am J Neuroradiol 2010;31:e33.
15. Braga FT, Rocha AJ, Gomes HR, et al. Noninvasive MR cisternography with FLAIR and 100% supplemental O_2 in the evaluation of neurocysticercosis. AJNR Am J Neuroradiol 2004;25:295–7.
16. Poeschl P, Janzen A, Schuierer G, et al. Calcified neurocysticercosis lesions trigger symptomatic inflammation during antiparasitic therapy. AJNR Am J Neuroradiol 2006;27:653–5.

17. Gupta RK, Prakash M, Mishra AM, et al. Role of diffusion weighted imaging in differentiation of intracranial tuberculoma and tuberculous abscess from cysticercus granulomas: a report of more than 100 lesions. Eur J Radiol 2005;55:384–92.

18. Pretell EJ, Martinot C Jr, Garcia HH, et al. Differential diagnosis between cerebral tuberculosis and neurocysticercosis by magnetic resonance spectroscopy. J Comput Assist Tomogr 2005;29:112–4.

19. Agarwal M, Chawla S, Husain N, et al. Higher succinate than acetate levels differentiate cerebral degenerating cysticerci from anaerobic abscesses on in-vivo proton MR spectroscopy. Neuroradiology 2004;46:211–5.

20. Umredkar A, Singla N, Mohindra S, et al. Giant intraparenchymal neurocysticercosis: report of surgical aspects two cases. Neurol India 2009;57:800–2.

21. Sabel M, Neuen-Jacob E, Vogt C, et al. Intracerebral neurocysticercosis mimicking glioblastoma multiforme: a rare differential diagnosis in Central Europe. Neuroradiology 2001;43:227–30.

22. de Souza A, Nalini A, Kovoor JM, et al. Natural history of solitary cerebral cysticercosis on serial magnetic resonance imaging and the effect of albendazole therapy on its evolution. J Neurol Sci 2010;288:135–41.

23. Govindappa S, Narayanan J, Krishnamoorthy V, et al. Improved detection of intraventricular cysticercal cysts with the use of three dimensional constructive interference in steady state MR sequences. AJNR Am J Neuroradiol 2000;21:679–84.

24. Araujo AL, Rodrigues RS, Marchiori E, et al. Migrating intraventricular cysticercosis: magnetic resonance imaging findings. Arq Neuropsiquiatr 2008;66:111–3.

25. Hauptman JS, Hinrichs C, Mele C, et al. Radiologic manifestations of intraventricular and subarachnoid racemose neurocysticercosis. Emerg Radiol 2005; 11:153–7.

26. Jayakumar PN, Chandrashekar HS, Srikanth SG, et al. MRI and in vivo proton MR spectroscopy in a racemose cysticercal cyst of the brain. Neuroradiology 2004;46:72–4.

27. Chang J, Chang J, Park Y, et al. Cysticercosis of cerebellopontine cistern: differential diagnosis using MRI. Acta Neurochir 2004;146:325–8.

28. Arriada-Mendicoa N, Celis-Lopez MA, Higuera-Calleja S, et al. Imaging features of sellar cysticercosis. AJNR Am J Neuroradiol 2003;24:1386–9.

29. Levy AS, Lillehei KO, Rubisttein D, et al. Subarachnoid neurocysticercosis with occlusion of the major intracranial arteries: case report. Neurosurgery 1995;36:183–8.

30. Shin DA, Shin HC. A case of extensive spinal cysticercosis involving the whole spinal canal in a patient with a history of cerebral cysticercosis. Yonsei Med J 2009;50:582–4.

31. Paterakis K, Kapsalaki E, Hadjigeorgiou G, et al. Primary spinal intradural extramedullary cysticercosis. Surg Neurol 2007;68:309–11.

32. Ciftçi E, Diaz-Marchan P, Hayman L. Intradural-extramedullary spinal cysticercosis: MR imaging findings. Comput Med Imaging Graph 1999;23:161–4.

33. Parmar H, Shah J, Patwardhan V, et al. MR imaging in intramedullary cysticercosis. Neuroradiology 2001; 43:961–7.

34. Lee GT, Antelo F, Mlikotic A. Best cases from the AFIP: cerebral toxoplasmosis. Radiographics 2009; 29:1200–5.

35. Batra A, Tripathi R, Gorthi S. Magnetic resonance evaluation of cerebral toxoplasmosis in patients with the acquired immunodeficiency syndrome. Acta Radiol 2004;45:212–21.

36. Thurnher MM, Donovan Post MJ. Neuroimaging in the brain in HIV-1-infected patients. Neuroimaging Clin N Am 2008;18:93–117.

37. Smith B, Smirniotopoulos G, Rushing E. Central nervous system infections associated with human immunodeficiency virus infection: radiologic-pathologic correlation. RadioGraphics 2008;28: 2033–58.

38. Chang L, Cornford ME, Chiang FL, et al. Radiologic-pathologic correlation. Cerebral toxoplasmosis and lymphoma in AIDS. AJNR Am J Neuroradiol 1995; 16:1653–63.

39. Kumar G, Mahadevan A, Guruprasad A, et al. Eccentric target sign in cerebral toxoplasmosis: neuropathological correlate to the imaging feature. J Magn Reson Imaging 2010;31:1469–72.

40. Masamed R, Meleis A, Lee E, et al. Cerebral toxoplasmosis: case review and description of a new imaging sign. Clin Radiol 2009;64:560–3.

41. Chaudhari VV, Yim CM, Hathout H, et al. Atypical imaging appearance of toxoplasmosis in an HIV patient as a butterfly lesion. J Magn Reson Imaging 2009;30:873–5.

42. Barcelo C, Catalaa I, Loubes-Lacroix F, et al. Interest of MR perfusion and MR spectroscopy for the diagnostic of atypical cerebral toxoplasmosis. J Neuroradiol 2010;37:68–71.

43. Schroeder P, Post M, Oschatz E, et al. Analysis of the utility of diffusion-weighted MRI and apparent diffusion coefficient values in distinguishing central nervous system toxoplasmosis from lymphoma. Neuroradiology 2006;48:715–20.

44. Camacho DLA, Smith JK, Castillo M. Differentiation of toxoplasmosis and lymphoma in AIDS patients by using apparent diffusion coefficients. AJNR Am J Neuroradiol 2003;24:633–7.

45. Chong-Han CH, Cortez SC, Tung GA. Diffusion-weighted MRI of cerebral toxoplasma abscess. AJR Am J Roentgenol 2003;181:1711–4.

46. Young R, Ghesani M, Kagetsu N, et al. Lesion size determines accuracy of thallium-201 brain

single-photon emission tomography in differentiating between intracranial malignancy and infection in AIDS patients. AJNR Am J Neuroradiol 2005;26: 1973–9.

47. Cabral RF, Valle Bahia PR, Gasparetto EL, et al. Immune reconstitution inflammatory syndrome and cerebral toxoplasmosis. AJNR Am J Neuroradiol 2010;31:E65–6.

48. Ionita C, Wasay M, Balos L, et al. MR imaging in toxoplasmosis encephalitis after bone marrow transplantation: paucity of enhancement despite fulminant disease. Am J Neuroradiol 2004;25:270–3.

49. Surendrababu N, Kuruvilla K, Jana A. Unusual pattern of calcification in congenital toxoplasmosis: the tram-track sign. Pediatr Radiol 2006;36:569.

50. Abdel Razek A, Shamam O, Abdel wahab N. MR appearance of cerebral cystic echinococcosis: WHO classification. Acta Radiol 2009;50:549–54.

51. Bukte Y, Kemanoglu S, Nazaroglu H, et al. Cerebral hydatid disease: CT and MRI findings. Swiss Med Wkly 2004;134:459–67.

52. Al Zain TJ, Al-Witry SH, Khalili HM, et al. Multiple intracranial hydatidosis. Acta Neurochir 2002;44: 1179–85.

53. Tuzun M, Altinors N, Arda IS, et al. Cerebral hydatid disease CT and MR findings. Clin Imaging 2002;26: 353–7.

54. El-Shamam O, Amer T, El-Atta MA. Magnetic resonance imaging of simple and infected hydatid cysts of the brain. Magn Reson Imag 2001;19:965–74.

55. Tüzün M, Hekimoglu B. Hydatid disease of the CNS: imaging features. AJR Am J Roentgenol 1998;171: 1497–500.

56. Topal U, Parlak M, Kihc C, et al. CT and MRI findings in cerebral hydatid disease. Eur Radiol 1995;5: 244–7.

57. Jayakumar PN, Srikanth SG, Chandrashekar HS, et al. Pyruvate: an in vivo marker of cestodal infestation of the human brain on proton MR spectroscopy. J Magn Reson Imaging 2003;18:675–80.

58. Chawla S, Kumar S, Gupta R. Marker of parasitic cysts on in vivo proton magnetic resonance spectroscopy: is it succinate or pyruvate? J Magn Reson Imaging 2004;20:1052–3.

59. Kalaitzoglou I, Drevelengas A, Petridis A, et al. Albendazole treatment of cerebral hydatid disease: evaluation of results with CT and MRI. Neuroradiology 1998;40:36–9.

60. Cemil B, Tun K, Gurcay A, et al. Cranial epidural hydatid cysts: clinical report and review of the literature. Acta Neurochir 2009;151:659–62.

61. Rumboldt Z, Jednacak H, Talan-Hranilovic J, et al. Unusual appearance of a cisternal hydatid cyst. Am J Neuroradiol 2003;24:112–4.

62. Lakhdar F, Arkha Y, Rifi L, et al. Spinal intradural extramedullary hydatidosis: report of three cases. Neurosurgery 2009;65:372–6.

63. Senturk S, Oguz K, Soylemezoglu F, et al. Cerebral alveolar echinoccosis mimicking primary brain tumor. AJNR Am J Neuroradiol 2006;27:420–2.

64. TunacH M, Tunac H A, Engin G, et al. MRI of cerebral alveolar echinococcosis. Neuroradiology 1999;41: 844–6.

65. Liu H, Lim C, Feng X, et al. MRI in cerebral schistosomiasis: characteristic nodular enhancement in 33 patients. AJR Am J Roentgenol 2008;191:582–8.

66. Sanelli PC, Lev MH, Gonzalez RG, et al. Unique linear and nodular MR enhancement pattern in schistosomiasis of the central nervous system. AJR Am J Roentgenol 2001;177:1471–4.

67. Mehta A, Teoh SK, Schaefer PW, et al. Cerebral schistosomiasis. AJR Am J Roentgenol 1997;168: 1322.

68. Joshi TN, Yamazaki MK, Zhao H, et al. Spinal schistosomiasis: differential diagnosis for acute paraparesis in a U.S. resident. J Spinal Cord Med 2010; 33:256–60.

69. Jiang Y, Zhang M, Xiang Z. Spinal cord schistosomiasis japonica: a report of 4 cases. Surg Neurol 2008; 69:392–7.

70. Saleem S, Belal A, El-Ghandour N. Spinal cord schistosomiasis: MR imaging appearance with surgical and pathologic correlation. AJNR Am J Neuroradiol 2005;26:1646–54.

71. Bennett G, Provenzale J. Schistosomal myelitis: findings at MR imaging. Eur J Radiol 1998;27:268–70.

72. Singh P, Kochhar R, Vashishta R, et al. Amebic meningoencephalitis: spectrum of imaging findings. AJNR Am J Neuroradiol 2006;27:1217–21.

73. Healy J. Balamuthia amebic encephalitis: radiographic and pathologic findings. AJNR Am J Neuroradiol 2002;23:486–9.

74. Sarica F, Tufan K, Cekinmez M, et al. A rare but fatal case of granulomatous amebic encephalitis with brain abscess: the first case reported from Turkey. Turk Neurosurg 2009;19:256–9.

75. Nickerson I, Tong K. Imaging cerebral malaria with a susceptibility-weighted MR sequence. AJNR Am J Neuroradiol 2009;30:e85–6.

76. Gamanagatti S, Kandpal H. MR imaging of cerebral malaria in a child. Eur J Radiol 2006;60:46–7.

77. Sakai O, Barest GD. Diffusion-weighted imaging of cerebral malaria. J Neuroimaging 2005;15:278–80.

78. Shirakawa K, Yamasaki H, Ito A, et al. Cerebral sparganosis: the wandering lesion. Neurology 2010;74:180.

79. Chiu C, Chiou T, Hsu Y, et al. MR spectroscopy and MR perfusion character of cerebral sparganosis: a case report. Br J Radiol 2010;83:e31–3.

80. Song T, Wang W, Zhou B, et al. CT and MR characteristics of cerebral sparganosis. AJNR Am J Neuroradiol 2007;28:1700–5.

81. Bo G, Xuejian W. Neuroimaging and pathological findings in a child with cerebral sparganosis. Case report. J Neurosurg 2006;105:470–2.

82. Rengarajan S, Nanjegowda N, Bhat D, et al. Cerebral sparganosis: a diagnostic challenge. Br J Neurosurg 2008;22:784–6.

83. Moon WK, Chang KH, Cho SY, et al. Cerebral sparganosis: MR imaging versus CT features. Radiology 1993;188:751–7.

84. Nomura M, Nitta H, Nakada M, et al. MRI findings of cerebral paragonimiasis in chronic stage. Clin Radiol 1999;54:622–4.

85. Zhang J, Huan Y, Sun L, et al. MRI features of pediatric cerebral paragonimiasis in the active stage. J Magn Reson Imaging 2006;23:569–73.

86. Joo EY, Kim JH, Tae WS, et al. Simple partial status epilepticus localized by single-photon emission computed tomography subtraction in chronic cerebral paragonimiasis. J Neuroimaging 2004;14:365–8.

87. Lury K, Castillo M. Chagas' disease involving the brain and spinal cord: MRI findings. AJR Am J Roentgenol 2005;185:550–2.

88. Gill D, Chatha D, Carpio-O'Donovan R. MR imaging findings in African trypansomiasis. AJNR Am J Neuroradiol 2003;24:1383–5.

89. Xinou E, Lefkopoulos A, Gelagoti M, et al. CT and MR imaging findings in cerebral toxocaral disease. AJNR Am J Neuroradiol 2003;24:714–8.

90. Dauriac-Le Masson V, Chochon F, Demeret S, et al. Toxocara canis meningomyelitis. J Neurol 2005;252:1267–8.

91. Duprez TPJ, Bigaignon G, Delgrange E, et al. MRI of cervical cord lesions and their resolution in Toxocara canis myelopathy. Neuroradiology 1996;38:792–5.

92. Feydy A, Touze E, Miaux Y, et al. MRI in a case of neurotrichinosis. Neuroradiology 1996;38:80–2.

93. Gelal F, Kumral E, Dirim Vidinli B, et al. Diffusion-weighted and conventional MR imaging in neurotrichinosis. Acta Radiol 2005;46:196–9.

Neuroimaging in Postinfectious Demyelination and Nutritional Disorders of the Central Nervous System

C.C. Tchoyoson Lim, MBBS, FRCR, MMed (DiagRadiol)[a,b,*]

KEYWORDS

- Myelin sheath • Oligodendrocytes • Encephalomyelitis
- Demyelination

The white matter of the brain may be damaged in a variety of conditions, including inflammatory demyelination. Apart from the leukodystrophies (also called dysmyelinating disorders), which are characterized by defective formation or maintenance of myelin in younger patients, demyelinating diseases in the central nervous system are typically classified as primary (of unknown cause, archetypically multiple sclerosis [MS]) or secondary (from other causes) (Box 1).[1] Although secondary white matter disease may have varied and sometimes doubtful causes, the underlying pathologic change seems to be damage to the myelin sheath and oligodendrocytes (the cells that form the myelin). This report focuses on postinfectious demyelination and nutritional disorders of the nervous system, and also discusses tumefactive demyelinating lesions that may mimic neoplasm on neuroimaging.

WHITE MATTER DISEASES ASSOCIATED WITH INFECTIONS

White matter diseases associated with infectious agents may be caused by autoimmune-mediated damage to the oligodendrocytes, myelin destruction by cross-reaction against viral antigens, or direct infection of the glial or neuronal cells of the brain.[1,2] The latter group, which includes subacute sclerosing panencephalitis, progressive rubella panencephalitis, HIV encephalitis, and progressive multifocal leukoencephalitis, typically manifest months or years later and are not discussed in this report.

Acute Disseminated Encephalomyelitis

Frequently described in children (Fig. 1), but also found in adult patients (Fig. 2), ADEM is thought to be a monophasic self-limited, autoimmune response to central nervous system antigen triggered by viral infections.[3,4] The virus is usually not recovered from the brain. Histologically, ADEM is similar to experimental allergic encephalomyelitis, with inflammatory cell (primarily lymphocytic) infiltration and demyelination. A wide range of conditions are associated with ADEM, including non-specific respiratory infection, specific viral illness (such as measles, rubella, mumps, and chickenpox), and vaccination (including diphtheria, smallpox, tetanus, and typhoid); ADEM may even arise spontaneously.[2–11]

Patients often present with an abrupt onset days to weeks (ranging from 2 to 31 days) after an infectious episode or vaccination with fever, headaches,

No funding support for this manuscript: the author has nothing to disclose.
a Department of Neuroradiology, National Neuroscience Institute, Singapore
b Department of Neurology, Duke-NUS Graduate Medical School, Singapore
* National Neuroscience Institute, 11 Jalan Tan Tock Seng, Singapore 308433.
E-mail address: Tchoyoson_Lim@nni.com.sg

Box 1
Causes of demyelinating white matter disease

Primary demyelinating disease

1. MS

2. Neuromyelitis optica

Secondary demyelinating disease

1. Associated with infectious agents

   a. Acute disseminated encephalomyelitis (ADEM)

   b. Acute hemorrhagic leukoencephalitis (AHLE)

   c. Acute necrotizing encephalopathy (ANE)

   d. Subacute sclerosing panencephalitis (SSPE)

   e. HIV encephalitis and progressive multifocal leukoencephalitis

2. Associated with nutritional deficiency

   a. Osmotic demyelination (central pontine and extrapontine myelinolysis)

   b. Wernicke encephalopathy

   c. Marchiafava-Bignami disease (MBD)

   d. Subacute combined degeneration of the spinal cord (SACD)

   e. Copper deficiency myelopathy

3. Associated with physical, chemical, toxic, or hypoxic/ischemic causes

   a. Radiotherapy and chemotherapeutic agents

   b. Chemicals (eg, toluene and mercury)

   c. Hypertensive encephalopathy and posterior reversible encephalopathy syndrome

   d. Cerebral autosomal dominant arteriopathy with subcortical infarcts and leukoencephalopathy

---

meningeal signs, focal neurologic deficits, or drowsiness.[10] Optic neuritis in the pediatric age group is not usually associated with MS, and ADEM should be considered in these patients, especially if accompanied by other symptoms.[2] The cerebrospinal fluid may be normal or show nonspecific pleocytosis. A favorable response to intravenous glucocorticoids is typical, with severe cases requiring plasmapheresis or immunoglobulin therapy.

MR imaging appearance of ADEM

ADEM lesions tend to be fewer, larger, and more asymmetric and more frequently involve the deep gray matter, such as the basal ganglia (see **Fig. 2**) and thalami, compared with MS (the archetypal white matter disease).[5–11] The subcortical rather than periventricular or corpus callosal sites

are typical (again compared with MS).[5,10] They usually show increased signal intensity on T2-weighted or fluid-attenuated inversion recovery (FLAIR) images and low signal intensity on T1-weighted images, without hemorrhage or calcification and with poorly defined margins and only mild mass effect. Contrast enhancement (typically in acute phase) is mild and may exhibit a similar pattern to that in MS.[7] On diffusion-weighted (DW) MR images, increased apparent diffusion coefficient (ADC) has been reported (see **Fig. 1**).[12] On MR spectroscopy, low N-acetylaspartate (NAA) and elevated lactate (see **Fig. 1D**) have been described without increase in choline.[13,14] The optic nerve may also be involved. Spinal cord involvement (up to 28%) usually affects the thoracic segments, but imaging features are nonspecific compared with other causes of myelitis, with single or multiple large lesions with variable enhancement rather than long segmental swelling.[10,11]

Sequential MR imaging plays an important role in establishing the monophasic nature of ADEM, but there are no clear guidelines on interval and duration of studies. On follow-up imaging after treatment with steroids, there is typically decrease in the size and number of lesions or complete resolution in conjunction with clinical improvement. Relapse with appearance on MR imaging of new lesions can occasionally be observed in ADEM.[4] Because there are no formal radiologic features that differentiate ADEM from MS and diagnosis is based on a monophasic and isolated clinical episode, it is difficult at initial MR imaging to predict future clinical relapses. If a relapse occurs and is thought to be part of the same acute monophasic process, the term, muliphasic disseminated encephalomyelitis is used, but if relapses are disseminated in site and time, some patients initially diagnosed as ADEM may be reclassified as having MS.[10,11] Clinical and radiologic discrimination may be difficult.

Acute Hemorrhagic Leukoencephalitis

Originally called Hurst disease,[15] AHLE (or acute hemorrhagic encephalomyelitis) is considered the most severe or fulminating form of ADEM, affecting approximately 2% of cases.[16–19] Victims are typically young, presenting with abrupt onset of fever, progressive neurologic deterioration to coma and death 1 to 5 days after viral infections, sepsis, or in association with allergic causes (including ulcerative colitis and asthma). Rarely, recovery after treatment with high-dose steroids has been reported.[16–18] Histologically, acute perivascular demyelination and hemorrhagic necrotizing angiitis are seen, ranging from petechiae to hematomas.

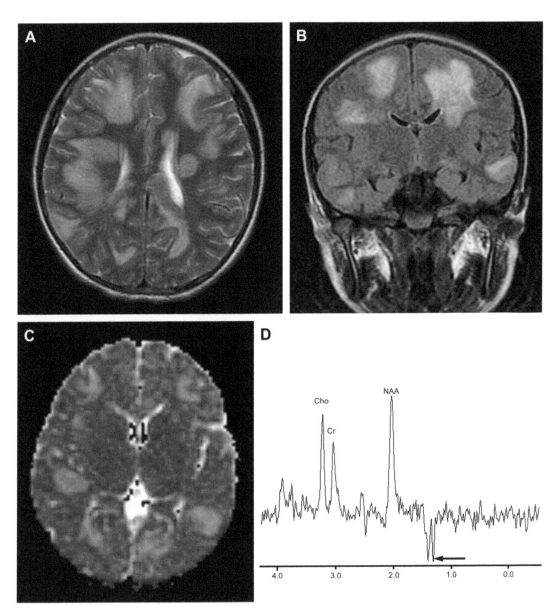

Fig. 1. A 14-year-old girl with ADEM complaining of fever and headache 12 days after upper respiratory tract infection. (*A*) Axial T2-weighted and (*B*) coronal FLAIR images showing bilateral asymmetric multifocal hyperintensities in the subcortical white matter. (*C*) ADC map shows increased ADC in lesions on DW MR imaging. (*D*) Long–echo time MR spectroscopy reveals the presence of lactate (inverted doublet at 1.3 ppm [*arrow*]), decreased NAA (at 2.0 ppm), and minimal higher choline (Cho at 3.2 ppm).

MR imaging appearance of AHLE

Multifocal but asymmetric focal areas of high signal intensity on T2-weighted images are typically seen in the white matter, especially centrum semiovale and internal capsule, but sparing the subcorital U-fibers. Lesions, which are typically described in the frontal and parietal lobes, tend to be larger with more edema, mass effect, and hemorrhage.[2,17–20] Petechial hemorrhage and larger hematomas are typically seen as areas of susceptibility

on spin-echo and gradient-recalled–echo images (**Fig. 3**). Restricted diffusion has been described on DW MR images.[20] Patients typically deteriorate rapidly, often with fatal outcomes.

Acute Necrotizing Encephalopathy

First described in 1995 in Japan and Taiwan, ANE, also known as ANE of childhood, affects predominantly infants and children, with a high rate of death

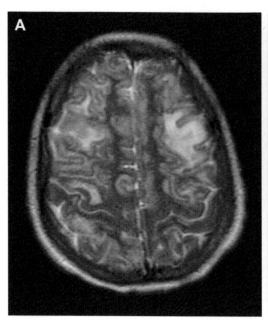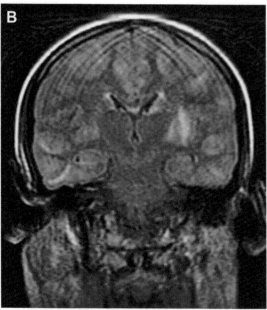

Fig. 2. An 18-year-old woman with ADEM presenting with seizures after an episode of nonspecific viral infection. (*A*) Axial T2-weighted and (*B*) FLAIR images show a few large lesions in the subcortical white matter and basal ganglia.

or irreversible neurologic sequelae.[21,22] Histologically, ANE shows severe necrosis, involving both the gray and white matter of the brain, with focal areas of breakdown of the blood-brain barrier.[21,23] The etiology and pathogenesis of the disease, however, remain mostly unknown, but viral infections, in particular influenza A, have been implicated, and ANE may be a monophasic postinfectious reaction similar to ADEM.[24] Although ANE is typically seen in the East Asia, it has been reported in other parts of the world,[25,26] and there are reports of a recurrent and familial, autosomal dominant form of ANE.[27] Recurrence is rare in sporadic ANE, but it is generally associated with poor clinical outcomes, although patients without cavitation or hemorrhage may have better outcomes.[28,29]

MR imaging appearance of ANE

Distinctive findings include multiple, bilateral, and symmetric brain lesions almost invariably affecting not only the thalamus (**Fig. 4**) but also the brainstem, cerebral white matter, and cerebellum.[21–30] Thalamic lesions may show a concentric structure on CT and MR images.[21,24] High density on CT and T1 shortening on MR imaging may represent hemorrhages in the thalamus, which tends to be more prominent deep in the brain.[23,24] The presence of hemorrhage, cavitation, or atrophy and extensive involvement, including the brainstem, may be associated with poorer outcome.[28,29] Elevated lactate and low ADC (in contrast to

ADEM) may be found on MR spectroscopy and DW MR images, respectively.[12,30] In some cases, a peculiar pattern of concentric layers of different ADC changes can be seen, which correlates with pathologic descriptions of central necrosis, outer cytotoxic edema (which corresponded with contrast enhancement) surrounded by peripheral vascogenic edema (see **Fig. 4**D).[25]

TUMEFACTIVE DEMYELINATION OR INFLAMMATORY DEMYELINATING PSEUDOTUMOR

Occasionally, a solitary focus of demyelination may mimic neoplasm clinically and on neuroimaging, and misdiagnosis is only recognized after biopsy or surgical resection. When histopathologic features of lymphocyte infiltration and macrophage infiltration with demyelination and preservation of axons are found, these lesions have been reported as inflammatory demyelinating pseudotumor, focal tumor-like demyelinating lesions, or tumefactive demyelination.[31–34] The literature definition of tumefactive lesions is hampered by lack of uniform nomenclature and small study size; it may refer to various combinations of large size (larger than 2 cm), presence of mass effect or edema, and/or atypical enhancement.[35] Although the diagnosis is made on pathology, histologic specimens may likewise be misinterpreted as neoplasm given their sometimes hypercellular nature.

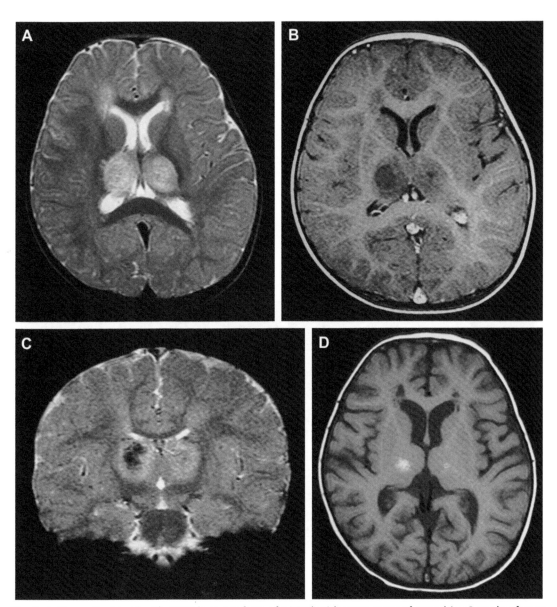

Fig. 3. A 14-month-old girl with AHLE (a severe form of ADEM) with acute onset of convulsion 3 weeks after an oral Sabin polio vaccine. (*A*) Axial T2-weighted MR imaging of the brain at the level of thalamus shows acute edema of the bilateral thalami and hyperintensity change of the frontal periventricular white matter. (*B*) Post-contrast T1-weighted (repetition time/echo time: 667/16) image at the same level shows necrosis of the T2-hyperintense lesions. (*C*) A coronal gradient-echo T2 star (repetition time/echo time/flip angle: 683/40/15) through the thalamus shows hemorrhage in the right thalamus. (*D*) A follow-up T1-weighted MR image 3 weeks later shows atrophy of the thalamus with a small old hematoma in the right central nucleic region. Also note cystic encephalomalacia of the frontal periventricular white matter. (*Reprinted from* Lo CP, Chen CY. Neuroimaging of viral infections in infants and young children. Neuroimag Clin North Am 2008;18[1]:119–32; with permission.)

In a large retrospective study of 168 patients with biopsy-confirmed inflammatory demyelinating disease, the clinical presentation was a first neurologic event in 61%, relapsing remitting clinical course in 29%, and progressive in 4%; at follow-up, 70% developed definite MS, and 14% had an isolated demyelinating syndrome.[35] If demyelinating pseudotumor is suspected, treatment with a course of steroids may be followed by dramatic clinical and neuroimaging improvement, obviating biopsy. Although clinical features may be monophasic and of acute onset, they may be ambiguous or

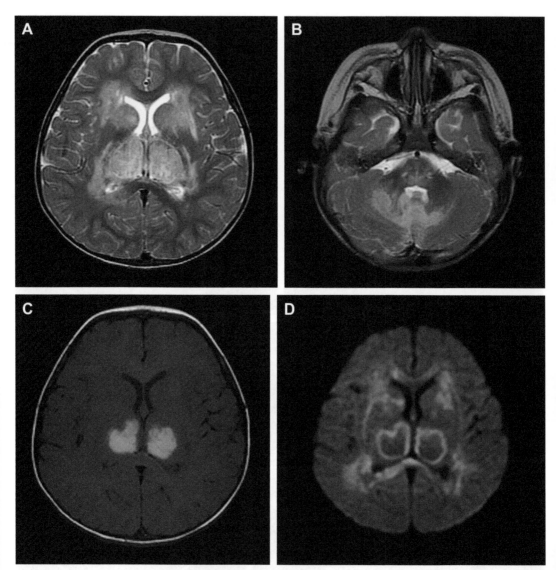

Fig. 4. A 2-year-old girl with ANE presenting with fever, cough, and altered consciousness. (*A, B*) Axial T2-weighted MR images showing bilaterally symmetric hyperintensity and swelling of the thalamus and also abnormal high signal in the cerebral white matter, corpus callosum corticospinal tract, brainstem and cerebellum. (*C*) Axial T1-weighted MR image shows the swollen thalami to be hyperintense. (*D*) Axial DW MR image reveals a concentric pattern of inner low signal and outer increased signal surrounded by another area of low signal in the thalamus. Hyperintensity is also noted in the white matter.

atypical, leading some investigators to suggest that this entity was intermediate between MS and ADEM.[33,36] Demyelinating lesions mimicking brain tumors are rare in the pediatric population and are considered comparatively benign, often with a monophasic course.[32,36]

MR imaging appearance of inflammatory demyelinating pseudotumor

On neuroimaging, inflammatory demyelinating lesions mimic neoplasms in that they tend to be solitary, large and ill defined; often enhance after contrast administration; and seem to occupy space and exert mass effect.[33–36] Frontal and parietal subcortical regions are most often affected (in up to half of patients), and a butterfly configuration involving the corpus callosum (**Fig. 5**) was observed in 12%; 38% of patients studied with spinal MRI also had spinal cord lesions.[35] Although the mass effect and edema tends to be minor relative to lesion size in comparison with tumors and abscesses, there still seems to be a strong association.[35]

MR imaging is sensitive but not specific: high signal on T2-weighted images and hemispheric

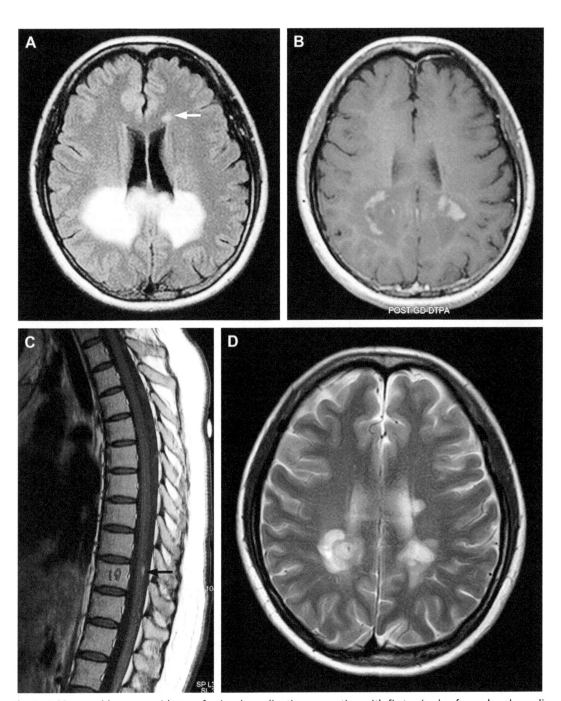

Fig. 5. A 32-year-old woman with tumefactive demyelination presenting with first episode of poor hand coordination. (*A*) Axial FLAIR image showing bilateral periventricular hyperintensity also affecting the corpus callosum. Note an additional periventricular lesion (*arrow*) oriented perpendicular to the frontal horn typical of Dawson finger of MS. (*B*) After contrast injection, the large low signal lesions on T1-weighted image shows patchy peripheral enhancement. (*C*) Sagittal T1-weighted image after contrast injection reveals a single enhancing silent lesion (*arrow*) in the T10 segment of the thoracic spinal cord. (*D*) Axial T2-weighted MR image after a course of steroids shows decrease in lesion size accompanied by clinical improvement.

location are typically nondiscriminatory between neoplasm and tumefactive demyelination. There may, however, be imaging features that might suggest non-neoplastic demyelinating disease, such as multiple other asymptomatic or silent white matter plaques, in up to 70% of prebiopsy MR images, which fulfill the Barkhof criteria for MS (see **Fig. 5**A).[35] Visualization of veins coursing through the lesion may also be helpful, because demyelination tends to be perivascular whereas neoplasms displace or engulf veins.[37,38] MR spectroscopy has been described in demyelinating lesions and the NAA, choline, and lactate findings may also mimic neoplasm and need to be interpreted with caution.[38–42] High level of glutamate/glutamine on short–echo time spectroscopy has been found and may be useful.[42] Lower relative cerebral blood volume detected on dynamic perfusion MR imaging studies might be helpful to characterize demyelinating lesions because neoplasms typically show increased perfusion from angioneogenesis.[38,43] The MR imaging discrimination between neoplasia and tumefactive demyelination remains a diagnostic challenge to radiologists.

WHITE MATTER DISEASES ASSOCIATED WITH NUTRITIONAL AND VITAMIN DEFICIENCY

Nutritional deficiencies, including beriberi from vitamin B_1 deficiency and pernicious anemia from vitamin B_{12} deficiency, are important health issues in the developing world, but central nervous system manifestations with MR imaging findings are less commonly reported. Alcohol misuse greatly contributes to nutritional deficiencies, resulting in disorders, such as osmotic demyelination, Wernicke encephalopathy, and MBD.

Osmotic Demyelination

Osmotic demyelination is associated with electrolyte imbalances (especially rapid correction of hyponatremia) and typically occurs in chronic alcoholics, the malnourished, or the chronically debilitated, such as patients with burns, organ transplantation, syndrome of inappropriate secretion of antidiuretic hormone, neoplasia, or severe lung, liver, or kidney disease.[44–49] The pathogenesis is poorly understood, but oligodendroglial cells are susceptible to osmotic stresses, and the distribution of neuroimaging changes parallels their distribution in the central pons, thalamus, and putamen.[49,50] Although initially thought to be a purely demyelinating disease sparing the nerves and axons, there may be more complex pathophysiologic processes involved.[49–51]

Central pontine myelinolysis (CPM) and extrapontine myelinolysis (EPM) are terms used to describe osmotic damage involving the pons and the extrapontine structures, respectively.[46] The clinical manifestations are variable and include spastic quadriparesis, pseudobulbar palsy, decreased levels of consciousness, locked-in syndrome, and coma; a significant number of patients die. Serial measurements of serum sodium levels are helpful for diagnosis.

MR imaging appearance of osmotic demyelination

In CPM, a symmetric trident, butterfly, or bat wing–shaped focus of increased signal intensity is typically detected in the central upper or middle pons on T2-weighted or FLAIR images, with low signal on T1-weighted images (**Fig. 6**). Characteristic sparing of the corticospinal tracts, the peripheral and ventrolateral aspects of the pons, is seen.[47] Contrast enhancement may occur occasionally at the lesion periphery.

EPM is less common and is detected as areas of T2 prolongation in the globus pallidus, putamen, thalamus, cerebellum, and cerebral cortex; EPM may occur in the absence of CPM.[44] The lesions may show hyperintensity on DW MR imaging, with elevated diffusion or restricted diffusion in the early stages of the disease process, possibly related to osmotic shifts in intracellular water.[51–54] The key feature to diagnosis is the bilaterally symmetric distribution of lesions.

Wernicke Encephalopathy

Wernicke encephalopathy is an acute, potentially fatal (in 17%) neuropsychiatric syndrome resulting from thiamine deficiency; the condition is often underdiagnosed.[55–57] Thiamine (vitamin B_1) is an important osmotic regulator, and deficiency may occur as a result of malnourished states ranging from chronic alcoholism, gastrointestinal surgery (including gastroplasty for obesity), bowel obstruction, hyperemesis gravidarum, systemic disease, magnesium depletion, and prolonged parenteral therapy without vitamin supplementation.[57] Malignancy is the most common cause in children. Histopathologically, demyelination, edema, petechial hemorrhages, and reactive astrocytosis have been described, affecting specific areas of the brain, eventually leading to atrophy.[55]

The classical clinical triad of Wernicke encephalopathy, including ocular dysfunction (nystagmus and ophthalmoplegia), altered consciousness, and ataxia, is seen in only 16% of patients, and the symptomatology may be confusing.[56] Wernicke encephalopathy is a medical emergency requiring intravenous thiamine replacement[58] and

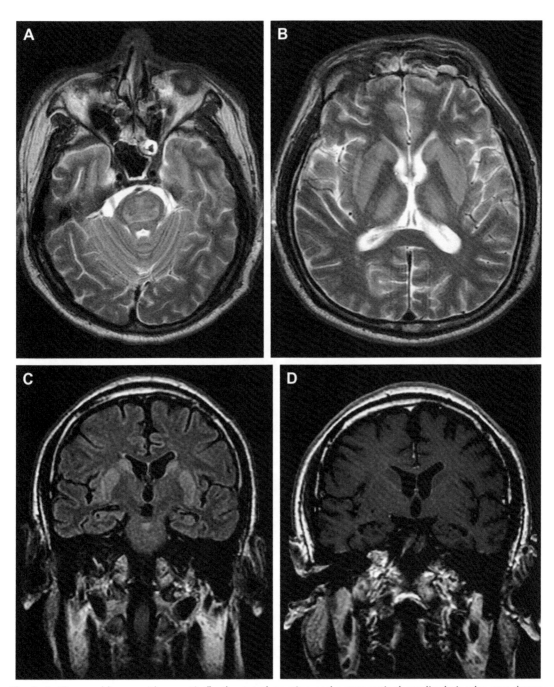

Fig. 6. A 48-year-old man with osmotic (both central pontine and extrapontine) myelinolysis who was drowsy and tetraplegic after correction of hyponatremia (sodium 90 mEq/L on admission, due to vomiting and antihypertensive medications). (A) Axial T2-weighted MR image showing symmetric trident-shaped area of abnormal high signal within the central pons sparing the corticospinal tracts and pontine periphery. (B) Axial T2-weighted and (C) coronal FLAIR image shows that the basal ganglia and thalamus are also involved in a bilaterally symmetric manner typical of a systemic disease. (D) Coronal T1-weighted image after contrast injection shows no abnormal enhancement of the basal ganglia.

is difficult to diagnose because of poorly recognized clinical signs and its similarity to drunkenness in known alcoholics. Hence, a high index of suspicion on neuroimaging is important, especially

because blood thiamine concentration and red blood cell transketolase activity are difficult tests to perform and lack specificity.[57] Left untreated, Korsakoff psychosis (a syndrome of severe memory impairment seen in up to 80% of survivors) or death may result.[55,59]

MR imaging appearance of Wernicke encephalopathy

MR imaging has sensitivity of only 53% but a high specificity of 93%.[60,61] On T2-weighted images, characteristic findings of bilateral hyperintensity of the medial dorsal thalamus (which are affected histologically in 100% of patients) (Fig. 7), mamillary bodies, hypothalamus, periaqueductal gray matter, floor of the fourth ventricle, and tectal plate may be seen.[60–63] Hyperintensity on DW MR imaging representing diffusion restriction may be seen.[64,65] MR

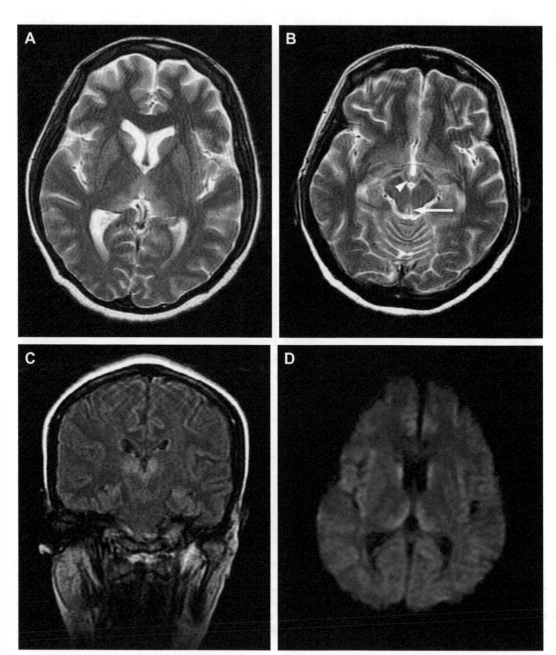

Fig. 7. A 26-year-old woman with Wernicke encephalopathy secondary to hyperemesis gravidarum presenting with decreased GCS and confusion. (A, B) Axial T2-weighted MR images showing bilaterally symmetric hyperintensity in the medial thalamus, mamillary bodies (arrowhead), and periaqueductal gray matter (arrow). The caudate heads and basal ganglia also seem involved. (C) Coronal FLAIR image shows typical medial thalamus hyperintensity. (D) Axial DW MR image showing medial thalamic and caudate hyperintensity. The ADC was slightly decreased.

spectroscopy reveals the presence of abnormal lactate and normal or decreased NAA.[66,67] Contrast enhancement of the thalamus and mamillary bodies is more common in chronic alcoholic abuse, whereas atypical involvement of the cerebral cortex, cerebellum, and cranial nerve nuclei (usually together with the more typical structures) is associated with nonalcoholic patients: these features may help distinguish these 2 groups of patients.[68,69] Cortical involvement may indicate poor prognosis even when thiamine is promptly administered.

Marchiafava-Bignami Disease

Initially described in male Italian alcoholics consuming large quantities of red wine, this rare condition is now recognized worldwide among poorly nourished alcoholics as well as nondrinkers with severe nutritional deficiency.[70–74] Patients present acutely with sudden altered consciousness, seizures, hypertonia, and pyramidal signs, progressing rapidly to unconsciousness and death. Subacute and chronic progressive forms of the disease over months to years have also been described, with dementia, clouded consciousness, and interhemispheric disconnection. Improved antemortem detection and survival have been reported,[72,73] with some cases attributed to partial rather than complete involvement of the corpus callosum.[74] The mainstay of treatment is supportive, with thiamine substitution and improvement of nutritional status. The pathogenesis of MBD is poorly understood, but demyelination of the corpus callosum with reduction of oligodendrocytes, abundant lipid-laden macrophages, and necrotic and cystic lesions have been described, predominantly affecting the central fibers with preservation of the upper and lower edges.

MR imaging appearance of MBD

The body of the corpus callosum (followed by genu and finally splenium) is characteristically affected, with extracallosal involvement sometimes reported.

In the acute fulminant form, there is swelling and hyperintensity on T2-weighted or FLAIR images; the lesions may enhance.[75] Central focal hypointensity on the T2-weighted may represent hemosiderin or lipid-laden macrophages.[76] On DW MR imaging, low ADC has been reported (Fig. 8), probably representing severe edema rather than merely demyelination.[77,78] MR spectroscopy has been described in a case report, where lactate was detected, with reduction in NAA/creatine ratio and increased choline/creatine ratio.[79]

The centrum semiovale, periventricular, and frontal lobe white matter may also be involved and may be detected as confluent areas of high signal on T2-weighted images.[72,73] Cerebral cortex, internal capsule (see Fig. 8C), and thalamus involvement has also been shown, and cortical involvement (attributed to Morel laminar necrosis) and low ADC may be related to poor prognosis.[78] Serial imaging in survivors or in the chronic mild progressive disease usually reveal focal cystic necrosis or atrophy and thinning of the corpus callosum.

Subacute Combined Degeneration of the Spinal Cord

Vitamin B_{12} (cyanocobalamine) deficiency can cause pernicious anemia and affect the central or peripheral nervous system, causing SACD, with demyelination and vacuolation of the posterior and lateral columns. Vitamin B_{12} deficiency may be due to dietary deficiency (particularly in breastfed infants of strict vegetarians), but gastric surgery and malabsorption syndromes are also important causes. In developed countries, pernicious anemia from autoimmune gastritis (where the gastric parietal cells are destroyed and fail to produce intrinsic factor, which is essential for intestinal absorption of normal dietary intake of vitamin B_{12}) is the most common cause, especially in the elderly.[80–86] Nitrous oxide, used as an inhalational anesthetic for dental and surgical procedure and also abused as an illegal euphoriant, irreversibly inactivates the cobalt core of vitamin B_{12} and can also cause SACD after single or prolonged exposure.[87]

Patients with SACD complain of generalized weakness, loss of position and vibration sense (particularly of the lower limbs), and paresthesias (pins and needles) of the hands and feet. It is thought that vitamin B_{12} deficiency results in elevation of methylmalonic acid, which is toxic to myelin, and elevated serum methylmalonic acid and total homocysteine levels may be more useful in diagnosis, because serum cobalamin measurement can be normal in some patients with SACD and deficiency.[88] If deficiency remains undiagnosed and vitamin B_{12} intramuscular injections are not instituted, patients may develop paraplegia with spasticity and contractures.

MR imaging appearance of SACD

Increased signal intensity on T2-weighted images involving the posterior and lateral white matter columns (Fig. 9) is typically seen, with the cervical and upper thoracic cord the most severely affected.[80–86] There may be mild expansion but the spinal cord usually does not enhance, and typically full-blown cord lesions appear as a continuous long segment, rarely also involving the anterior columns.[81,82,86]

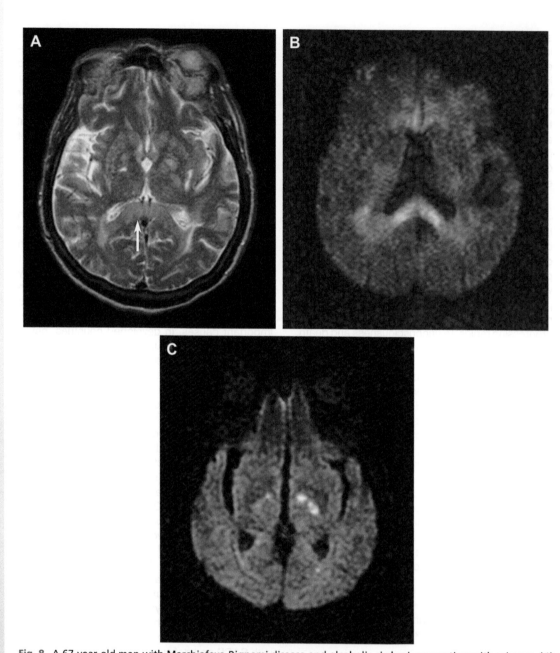

Fig. 8. A 67-year-old man with Marchiafava-Bignami disease and alcoholic cirrhosis presenting with seizures. (A) Axial T2-weighted MR images showing hyperintensity and thickening of the corpus callosum (*arrow*). Axial DW MR images showing hyperintensity of the corpus callosum (*B*) and corticospinal tract (*C*).

In some patients, MR imaging findings may precede clinical symptoms, and radiologists play an important role in early diagnosis of SACD, because timely treatment may prevent or reverse neurologic symptoms.[85] Spinal cord lesions may resolve after treatment, but in long-standing cases the cord may atrophy.[82,85] Uncommonly, abnormality of the white matter of the brain has been reported.[83,84]

MR IMAGING FINDINGS IN OTHER NUTRITIONAL ABNORMALITIES

Acquired copper deficiency can cause a clinical and MR image identical to SACD, and both conditions may coexist.[89,90] Neurologic manifestations of vitamin E deficiency include a progressive spinocerebellar syndrome with corticospinal tract dysfunction and peripheral neuropathy or findings

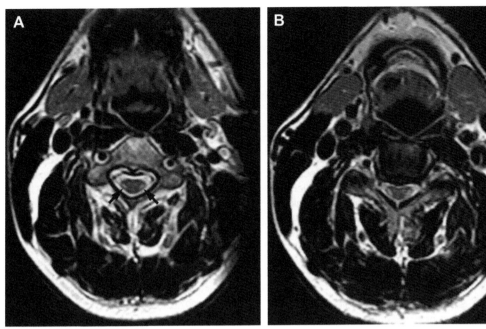

Fig. 9. A 53-year-old man with SACD after gastric surgery. (*A, B*) Axial T2-weighted image shows nonenhancing bilaterally symmetric high signal intensity in the lateral columns of the cervical spinal cord (*arrows*). The posterior columns in this patient are normal; this region would also be involved in classical SACD.

similar to SACD. It is unclear if folate deficiency in isolation can cause myeloneuropathy.[88]

THE RADIOLOGIST'S ROLE IN POSTINFECTIOUS AND NUTRITIONAL ABNORMALITIES

MR imaging is the best imaging method for evaluating demyelinating diseases and provides better visualization of lesions compared with CT. Enhancement of demyelinating lesions is highly variable in postinfectious and nutritional abnormalities, usually occurring in the acute phase, with breakdown of the blood-brain barrier. DW MR imaging may be helpful in differentiating ADEM from ANE but there is much overlap, and MR spectroscopy may not be helpful in distinguishing the various causes of demyelination.[12] Likewise, MR spectroscopy may be limited in distinguishing neoplasm from tumefactive demyelination, although perfusion imaging may be helpful in this respect.[38,91] Other advanced MR imaging techniques, such as diffusion tensor imaging, functional MR imaging, and higher field strength (7T) MR imaging scanners may be helpful to provide information about these uncommon demyelinating processes.

Because the MR imaging features of postinfectious and nutritional abnormalities may not be specific, radiologists need to consider a wide range of demyelinating diseases, particularly of bilaterally symmetric lesions in the thalamus, which can be affected by ANE, EPM, Wernicke encephalopathy, and ADEM or AHLE. Other considerations in the differential diagnosis include thalamic infarction, primary cerebral lymphoma, Behçet disease, deep venous occlusion, Leigh disease, Wilson disease, and variant Creutzfeldt-Jakob disease; many of these conditions may also involve the basal ganglia and/or the white matter.[57,92,93] Furthermore, nutritional abnormalities, such as MBD, may be associated with additional MR imaging findings of Wernicke encephalopathy and osmotic myelinolysis, given that the risk factors of alcoholism and poor nutrition may predispose a single patient to more than one disease.

In MS, there is evidence that myelin is not the only tissue damaged and that axons and neurons are harmed as well. Similarly, secondary demyelinating diseases associated with infection and nutritional abnormalities may also be affected by more complex pathologic processes. The fact that different infections can produce the same phenotype suggests that demyelinating disorders may be mediated by host factors. Furthermore, the discovery of RANBP2 mutations in familial and recurrent cases of ANE suggests that the necrotizing encephalopathies, which include such disparate diseases as ANE, Wernicke encephalopathy, and Leigh syndrome, may share similarities but have distinct pathogenesis and MR imaging phenotypes.[27]

The diagnosis of many postinfectious and nutritional demyelinating diseases is primarily based on characteristic neuroradiologic findings, and radiologists play an important role in alerting attending physicians to the possibility of unsuspected postinfectious demyelinating complications when patients undergo neuroimaging for nonspecific clinical deterioration. When evaluating these patients, the lesion location, imaging features, history, and laboratory evaluation can help narrow the differential diagnosis. Because the imaging findings of these conditions frequently overlap, however, knowledge of patients' clinical condition and good communication between radiologists and clinicians remain essential for correct interpretation.

REFERENCES

1. Smith AB, Smirniotopoulos JG. Imaging evaluation of demyelinating processes of the central nervous system. Postgrad Med J 2010;86:218–29.

2. Lo CP, Chen CY. Neuroimaging of viral infections in infants and young children. Neuroimaging Clin N Am 2008;18(1):119–32.

3. Hart MN, Earle KM. Haemorrhagic and perivenous encephalitis: a clinical-pathological review of 38 cases. J Neurol Neurosurg Psychiatry 1975;38(6): 585–91.

4. Saito H, Endo M, Takase S, et al. Acute disseminated encephalomyelitis after influenza vaccination. Arch Neurol 1980;37(9):564–6.

5. Atlas SW, Grossman RI, Goldberg HI, et al. MR diagnosis of acute disseminated encephalomyelitis. J Comput Assist Tomogr 1986;10(5):798–801.

6. Kesselring J, Miller DH, Robb SA, et al. Acute disseminating encephalomyelitis; MRI findings and the distinction from multiple sclerosis. Brain 1990; 113:291–302.

7. Caldemyer KS, Smith RR, Harris TM, et al. MRI in acute disseminating encephalomyelitis. Neuroradiology 1994;36:216–20.

8. Baum PA, Barkovich AJ, Koch TK, et al. Deep gray matter involvement in children with acute disseminating encephalomyelitis. AJNR Am J Neuroradiol 1994;15:1275–83.

9. Singh S, Alexander M, Korah IP. Pictorial essay— acute disseminated encephalomyelitis: MR imaging features. Am J Roentgenol 1999;173:1101–7.

10. Dale RC, de Sousa C, Chong WK, et al. Acute disseminated encephalomyelitis, multiphasic disseminated encephalomyelitis and multiple sclerosis in children. Brain 2000;123:2407–22.

11. Tenembaum S, Chitnis T, Ness J, et al. Acute disseminated encephalomyelitis. Neurology 2007; 68:S23–36.

12. Harada M, Hisaoka S, Mori K, et al. Differences in water diffusion and lactate production in two different types of postinfectious encephalopathy. J Magn Reson Imaging 2000;11:559–63.

13. Bizzi A, Uluğ AM, Crawford TO, et al. Quantitative proton MR spectroscopic imaging in acute disseminated encephalomyelitis. ANJR Am J Neuroradiol 2001;22(6):1125–30.

14. Mader I, Wolff M, Nägele T, et al. MRI and proton MR spectroscopy in acute disseminated encephalomyelitis. Childs Nerv Syst 2005;21(7):566–72.

15. Hurst EW. Acute haemorrhagic leucoencephalitis: a previously undefined entity. Med J Aust 1941;2:1–6.

16. Huang CC, Chu NS, Chen TJ, et al. Acute haemorrhagic leucoencephalitis with a prolonged clinical course. J Neurol Neurosurg Psychiatry 1988;51(6): 870–4.

17. Markus R, Brew BJ, Turner J, et al. Successful outcome with aggressive treatment of acute haemorrhagic leukoencephalitis. J Neurol Neurosurg Psychiatry 1997;63:551–2.

18. Seales D, Greer M. Acute hemorrhagic leukoencephalitis—a successful recovery. Arch Neurol 1991; 48:1086–8.

19. Kuperan S, Ostrow P, Landi MK, et al. Acute hemorrhagic leukoencephalitis vs ADEM: FLAIR MRI and neuropathology findings. Neurology 2003;60:721–2.

20. Mader I, Wolff M, Niemann G, et al. Acute haemorrhagic encephalomyelitis (AHEM)—MRI findings. Neuropediatrics 2004;35:143–6.

21. Mizuguchi M, Abe J, Mikkaichi K, et al. Acute necrotizing encephalopathy of childhood—a new syndrome presenting with multifocal, symmetric brain lesions. J Neurol Neurosurg Psychiatry 1995;58: 555–61.

22. Mizuguchi M. Acute necrotizing encephalopathy of childhood presenting with multifocal, symmetric brain lesions occurring outside Japan—letter to Wang HS. J Neurol Neurosurg Psychiatry 1995;59: 661–3.

23. Mizuguchi M, Hayashi M, Nakano I, et al. Concentric structure of thalamic concentric structure of thalamic lesions in acute necrotizing encephalopathy. Neuroradiology 2002;44:489–93.

24. Yagishita A, Nakano I, Ushioda T, et al. Acute encephalopathy with bilateral thalamotegmental involvement in infants and children: imaging and pathology findings. AJNR Am J Neuroradiol 1995; 16:439–47.

25. Albayram S, Bilgi Z, Selcuk H, et al. Diffusion-weighted MR imaging findings of acute necrotizing encephalopathy. AJNR Am J Neuroradiol 2004;25: 792–7.

26. Campistol J, Gassio R, Pineda M, et al. Acute necrotizing encephalopathy of childhood (infantile bilateral thalamic necrosis): two non-Japanese chases. Dev Med Child Neurol 1997;40:771–4.

27. Neilson DE, Eiben RM, Waniewski S, et al. Autosomal dominant acute necrotizing encephalopathy. Neurology 2003;61:226–30.

28. Kim JH, Kim IO, Lim MK, et al. Acute necrotizing encephalopathy in korean infants and children: imaging findings and diverse clinical outcome. Korean J Radiol 2004;5(3):171–7.

29. Wong AM, Simon EM, Zimmerman RA, et al. Acute necrotizing encephalopathy of childhood: correlation of MR findings and clinical outcome. AJNR Am J Neuroradiol 2006;27:1919–23.

30. Goo HW, Choi CG, Yoon CH, et al. Acute necrotizing encephalopathy: diffusion MR imaging and localized proton MR spectroscopic findings in two infants. Korean J Radiol 2003;4:61–5.

31. Prockop LD. Demyelinating disease presenting as an intracranial mass lesion. Arch Neurol 1965; 13(5):559.

32. Hunter SB, Ballinger WE, Rubin JJ. Multiple sclerosis mimicking primary brain tumor. Arch Pathol Lab Med 1987;111:464–8.

33. Kepes JJ. Large focal tumor-like demyelinating lesions of the brain: intermediate entity between multiple sclerosis and acute disseminated encephalomyelitis? A study of 31 patients. Ann Neurol 1993; 33:18–27.

34. Zagzag D, Miller DC, Kleinman GM, et al. Demyelinating disease versus tumor in surgical neuropathology. Clues to a correct pathological diagnosis. Am J Surg Pathol 1993;17:537–45.

35. Lucchinetti CF, Gavrilova RH, Metz I, et al. Clinical and radiographic spectrum of pathological confirmed tumefactive multiple sclerosis. Brain 2008; 131:1759–75.

36. Dagher AP, Smirniotopoulos J. Tumefactive demyelinating lesions. Neuroradiology 1996;38:560–5.

37. Malhotra HS, Jain KK, Agarwal A, et al. Characterization of tumefactive demyelinating lesions using MR imaging and in-vivo proton MR spectroscopy. Mult Scler 2009;15:193–203.

38. Cha S, Pierce S, Knopp EA, et al. Dynamic contrast-enhanced T2-weighted MR imaging of tumefactive demyelinating lesions. AJNR Am J Neuroradiol 2001;22:1109–16.

39. Ernst T, Chang L, Walot I, et al. Physiologic MRI of a tumefactive multiple sclerosis lesion. Neurology 1998;51:1486–8.

40. De Stefano N, Caramanos Z, Preul MC, et al. In vivo differentiation of astrocytic brain tumors and isolated demyelinating lesions of the type seen in multiple sclerosis using 1H magnetic resonance spectroscopic imaging. Ann Neurol 1998;44:273–8.

41. Saindane AM, Cha S, Law M, et al. Proton MR Spectroscopy of Tumefactive Demyelinating Lesions. AJNR Am J Neuroradiol 2002;23:1378–86.

42. Cianfoni A, Niku S, Imbesi SG. Metabolite findings in tumefactive demyelinating lesions utilizing short echo time proton magnetic resonance spectroscopy. AJNR Am J Neuroradiol 2007;28:272–7.

43. Cheong LH, Lim CCT, Koh TS. Dynamic contrast-enhanced CT imaging of intracranial meningioma: a comparison of distributed and compartmental tracer-kinetic models. Radiology 2004;232(3):921–30.

44. Adams RD, Victor M, Mancall EL. Central pontine myelinolysis: a hitherto undescribed disease occurring in alcoholic and malnourished patients. AMA Arch Neurol Psychiatry 1959;81:154–72.

45. Rippe DJ, Edwards MK, D'Amour PG, et al. MR imaging of central pontine myelinolysis. J Comput Assist Tomogr 1987;11(4):724–6.

46. Gerard E, Healy ME, Hesselink JR. MR demonstration of mesencephalic lesions in osmotic demyelination syndrome (central pontine myelinolysis). Neuroradiology 1987;29(6):582–4.

47. Miller GM, Baker HL, Okazaki H, et al. Central pontine myelinolysis and its imitators: MR findings. Radiology 1988;168:795–802.

48. Mascalchi M, Cincotta M, Piazzini M. Case report—MRI demonstration of pontine and thalamic myelinolysis in a normonatremia alcoholic. Clin Radiol 1993; 47(2):137–8.

49. Lampl C, Yazdi K. Central pontine myelinolysis. Eur Neurol 2002;47:3–10.

50. Abbott R, Silber E, Felber J, et al. Osmotic demyelination syndrome. BMJ 2005;31:829–30.

51. Chua GC, Sitoh YY, Lim CC, et al. MRI findings in osmotic myelinolysis. Clin Radiol 2002;57(9):800–6.

52. Chu K, Kang DW, Ko SB. Diffusion-weighted MR findings of central pontine and extrapontine myelinolysis. Acta Neurol Scand 2001;104:385–8.

53. Cramer SC, Stegbauer KC, Schneider A. Decreased diffusion in central pontine myelinolysis. AJNR Am J Neuroradiol 2001;22:1476–9.

54. Ruzek KA, Campeau NG, Miller GM. Early diagnosis of central pontine myelinolysis with diffusion-weighted imaging. AJNR Am J Neuroradiol 2004;25:210–3.

55. Victor M, Adams RD, Collins GH. The Wernicke-Korsakoff syndrome: a clinical and pathological study of 245 patients, 82 with post-mortem examinations. Contemp Neurol Ser 1971;7:1–206.

56. Harper CG, Giles M, Finlay-Jones R. Clinical signs in the Wernicke-Korsakoff complex: a retrospective analysis of 131 cases diagnosed at necropsy. J Neurol Neurosurg Psychiatry 1986;49:341–5.

57. Sechi GP, Serra A. Wernicke's encephalopathy: new clinical settings and recent advances in diagnosis and management. Lancet Neurol 2007;6:442–55.

58. Ogershok PR, Rahman A, Nestor S, et al. Wernicke encephalopathy in nonalcoholic patients. Am J Med Sci 2002;323:107–11.

59. Kopelman MD. The Korsakoff syndrome. Br J Psychiatry 1995;166:154–73.

60. Antunez E, Estruch R, Cardenal C, et al. Usefulness of CT and MR imaging in the diagnosis of acute

Wernicke's encephalopathy. AJR Am J Roentgenol 1998;171:1131–7.

61. Chung SP, Kim SW, Yoo IS, et al. Magnetic resonance imaging as a diagnostic adjunct to Wernicke's encephalopathy in the ED. Am J Emerg Med 2003;21:497–502.

62. Mascalchi M, Simonelli P, Tessa C, et al. Do acute lesions of Wernicke's encephalopathy show contrast enhancement? Report of three cases and review of literature. Neuroradiology 1999;41:249–54.

63. Zuccoli G, Gallucci M, Capellades J, et al. Wernicke encephalopathy: MR findings at clinical presentation in twenty-six alcoholic and nonalcoholic patients. AJNR Am J Neuroradiol 2007;28:1328–31.

64. Tajima Y, Yoshida A, Ura S. Diffusion weighted MR imaging of Wernicke encephalopathy. No To Shinkei 2000;52:840–1.

65. Chu K, Kang DW, Kim HJ, et al. Diffusion-weighted imaging abnormalities in Wernicke encephalopathy—reversible cytotoxic edema? Arch Neurol 2002;59:123–7.

66. Rugilo CA, Uribe Rocca MC, Zurru MC, et al. Proton MR spectroscopy in Wernicke's encephalopathy. AJNR Am J Neuroradiol 2003;24:952–5.

67. Murata T, Fujito T, Kimura H, et al. Serial MRI and (1) H-MRS of Wernicke's encephalopathy: report of a case with remarkable cerebellar lesions on MRI [abstract]. Psychiatry Res 2001;108:49–55.

68. Fei G, Zhong C, Lin J, et al. Clinical characteristics and MR imaging features of nonalcoholic wernicke encephalopathy. AJNR Am J Neuroradiol 2008;29:164–9.

69. Zuccoli G, Santa Cruz D, Bertolini M, et al. MR imaging findings in 56 patients with wernicke encephalopathy: nonalcoholics may differ from alcoholics. AJNR Am J Neuroradiol 2009;30:171–6.

70. Leong AS. Marchiafava-Bignami disease in a nonalcoholic Indian male. Pathology 1979;11(2):241–9.

71. Izquierdo G, Quesada MA, Chacon J, et al. Neuroradiological abnormalities in Marchiafava-Bignami disease of benign evolution. Eur J Radiol 1992;15(1):71–4.

72. Arbelaez A, Pajon A, Castillo M. Acute Marchiafava-Bignami disease: MR findings in two patients. AJNR Am J Neuroradiol 2003;24:1955–7.

73. Ruiz-Martinez J, Perez-Balsa AM, Ruibal M, et al. Marchiafava-Bignami disease with widespread extracallosal lesions and favourable course. Neuroradiology 1999;41(1):40–3.

74. Heinrich A, Runge U, Khaw AV. Clinicoradiologic subtypes of Marchiafava-Bignami disease. J Neurol 2004;251:1050–9.

75. Yamamoto T, Ashikaga R, Araki Y, et al. Case report—a case of Marchiafava-Bignami disease: MRI findings on spin-echo and fluid attenuated inversion recovery (FLAIR) images. Eur J Radiol 2000;34:141–3.

76. Chang KH, Cha SH, Han MH, et al. Marchiafava-Bignami disease—serial changes in corpus callosum on MRI. Neuroradiology 1992;34(6):480–2.

77. Hlaihel C, Gonnaud PM. Champin. Diffusion-weighted magnetic resonance imaging in Marchiafava–Bignami disease: follow-up studies. Neuroradiology 2005; 47:520–4.

78. Menegon P, Sibon I, Pachai C, et al. Marchiafava–Bignami disease: diffusion weighted MRI in corpus callosum and cortical lesions. Neurology 2005;65: 475–7.

79. Gambini A, Falini A, Moiola L, et al. Marchiafava-Bignami disease: longitudinal MR imaging and MR spectroscopy study. AJNR Am J Neuroradiol 2003; 24:249–53.

80. Timms SR, Curé JK, Kurent JE. Subacute combined degeneration of the spinal cord: MR findings. AJNR Am J Neuroradiol 1993;14:1224–7.

81. Larner AJ, Zeman AZ, Allen CM, et al. MRI appearances in subacute combined degeneration of the spinal cord due to vitamin B12 deficiency. J Neurol Neurosurg Psychiatry 1997;62(1):99–100.

82. Ravina B, Loevner LA, Bank W. MR findings in subacute combined degeneration of the spinal cord: a case of reversible cervical myelopathy. Am J Roentgenol 2000;174(3):863–5.

83. Stojsavljevic N, Levic Z, Drulovic J, et al. A 44-month clinical-brain MRI follow-up in a patient with B-12 deficiency. Neurology 1997;49(3):878–81.

84. Katsaros VK, Glocker FX, Hemmer B, et al. MRI of spinal cord and brain lesions in subacute combined degeneration. Neuroradiology 1998;40(11):716–9.

85. Yamada K, Shrier DA, Tanaka H, et al. A case of subacute combined degeneration: MRI findings. Neuroradiology 1998;40(6):398–400.

86. Karantanas AH, Markonis A, Bisbiyiannis G. Subacute combined degeneration of the spinal cord with involvement of the anterior columns: a new MRI finding. Neuroradiology 2000;42(2):115–7.

87. Kinsella LJ, Green R. 'Anesthesia paresthetica': nitrous oxide-induced cobalamin deficiency. Neurology 1995;45(8):1608–10.

88. Kumar N. Pearls: myelopathy. Semin Neurol 2010; 30(1):38–43.

89. Kumar N, Gross JB Jr, Ahlskog JE. Copper deficiency myelopathy produces a clinical picture like subacute combined degeneration. Neurology 2004;63(1):33–9.

90. Kumar N, Ahlskog JE, Klein CJ, et al. Imaging features of copper deficiency myelopathy: a study of 25 cases. Neuroradiology 2006;48(2):78–83.

91. Nagar VA, Ye J, Xu M, et al. Multivoxel MR spectroscopic imaging - distinguishing intracranial tumors from non-neoplastic disease. Ann Acad Med Singapore 2007;36:309–13.

92. Lim CCT. Magnetic resonance imaging findings in bilateral basal ganglia lesions. Ann Acad Med Singapore 2009;38(9):795–802.

93. Hegde AN, Mohan S, Lath N, et al. Differential diagnosis for bilateral abnormalities of the basal ganglia and thalamus. Radiographics 2011;31(1):5–30.

Central Nervous System Fungal Infections in Tropics

N. Khandelwal, MD, Dip NBE, FICR*, Vivek Gupta, MD,
Paramjeet Singh, MD

KEYWORDS

- Central nervous system • Fungal infections
- Immunocompromised patients • Tropical medicine

Fungal infections of the central nervous system (CNS) are rare although relatively more frequent in the tropics. Fungi can be grouped broadly into filamentous fungi, dimorphic fungi, and yeasts. Clinically common fungi that invade the CNS, such as *Aspergillus* and *Mucor*, are classified as filamentous fungi. *Cryptococcus* and *Candida* are yeasts. Other fungi, such as *Blastmyces*, *Histoplasma*, *Coccidioides*, and *Paracoccidioides*, fall under dimorphic fungi.

CNS fungal infections occur mostly in immunocompromised patients, especially those with HIV infection and those with solid-organ transplantation. In the general population, however, CNS fungal infections are seen more frequently in patients with long-standing diabetes. These infections are generally secondary in nature, with the primary focus elsewhere in body. Primary CNS fungal infections are rare.

The region of brain affected by a particular fungus largely depends on its size, which in turn decides the site of lodgment in the brain. The smaller fungi, such as *Candida* and *Cryptococcus*, can reach the cerebral microcirculation causing meningitis and microabscesses. The larger ones, such as *Aspergillus* and *Mucor*, occlude the large arteries or their major branches resulting in large areas of bland infarction. These areas of infarction then secondarily may change into abscesses.

Most people affected by fungal infections, being immunocompromised, lack cellular reactions and thus neuroimaging findings are often nonspecific. These patients may manifest with a host of features pointing toward underlying chronic meningitis, acute meningoencephalitis brain abscesses, or stroke. The correct diagnosis of fungal infections thus is based on combined approach of imaging, clinical settings, and cerebrospinal fluid findings.

Although almost any fungus may cause encephalitis, those common to the tropics are cryptococcal meningoencephalitis, aspergillosis, mucormycosis, and more rarely candidiasis. Other fungal infections, such as blastomycosis, coccidioidomycosis, and histoplasmosis, are not generally seen in tropics.

COMMON IMAGING FEATURES

Fungal abscesses appear as solid or ring-enhancing lesions. MRI shows patchy or punctate T2-hyperintensity with frequently absent enhancement on postcontrast images. Conventional MRI may show similar features in the pyogenic, tubercular, and fungal abscesses. On diffusion-weighted imaging (DWI), low apparent diffusion coefficient (ADC) has been found in fungal similar to pyogenic abscesses. More specifically, the fungal abscesses may show restriction of diffusion in the intracavitary projections and the wall, with center of the abscess showing no restriction of diffusion.[1]

On MR spectroscopy fungal lesions are known to show lipids (1.2–1.3 ppm), lactate (1.3 ppm), alanine (1.5 ppm), acetate (1.9 ppm), succinate (2.4 ppm), and choline (3.2 ppm), and unidentified multiple signals are also seen between 3.6 and 3.8 ppm. These peaks are caused by trehalose sugar present in the fungal wall.[2]

Department of Radiodiagnosis, Post Graduate Institute of Medical Education and Research, Sector-12, Chandigarh 160012, India
* Corresponding author.
E-mail address: khandelwaln@hotmail.com

Neuroimag Clin N Am 21 (2011) 859–866
doi:10.1016/j.nic.2011.07.006

neuroimaging.theclinics.com

SPECIFIC FUNGAL INFECTIONS
Aspergillosis

Aspergillus is a ubiquitous saprophytic fungus found in soil and plants. It has regularly septate hyphae and produces spores. Individuals are infected by inhaling these spores, which settle in lungs and paranasal sinuses.

Invasive aspergillosis is an increasing problem in patients treated with intensive chemotherapy and immunosuppressive therapy after solid organ or bone marrow transplantation. Intracranial spread of aspergillosis occurs in 10% to 20% of cases.

Two forms of *Aspergillus* infections in the brain have been recognized. The rhinocerebral form results from direct spread of fungi from paranasal sinuses into the brain. Cerebrovascular aspergillosis results from hematogenous spread of the fungi leading to occlusion of large and middle-size arteries.[3] MRI features of both are quite varied.

Imaging features

Imaging studies of patients with cerebral aspergillosis reveal three general patterns: (1) single or multiple infarcts; (2) ring lesions (single or multiple) consistent with abscess formation; and (3) dural or vascular infiltration arising from the paranasal sinuses or orbits. Other findings on imaging include mycotic aneurysm and contrast enhancement of affected parenchyma, and hemorrhagic transformation of infarcted areas.

In the hematogenous type of spread because of angioinvasive character of the fungi, early manifestations include ischemic lesions, which are detected by using DWI. Involvement of the basal ganglia is a characteristic finding, indicating a predominant affection of the lenticulostriate and thalamoperforator arteries (**Fig. 1**).[4] A cerebral infarction is followed in most cases by a conversion to an infected area, with associated abscess formation.[5]

Fungal cerebritis lesions are nonenhancing and are usually located in the basal ganglia and deep white matter. Peripheral rim enhancement has been reported in mature pyogenic and fungal abscesses. In pyogenic and tubercular abscesses, the outer margin of the wall is either smooth or lobulated in contrast to the fungal lesions, which have a crenated wall in most cases.[1]

In one study, fungal abscesses showed nonenhancing intracavitary projections that were not seen in other types of abscesses. The DWI images and ADC values showed restricted diffusion in these projections and the wall of the fungal abscess (**Fig. 2**). The study inferred that the presence of irregular projections in abscesses with ADC values less than those of the wall is probably because of the presence of fungal elements containing paramagnetic substances.[6] One uncommon complication of vascular wall erosion is fungal vasculitis, which may lead to mycotic aneurysm formation.[7]

In the Rhinocerebral pattern of spread, initial involvement of the paranasal sinuses and the orbits exists, which presents in most cases as a nonspecific, contrast-enhancing mucosal thickening of the sinuses on CT or MRI. A serious complication of this localized infection is the infiltration and erosion of the adjacent bony structures leading to localized meningitis.[8]

In the brain, a well-defined granuloma is usually seen in the basifrontal or anterior temporal region often having continuity with the adjacent sinus disease. The gramulomas are virtually indistinguishable from tubercular granulomas or other chronic granulomas. It is well defined in nature with T1-hypointensity, T2 hyperintense center with hypointense wall, and showing mild to moderate ring-like contrast enhancement. Presence of a concomitant sinonasal disease points toward fungal etiology. Dural enhancement is generally seen in lesions adjacent to involved sinuses (**Fig. 3**).

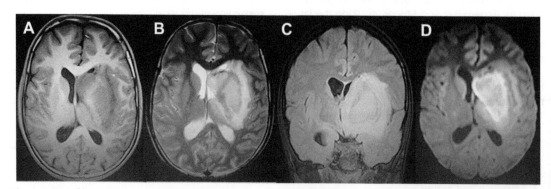

Fig. 1. MRIs of hematogenous spread of aspergillosis. T1-weighted (*A*), T2-weighted (*B*), FLAIR (*C*), and diffusion-weighted (*D*) images done on a 3-T scanner showing a large acute infarct involving the left basal ganglia and internal capsule with mild edema and mass effect. Biopsy from lung granuloma confirmed aspergillosis.

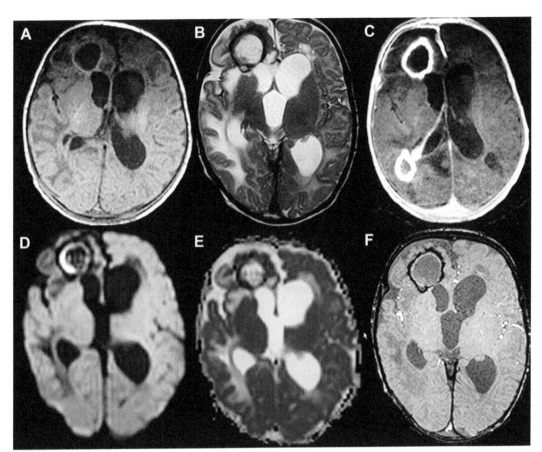

Fig. 2. MRIs of aspergilloma. T1-weighted (*A*), T2-weighted (*B*), contrast-enhanced T1 (*C*), DWI (*D*), ADC map (*E*), and susceptibility-weighted (*F*) images showing a well-defined aspergilloma in right frontal lobe. The center of the lesion is hypointense on T1-weighting, is hyperintense on T2-weighting, and is nonenhancing. No diffusion restriction is noted in the cavity (*D*, *E*). The wall, however, shows blooming of hypointense rim on susceptibility weighted imaging (SWI) (*F*) suggestive of microhemorrhages. There is restriction of diffusion in the wall (*D*, *E*). Another smaller granuloma is appreciated in the right parietal lobe on the contrast-enhanced image (*C*). Both the lesions show perilesional edema. Biopsy from the right frontal lesion confirmed the diagnosis.

To identify all relevant MRI features in intracerebral aspergillosis, MRI protocol should include DWI and contrast-enhanced T1-weighted images and T2-weighted sequences. For an early detection of hemorrhage, T2*-weighted sequences play an important role in clinical practice.

On MR spectroscopy fungal abscesses show cytosolic amino acids, lipids, and lactate, which

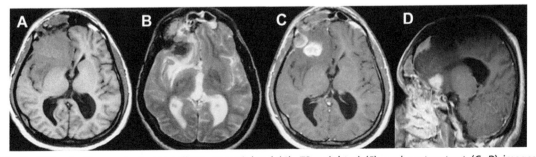

Fig. 3. MRIs of rhinocerebral aspergillosis. T1-weighted (*A*), T2-weighted (*B*), and postcontrast (*C*, *D*) images showing a solid lesion in the right basifrontal region, which is isointense on T1-weighting, hypointense on T2-weighting, and shows solid enhancement (*C*). Similar signal intensity lesion is present in the adjacent right frontal sinus, which is seen to erode its posterior wall and extend into the cerebral parenchyma. Note prominent dural enhancement seen better on the saggital image (*D*).

are similar to that of pyogenic abscesses; however, the presence of multiple signals seen between 3.6 and 3.8 ppm because of the disaccharide trehalose is a distinguishable feature of fungal abscesses.

Cryptococcosis

Cryptococcus neoformans is an encapsulated yeast-like fungus found in mammal and bird feces, particularly in pigeon droppings. *C neoformans* is the most common opportunistic fungal infection that affects the CNS in HIV and other immunocompromised patients. However, in approximately 30% patients, no definite predisposing disease may be seen.[9]

Infection is usually acquired by inhalation and then spreads hematogenously to the CNS. The CNS infection can be either meningeal or parenchymal.[10] Infection usually starts as meningitis and is more pronounced at the base of the brain.

Parenchymal involvement is seen as cryptococcomas, dilated Virchow-Robin spaces, or enhancing cortical nodules.[11] The most common parenchymal sites are the midbrain and the basal ganglia. As the infection spreads along the Virchow-Robin spaces, the perivascular spaces may dilate with mucoid gelatinous material that is produced by the capsule of the organism and looks like cysts. These cysts are also called "gelatinous pseudocysts."

Imaging features

The imaging manifestations of cryptococcosis are varied and frequently minimal. The imaging findings may consist of meningoencephalitis, intraventricular or intraparenchymal cryptococcomas, gelatinous pseudocysts, or hydrocephalus (Fig. 4). Communicating hydrocephalus occurs because of the acute meningeal exudates and also may occur late in the course of the infection because of meningeal adhesions. It is the most frequent finding of cryptococcal infection.[12]

On CT, cryptococcal lesions may have high or low attenuation. MRIs demonstrate T1 and T2 prolongation. Enhancement varies, but it is more likely to occur in immunocompetent hosts, because they can build up an effective inflammatory response. Cryptococcal lesions do not have restriction of diffusion, which distinguishes them from pyogenic abscesses.[13] Meningoencephalitis results in T2 hyperintensity within the region of involvement and meningeal enhancement may be seen (Fig. 5). The cryptococcomas are more common in immunocompetent patients and these may show enhancement because of high immune response of the host.[14] MR spectroscopy shows marked increase in lactate with decrease in *N*-acetyl aspartate, choline, and creatine.[15]

Mucormycosis

Mucormycosis is an acute and often lethal opportunistic infection, typically affecting immunocompromised patients or those with diabetes.[16] It is caused by one of the members of the mucoraceal family, including *Absidia*, *Mucor*, and *Rhizopus*.[17] After infection of the nasal cavity and paranasal sinuses, the fungi cause a necrotizing vasculitis that extends rapidly into deep face, orbits, cranial cavity, and brain through skull base partitions and foramina.

In particular, the fungus has an affinity for the internal elastic lamina of the arteries, through which it can hematogenously disseminate to distant sites.[18] This process of cerebral angioinvasion produces extensive endothelial damage that can lead to mycotic aneurysms, dissection,

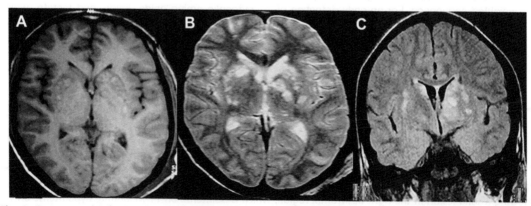

Fig. 4. Cryptococcal infection in an immunosuppressed patient. (*A–C*) Multiple well-defined round T1, T2, and FLAIR hyperintense lesions in bilateral basal ganglia suggestive of gelatinous pseudocysts. Cerebrospinal analysis confirmed the diagnosis.

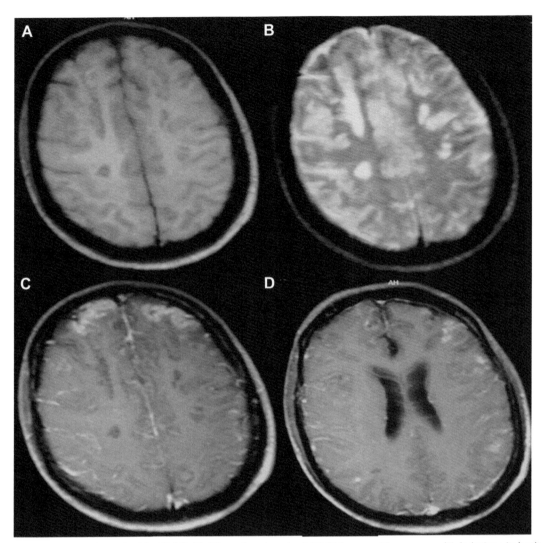

Fig. 5. Cryptococcal meningitis. T1 (*A*), T2 (*B*), and postcontrast (*C, D*) images. There are multiple lesions in both cerebral hemispheres isointense to hypointense on T1- and hyperintense on T2-weighted imaging. Postcontrast images showing diffuse abnormal meningeal enhancement with regions of nodularity over bilateral frontal regions. The nonenhancing deep white matter foci represent dilated Virchow-Robin spaces.

or thrombosis of the internal carotid artery with subsequent cerebral infarction.[19]

Imaging features

Imaging modalities include CT and MRI. In early stage disease both CT and MRI may be normal because radiologic findings lag behind clinical progression.[18] CT is useful in assessing the disease extent and typically shows mucosal thickening, opacification of the affected paranasal sinuses, and periorbital tissue destruction. CT is the optimal imaging modality to assess for bony destruction.

On MRI, hypointensity of the sinuses may be present on T1- and T2-weighted images. Intracranially, high T2-weighted imaging signal in the basal portions of the frontal and temporal lobe with mild mass effect is seen; this likely represents a combination of inflammation and infarction secondary to vascular invasion.[20]

MRI is superior in visualizing and evaluating intracranial and intradural extent of the disease. Thrombosis of the cavernous portion of the internal carotid artery is well detected on MR angiography (**Fig. 6**). Less commonly a hematogenous pattern of spread leading to central infarcts or

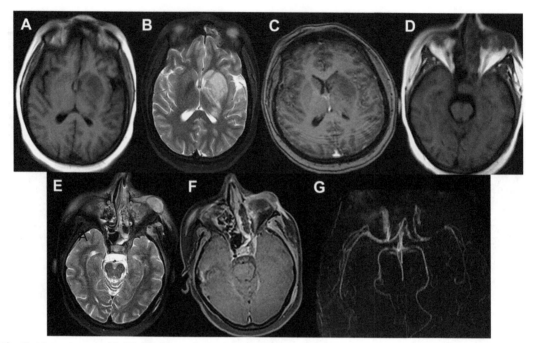

Fig. 6. Mucormycosis. T1 (*A*), T2 (*B*), and postcontrast T1 (*C*) axial MRIs show a bland infarct involving the left basal ganglion. T1 (*D*), T2 fat-suppressed (*E*), and postcontrast T1 fat-suppressed (*F*) axial MRIs at the level of cavernous sinus shows hypointense soft tissue on T1-weighting and T2-weighting, which is enhanced and involves the paranasal sinuses, left orbit with posterior extension, and left cavernous sinus. MR angiography (*G*) shows subtotal occlusion of left cavernous internal carotid artery and proximal middle cerebral artery leading to infarction in lenticulostriate arterial distribution.

granulomas may be seen in the brain secondary to *Mucor* infection (**Fig. 7**).

Candidiasis

Candidiasis is caused by a yeast fungus. *Candida albicans* is the most common species that causes disease. *Candida glabrata* may also be the organism seen mainly in adults causing candidemia.[21,22]

Candida albicans forms part of the normal flora in healthy persons present in mucous membranes and the gastrointestinal tract. The gastrointestinal tract is the site of entry for systemic infection mainly in patients with diabetes and lymphoproliferative disease. Intravenous drug abusers and patients in intensive care units show iatrogenic inoculation by way of indwelling catheters.

Primary CNS candidiasis is rare, mostly seen as secondary to hematogeneous dissemination. Clinical presentations may include features of meningitis, artery thrombosis, and subarachnoid hemorrhages. Meningitis is the most common clinical manifestation of CNS candidiasis in neonates and shows an acute progression. In adults, the disease may show a chronic and indolent course.

Other patterns of CNS involvement are brain microabscesses, small hemorrhagic infarcts, arterial thrombosis, and aneurysms.

Imaging features
CT may show foci of hypodensities, which on contrast examination may show nodular or ring-enhancing lesions. MRI shows abnormal meningeal enhancement, which appears as thicker, lumpy, or nodular enhancement in the subarachnoid space.[23] The microabscesses are seen as areas of hypointensities on T1-weighted images, which shows nodular or ring-enhancing lesions. The lesions are more common in the areas of the anterior or middle cerebral arteries and present at the gray–white junctions.[24]

Blastomycosis

Very rarely, CNS fungus infections in the tropics may be caused by *Blastomyces*. Blastomycosis is caused by *Blastomyces dermatitidis*, which is a dimorphic fungus. Route of infection is by inhalation of the fungal spores. Most cases present as features of chronic meningitis but in a few cases extra-axial plaque-like lesions have been reported,

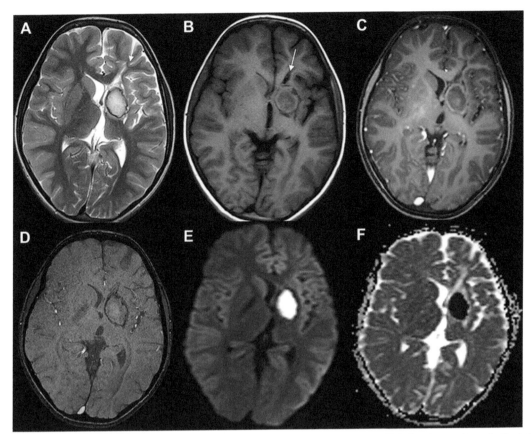

Fig. 7. Mucormycosis. T2 (*A*), T1 (*B*), and postcontrast T1 (*C*) axial MRIs show a well-defined granuloma in the left basal ganglion having a liquefied center and irregular T2-hypointense wall and virtually no edema. Wall shows blooming on SWI (*D*) and center shows diffusion restriction on DWI and ADC map (*E, F*). A linear gliotic tract is seen anterior to the lesion (*arrow* in *A* and *B*), secondary to biopsy, which was done to confirm the diagnosis.

which are hypointense on T1- and T2-weighted images and show significant enhancement on postcontrast images. These lesions mimic en-plaque meningiomas on imaging.[25]

SUMMARY

The CNS fungal infections range from chronic indolent forms to acute fulminant forms causing significant morbidity and mortality. They often show atypical and variable neuroradiologic findings because of the absence of typical inflammatory response. The major role of the neuroradiologist is to have a high degree of suspicion in immunocompromised patients regarding the possibility of CNS fungal infections and to keep in mind the appearances of various fungi even when immune response is intact. Next is to identify the pattern of involvement, whether hematogenous or direct sinonasal, and then to make a well-informed speculation regarding the type of the pathogen based on the clinical features and imaging appearance.

REFERENCES

1. Luthra G, Parihar A, Nath K, et al. Comparative evaluation of fungal, tubercular, and pyogenic brain abscesses with conventional and diffusion MR imaging and proton MR spectroscopy. AJNR Am J Neuroradiol 2007;28:1332–8.
2. Himmelreich U, Dzendrowoskyj TE, Allen C, et al. Cryptococcomas distinguished from gliomas with MR spectroscopy: an experimental rat and cell culture study. Radiology 2001;220:122–8.
3. Nadkarni T, Goel A. Aspergilloma of the brain: an overview. J Postgrad Med 2005;51:S37–41.
4. Gabelmann A, Klein S, Kern W, et al. Relevant imaging findings of cerebral aspergillosis on MRI: a retrospective case-based study in immunocompromised patients. Eur J Neurol 2007;14(5):548–55.
5. Shuper A, Levitsky HI, Cornblath DR. Early invasive CNS aspergillosis. An easily missed diagnosis. Neuroradiology 1991;33:183–5.
6. Haris M, Gupta RK, Husain N, et al. Measurement of DTI metrics in hemorrhagic brain lesions: possible

implication in MRI interpretation. J Magn Reson Imaging 2006;24:1259–68.

7. Ho CL, Deruytter MJ. CNS aspergillosis with mycotic aneurysm, cerebral granuloma and infarction. Acta Neurochirurgica (Wien) 2004;146:851–6.

8. Chang T, Teng MM, Wang SF, et al. Aspergillosis of the paranasal sinuses. Neuroradiology 1992;34:520–3.

9. Peretz JA, Kliot D, Finkelstein R, et al. Cryptococcal meningitis mimicking vascular dementia. Neurology 2004;62:2135.

10. Saigal G, Post MJD, Lolayekar S, et al. Unusual presentation of central nervous system cryptococcal infection in an immunocompetent patient. AJNR Am J Neuroradiol 2005;26:2522–6.

11. Tien RD, Chu PK, Hessellink JR, et al. Intracranial cryptococcosis in immunocompromised patients: CT and MR findings in 29 cases. AJNR Am J Neuroradiol 1991;12:283–9.

12. Takasu A, Taneda M, Otuki H, et al. Gd-DTPA-enhanced MR imaging of cryptococcal meningoencephalitis. Neuroradiology 1991;33:443–6.

13. Ho TL, Lee HJ, Lee KW, et al. Diffusion weighted and conventional magnetic resonance imaging in cerebral cryptococcoma. Acta Radiol 2005;46:411–4.

14. Vender JR, Miller DM, Roth T, et al. Intraventricular cryptococcal cysts. AJNR Am J Neuroradiol 1996;17:110–3.

15. Chang L, Miller BL, McBride D, et al. Brain lesions in patients with AIDS: H-1 MR spectroscopy. Radiology 1995;197:525–31.

16. Rumboldt Z, Castillo M. Indolent intracranial mucormycosis: case report. AJNR Am J Neuroradiol 2002;23:932–4.

17. Chan LL, Singh S, Jones D, et al. Imaging of mucormycosis skull base osteomyelitis. AJNR Am J Neuroradiol 2000;21:828–31.

18. Spellberg B, Edwards J Jr, Ibrahim A. Novel perspectives on mucormycosis: pathophysiology, presentation, and management. Clin Microbiol Rev 2005;18:556–69.

19. Rapidis AD. Orbitomaxillary mucormycosis (zygomycosis) and the surgical approach to treatment: perspectives from a maxillofacial surgeon. Clin Microbiol Infect 2009;15(5):98–102.

20. McLean FM, Ginsberg LE, Stanton CA. Perineural spread of rhinocerebral mucormycosis. AJNR Am J Neuroradiol 1996;17:114–6.

21. Pappas PG, Rex JH, Lee J, et al. A prospective observational study of candidemia: epidemiology, therapy, and influences on mortality in hospitalized adult and pediatric patients. Clin Infect Dis 2003;37(5):634–43.

22. Fridkin SK, Kaufman D, Edwards JR, et al. Changing incidence of Candida bloodstream infections among NICU patients in the United States: 1995–2004. Pediatrics 2006;117(5):1680–7.

23. Sage MR, Wilson AJ, Scroop R. Contrast media and the brain: the basis of CT and MR imaging enhancement. Neuroimaging Clin N Am 1998;8:695–707.

24. Kirkpatrick JB. Neurologic infections due to bacteria, fungi and parasites. In: Davis RL, Robertson DM, editors. Textbook of neuropathology. 3rd edition. Baltimore (MD): Williams and Wilkins; 1997. p. 845–53.

25. Kale HA, Narlawar RS, Maheswari S, et al. CNS blastomycosis, mimic of meningioma. Indian J Radiol Imaging 2002;12:483–4.

Neuroimaging in Epilepsy in Tropics

Swati Chinchure, MD, Chandrasekharan Kesavadas, MD*

KEYWORDS

• Epilepsy • Tropical countries • Imaging • Lesion

Epilepsy is a major public health problem in many tropical countries. Also, some of the tropical diseases are major contributors to the higher prevalence of epilepsy in these countries. The tropics have a relatively uniform hot climate present throughout the year associated with heavy rainfall causing higher humidity. Higher temperatures and humidity may favor replication of pathogenic agents both inside and outside the biological system. Infectious endemic tropical diseases disproportionately affect poor and marginalized populations in developing regions of Africa, Asia, Central America, and South America, resulting in a major public health hazard. Poor socioeconomic status promotes disease through undernutrition, poor sanitation, breeding of insects and rodents, and inaccessibility to medical care.[1] Hence, many tropical countries fall into the category of resource-poor countries. Prenatal risk factors, traumatic brain injuries (TBIs), various parasitic infestations, and infections of the central nervous system (CNS) are much more common in tropical countries.[2] The International League against Epilepsy (ILAE) has established a separate Commission on Tropical Diseases to study the epidemiology, etiology, and prognosis and to seek solutions to the problems faced by the population in the tropics.[1]

EPIDEMIOLOGY

Incidence and prevalence rates of epilepsy tend to be higher in resource-poor, tropical, and developing countries. Placencia and colleagues[3] in 1992 reported an incidence of 122 per 100,000 per year in Ecuador, South America. In general, prevalence figures from studies in Latin America have been higher than those in the developed world.[1] Incidence rates from 28.8 per 100,000 to 35.0 per 100,000 per year have been reported in the general population in China.[4,5] The results from India are higher and have been reported as 60 per 100,000 per year.[6] China and India, the 2 most populous nations in the world, together contribute approximately 20% of the people with epilepsy worldwide.[7] The age-adjusted incidence of epilepsy reported from the developed countries is 24 to 53 per 100,000 per year.[8] The annual incidence rates for epilepsy in Asia did not differ significantly from the rates in developed countries,[7,9] but the incidence rates were higher in sub-Saharan Africa and Latin America (63–158 and 78–190 per 100,000 person-years, respectively).[10,11]

A higher prevalence is seen in rural areas.[12] Although there is a steady increase in epilepsy prevalence rates with advancing age in the developed countries, the rates seem to peak in the second decade in tropical and resource-poor countries.[9–11]

DIAGNOSIS

Diagnosis of epilepsy is based on clinical judgment, findings on electroencephalography (EEG), and imaging. The skill and experience of the physician and the information provided by witness are important in making the proper clinical judgment. The neurologists and physicians managing epilepsy are fewer in most of these countries.[13] Although EEG facilities are available, there are no minimum standards and no governmental or professional authorities to ensure quality control.[14,15] Imaging facilities are few, along with

Department of Imaging Sciences and Interventional Radiology, Sree Chitra Tirunal Institute for Medical Sciences and Technology, Medical College Campus, Trivandrum 695011, Kerala, India
* Corresponding author.
E-mail addresses: chandkesav@yahoo.com; kesav@sctimst.ac.in

Neuroimag Clin N Am 21 (2011) 867–877
doi:10.1016/j.nic.2011.07.013
1052-5149/11/$ – see front matter © 2011 Elsevier Inc. All rights reserved.

low affordability of imaging. In a 2006 survey of the diagnostic facilities for epilepsy care around the world, magnetic resonance imaging (MRI) facilities were available in almost all European and North American countries compared with only 26% of African, 48% of western Pacific, and 56% of Southeast Asian countries.[14]

Moreover, most MRIs performed outside comprehensive epilepsy care facilities do not conform to the specification laid down for patients with chronic epilepsy.[16] Repeating MRI and performing more costly investigations, such as single photon emission computed tomography and positron emission tomography, can add to the cost of diagnosis and management.[17]

EPILEPSY CARE AND TREATMENT

There is great variability in the disease management of epilepsy among different countries, more so between tropical countries and countries in North America and Europe.

Treatment Gap

The treatment gap is defined as the number of people with active epilepsy not on treatment or on inadequate treatment expressed as a percentage of the total number of people with active epilepsy.[17] A recent systematic analysis that investigated the magnitude of the treatment gap in resource-poor countries found an overall rate of 56%.[18] A large proportion of patients with epilepsy discontinue the treatment despite being diagnosed and initiated on antiepileptic drug (AED) treatment. The main reasons cited for AED discontinuation were the inability to afford the treatment and a lack of information about the consequences of medication nonadherence.[7] Similar to the medical treatment gap, surgical treatment gap also exists in many of these countries. Despite the total direct cost of presurgical evaluation and surgery in most tropical countries amounting to a small fraction of the cost incurred in North America and Europe, this expenditure is still beyond the reach of most patients.[19]

Knowledge, Attitudes, and Practice

Numerous studies on knowledge, attitudes, and practice of epilepsy have been done in the tropical population.[20–22] Misunderstanding of epilepsy is quite common. Social stigma to epilepsy often causes more distress to a person with epilepsy than the seizures themselves. Lack of awareness is one of the most important factors for this social stigma. There is an increased need for health education campaigns to rehabilitate patients with

epilepsy in these communities and to improve their quality of life.

ETIOLOGY AND IMAGING

The Commission on Epidemiology and Prognosis of the ILAE has suggested that seizures should first be classified etiologically according to the presence or absence of a presumed causative or precipitating insult.[23] Before the computed tomography (CT) era, a large number of patients were classified to have epilepsy of unknown origin.[24] This number has reduced after the advent of CT and MRI. There is a difference in the cause of epilepsy that is noted in studies from developed countries and tropical countries. In developed countries, the common causes are vascular, traumatic, or neoplastic,[25] whereas studies from Latin America and Asian tropical countries have found a large number of patients in the symptomatic group with neurocysticercosis (NCC).[1,26] The other causes included in the developing countries are perinatal damage, head injuries, cerebrovascular diseases, and other brain infections.[1] Neuroinfections can present acutely with seizures as is seen in cerebral malaria or Japanese encephalitis. Neuroinfections can also present chronically as an epilepsy syndrome secondary to the presence of focal granulomatous lesions or gliosis and calcification secondary to NCC.

SINGLE RING-ENHANCING LESION

One of the common imaging finding in a patient from tropical country presenting with seizure is a single ring-enhancing lesion (SREL). SREL may occur in several infectious and neoplastic diseases of the CNS and is the most common radiologic abnormality seen in patients with acute-onset seizures in developing tropical countries. Most common differential for single enhancing lesion on CT or single hyperintense lesion on MRI in endemic areas is NCC versus tuberculosis (TB). Clinical presentation and CT remains the mainstay of diagnosis in the developing world. The clinicoradiologic picture forms the basis of diagnostic criteria for evaluation of SREL as proposed by Rajshekhar and colleagues.[27] These investigators made an attempt to differentiate between these 2 entities on the basis of clinical and imaging features. Rajshekhar and Chandy[28] noted that

1. Cysticerci are usually round in shape.
2. Cysticerci are usually 20 mm or less in size with ring enhancement or visible scolex.
3. The cerebral edema is not severe enough to produce midline shift or focal neurologic deficit.

In contrast, tuberculomas are usually irregular, solid, and larger than 20 mm in size. They are often associated with severe perifocal edema and focal neurologic deficit. These diagnostic criteria according to Rajshekhar and colleagues[27] showed high sensitivity and specificity and high positive and negative predictive values. However, it has been noticed that even if a patient does not fulfill these diagnostic criteria, it does not exclude the possibility of a cysticercal cause and vice versa.[29] Most of these solitary enhancing lesions disappear within weeks or months (**Fig. 1**).[30–32] These patients require only antiepileptic therapy, and medication may be withdrawn safely after the resolution of the lesion. Only a few patients, atypically, experience seizures even after disappearance of the lesion. Studies have shown that neither albendazole nor antituberculous therapy is helpful in modifying the natural course of these lesions or associated seizure disorder.[30,32] If the lesion increases in size and if focal neurologic

deficits manifest or seizures are uncontrolled, then brain biopsy may be required to establish final diagnosis.[31]

Advanced imaging is well exploited to further characterize these SREL and to differentiate between NCC and TB. Magnetization transfer (MT) can help differentiate between T2 hypointense NCC and tuberculomas. Cysticercus granulomas have a significantly higher MT ratio than similar-appearing tuberculomas[33] because of the presence of lipid-containing caseous necrosis in T2 hypointense tuberculomas. MT also helps in delineating perilesional gliosis in treated cases, which may be responsible for persistent seizures in few cases. Perilesional gliosis visible on MT spin echo MRI correlates with seizure recurrence.[34] Three-dimensional constructive interference into steady state/3-dimensional fast imaging employing steady-state acquisition and fluid-attenuated inversion recovery are good sequences for visualizing the scolex, which is

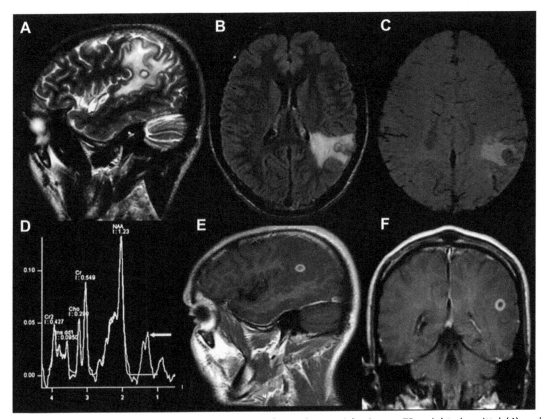

Fig. 1. SREL in a 39-year-old man with recent onset of complex partial seizures. T2-weighted sagittal (A) and fluid-attenuated inversion recovery axial (B) images show well-defined, thin-walled, low–signal intensity ring lesion with perilesional edema in left parietal region. Susceptibility-weighted axial image (C) shows the hypointensity within the lesion. Magnetic resonance spectroscopy (D) at short echo time (30 millisecond) shows a small lactate peak (arrow). Postcontrast T1 sagittal and coronal (E, F) images show ring enhancement. This patient was managed with antiepileptic medication for a month. Follow-up images (not shown) showed complete resolution of ring-enhancing lesion.

pathognomonic for NCC. Differentiation between NCC and tuberculoma is also possible on magnetic resonance spectroscopy. Tuberculomas show higher lipid peaks, more choline levels, less N-acetylaspartate levels, and less creatine levels than NCC, with choline to creatine ratio always greater than 1 in tuberculomas.[35] T2 hyperintense tuberculomas (tuberculomas with liquid caseation) can show diffusion restriction (**Fig. 2**) and can be differentiated from NCC, whereas T2 hypointense tuberculomas (tuberculomas with solid caseation) do not show diffusion restriction.[36]

The other differentials for SREL are cerebral abscess, metastasis, glioma, subacute infarct, and demyelination. Thick and nodular enhancing walls with increased perfusion favor neoplasm, whereas thin regular enhancing walls, perilesional edema, low T2 signal, and diffusion restriction favor abscess. Incomplete ring with minimal perilesional edema favors demyelination. In endemic regions, differentials of fungal infection, such as cryptococcal granulomas, also need to be considered irrespective of the immune status of the patient. Magnetic resonance spectroscopy detection of alpha, alpha-trehalose, which is specific but less sensitive, could help in differentiating cryptococcoma from tuberculoma.[37]

FEBRILE CONVULSIONS AND MESIAL TEMPORAL SCLEROSIS

Febrile seizures are defined as seizures that occur in infants and children aged between 6 months and 6 years, accompanied by fever (at least 38°C before the onset of seizure). Febrile convulsions (FC) are among the most frequent seizure disorders in children. Lifetime risk for FC is relatively high in developing countries.[38] Lower socioeconomic status and lack of knowledge about FC are the main factors related to this risk. Retrospective studies have shown that prolonged febrile seizures are a causative factor for the later development of mesial temporal sclerosis (MTS) and temporal lobe epilepsy.[39–41] Prolonged febrile seizures can produce acute hippocampal injury that evolves to hippocampal atrophy and subsequent temporal lobe epilepsy.

MTS is one of the most common causes of intractable epilepsy in tropical and developing countries. MRI shows volume loss and signal

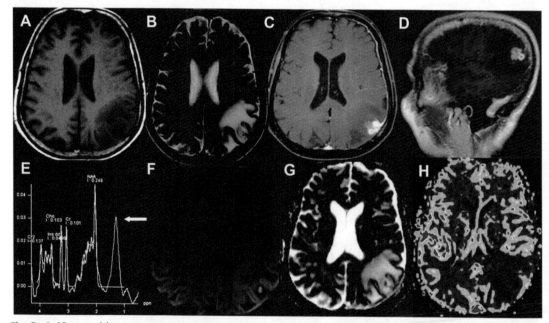

Fig. 2. A 46-year-old woman presented with right focal seizures. T1- and T2-weighted axial images (*A, B*) show signal changes suggestive of focal edema involving the gray matter and underlying white matter in the left parietal cortex. Postcontrast T1 fat-saturated axial and sagittal images (*C, D*) showing multiple conglomerate rings and nodular lesions with adjoining pachymeningeal enhancement along left cerebral convexity. Magnetic resonance spectroscopy at short echo time (*E*) shows lipid lactate peaks (*arrow*) at 1.3 ppm. Diffusion-weighted image and apparent diffusion coefficient map (*F, G*) reveal a central focus of diffusion restriction, suggesting liquid caseous necrosis within the lesion. T2* perfusion imaging shows low perfusion on relative cerebral blood volume map. (*H*) Based on the imaging findings, the patient received antituberculous medication for 9 months, which resulted in complete resolution of the lesion.

changes in the hippocampus and mesial temporal structures reflecting gliosis. In few patients with MTS, there can be associated malformation of cortical development, gliosis, or calcified granuloma (**Fig. 3**). This association is sometimes referred to as dual pathology. The best conventional magnetic resonance sequences to show alterations in the normal cytoarchitecture within

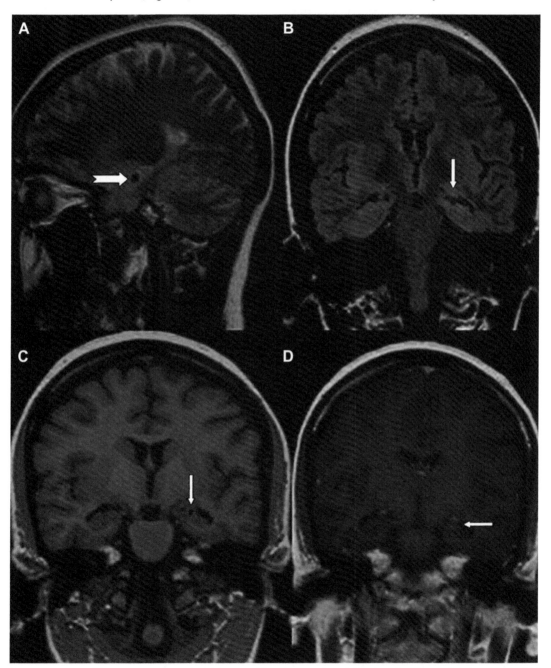

Fig. 3. A 28-year-old woman presented with intractable seizures. T2-weighted sagittal image (*A*) shows a small T2 hypointense nodular lesion in the left amygdala (*notched arrow*). In the coronal fluid-attenuated inversion recovery (FLAIR) image (*B*), the lesion is showing a hyperintense rim (*white arrow*). FLAIR coronal image (*B*) also reveals increased signal with volume loss involving left hippocampus, suggesting hippocampal sclerosis. T1-weighted spoiled gradient image (*C*) shows hypointense cystic lesion with peripheral rim isointensity (*white arrow*). Hippocampal volume loss is better appreciated on this sequence. Note that the lesion is showing minimal postcontrast enhancement (*white arrow*) in the postcontrast T1-weighted coronal image (*D*). Histopathology showed cysticercal granuloma with hippocampal sclerosis, a case of dual pathology.

hippocampus are inversion recovery and high-resolution fast-spin echo images. The 3-dimensional spoiled gradient echo imaging provides good information regarding hippocampal volume loss on the side of sclerosis. A smaller degree of asymmetry in volume and T2 signal is best detected by volumetric quantification and T2 relaxometry, respectively.[42] Measurement of apparent diffusion coefficient can also help lateralize the lesion side reflecting neuronal loss and gliosis. Secondary imaging criteria, such as atrophy of ipsilateral mammillary body and fornix, atrophy of collateral white matter, atrophy of ipsilateral temporal lobe/hemisphere, and prominence of temporal horn, increase diagnostic confidence.[42]

HEAD INJURY AND EPILEPSY

TBIs remain an important public health problem in most developing countries. Road traffic injuries are a leading cause of TBIs. Less strict policy interventions with inadequate traffic administration and poor vehicle and road maintenance are the main causes of road accidents in most developing countries in tropics. TBI, especially penetrating brain injury, carries a high risk of epilepsy decades after the injury.[43] Posttraumatic lesion location, lesion size, and lesion type were predictors of posttraumatic epilepsy.[43] Neuroimaging findings may provide useful predictors of the individual risk of developing posttraumatic epilepsy (Fig. 4).

EPILEPSY AND PERINATAL INSULT

Poor antenatal education, substandard care, poor organization of work, and lack of medical training are the main causes of high perinatal, maternal, and fetal morbidity and mortality in developing countries. Developing countries are constrained by limited financial and human resources. Low birth weight, feeding difficulties, and neonatal hypoglycemia are other fetal risk factors. Even though the survival rates have improved in recent

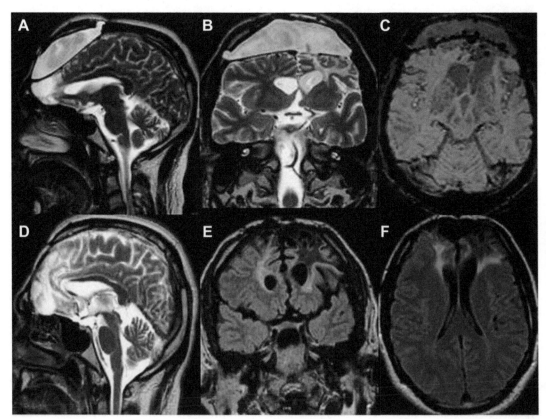

Fig. 4. A young male patient with previous road traffic accident presenting with seizures. T2-weighted sagittal (A) and coronal (B) images show large subdural collection with mass effect on bilateral frontal lobes. Foci of blooming suggesting hemorrhages noted on susceptibility-weighted image (C). The old subdural hematoma was removed. The patient continued to have seizures. A follow-up MRI using T2-weighted sagittal (D) and fluid-attenuated inversion recovery axial (E, F) images showed areas of gliosis involving bilateral frontal lobes and thinned out corpus callosum anteriorly. Note ex vacuo dilatation of bilateral frontal horns.

years for infant viability, these perinatal insults leave long-term morbidity in the form of seizures.

The loss of oxygen and glucose supply to the developing brain leads to excitotoxic neuronal cell damage by decreasing the reuptake of glutamate secondary to energy failure. This overexcitation of nerve cells can also manifest as seizures and can result in long-term neurodevelopmental disability.[44] Preterm infants with severe hypoxic ischemic insult (HII) show deep gray matter signal abnormalities involving thalami, basal ganglia, hippocampi, and corticospinal tract with sparing of perirolandic cortex. Mild to moderate HII in preterm infants show more vulnerability of the

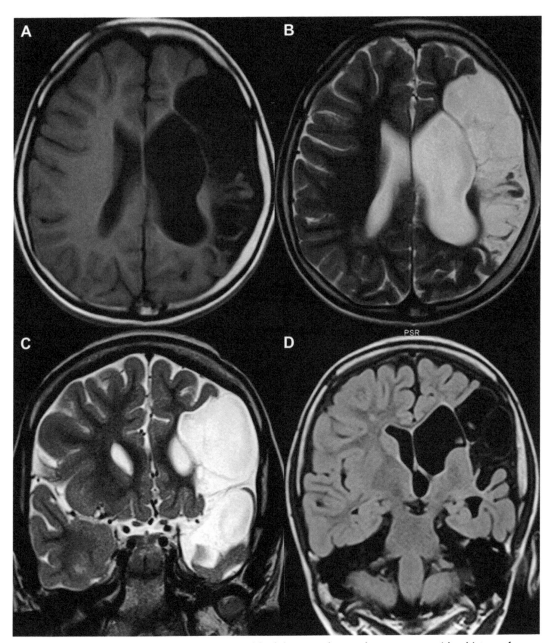

Fig. 5. Multicystic encephalomalacia in a 13-year-old adolescent who was born preterm with a history of severe and prolonged perinatal insult. T1- and T2-weighted axial images (A, B) show multiple cystic cavities with multiple thin septations in left frontoparietal region. Note volume loss involving the entire left cerebral hemisphere with dilatation of left lateral ventricle. Coronal T2 and fluid-attenuated inversion recovery images (C, D) show involvement of left temporal lobe along with frontal lobe and enlarged temporal horn. The lesion is limited to left middle cerebral artery territory and involves gray as well as white matter.

white matter and hence germinal matrix hemorrhage and periventricular leukomalacia. Term infants with severe HII show signal abnormalities in putamen, ventrolateral thalami, dorsal brainstem, hippocampal formation, and auditory and perirolandic cortices. When the hypoxic insult is particularly severe and prolonged, diffuse damage to the brain ensues, leading to multicystic encephalomalacia (Fig. 5). This differential involvement depends on (1) brain maturity and (2) time, severity, and duration of insult.[45]

Mild to moderate HII results in watershed infarcts in term infants. These patients can present with epilepsy later in life, and HII is a common substrate for epilepsy in developing tropical countries. There can be associated neonatal hypoglycemia. MRI shows posterior cortex (predominantly parietooccipital) gliosis and ulegyria (Fig. 6). Ulegyria is the term given to mushroom-shaped gyri that result as a result of greater perfusion at the apices of the gyri than at the depth of the sulci. The ulegyric cortex is thought to be epileptogenic.[46] The predominant posterior cortex involvement is thought to be because of (1) the region being watershed of middle cerebral and posterior cerebral arteries and (2) the region being an area of high degree of metabolic rate in the newborn. These lesions are usually bilateral and diffuse and show nonlocalizing ictal and interictal EEG. Moreover these patients can have associated MTS and compromised visual fields, making them difficult candidates for epilepsy surgery. However, surgery offers only hope in selected patients with intractable epilepsy.

EPILEPSY AND MALNUTRITION

Both epilepsy and malnutrition are important public health problems, and previous studies confirm the association between malnutrition and epilepsy.[47] Malnutrition and other related disorders are common in tropics because of complex

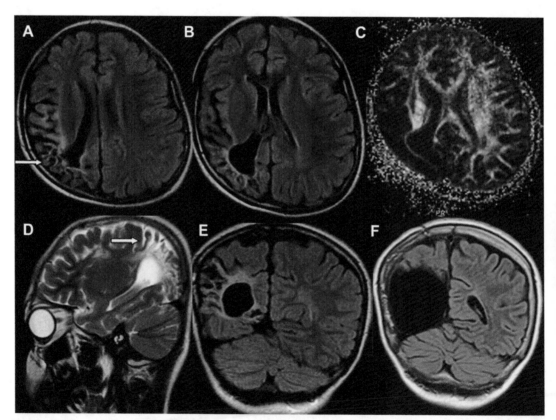

Fig. 6. A 10-year-old boy who was born full term and had perinatal hypoxic insult presented with intractable epilepsy. Fluid-attenuated inversion recovery (FLAIR) axial images (A, B) show right parietooccipital gliosis with ulegyria (white arrow). There is ex vacuo dilatation of trigone of right lateral ventricle. Fractional anisotropy map obtained by diffusion tensor imaging (C) shows severe reduction of peritrigonal white matter volume. T2 sagittal (D) and FLAIR coronal (E) images show mushroom-shaped gyri of involved cortex (arrow in D). Involved region was surgically excised. Postoperative FLAIR coronal image (F) shows postoperative cerebrospinal fluid collection. Seizure frequency was reduced after surgery.

relation among various factors such as poverty, illiteracy, medical negligence, alcoholism, substance abuse, and human immunodeficiency virus infection. In developing countries, alcoholism, malnutrition, and ileocecal TB are the common causes of vitamin B12 deficiency. Seizures rarely occur in patients with vitamin B12 deficiency.[48] The exact mechanism involved in epileptogenesis due to cobalamin deficiency is not clear. It is likely that cerebral neurons with destroyed myelin sheaths are more susceptible to the excitatory effects of glutamate.[49] Alcoholism, which acts as a triggering factor for seizures, is common in this population.

DRUGS AS A CAUSE OF EPILEPSY

Epileptogenic potential of antimalarial drugs is well known. Chloroquine and mefloquine are known to cause seizures and mental abnormalities. Quinine, the mainstay of therapy for falciparum malaria, causes hypoglycemia and may lead indirectly to seizures. Isoniazid, used to treat TB, has an effect on glutamate decarboxylase and can cause seizures. Although infections are a major preventable cause of epilepsy, some antimicrobials used for treatment have proconvulsant activity and may also interact adversely with AEDs.[50]

GENETIC FACTORS

Genetic factors play an important role in the causation of idiopathic epilepsy. Chromosomal, single gene (autosomal dominant, autosomal recessive, X-linked), mitochondrial, and polygenic/multifactorial disorders have been associated with epilepsy.[51] Consanguineous marriages and marriages among close relatives are more common among the people living in the developing countries, thus predisposing them to more genetic diseases. In recent years, even in the tropical and developing countries, better obstetric and neonatal care and liberal use of antibiotics have reduced the environmental causes of epilepsy, although leaving genetic causes unaltered.[52]

SUMMARY

There has been significant understanding of the epidemiology of epilepsy in some of the tropical countries of the world. It has to be recognized that etiologic factors responsible for epilepsy in these countries are quite different from those in the developed world. More important is to know that public understanding and attitudes, patients' concepts of disease, and the treatment gap are so different from that in North America and Europe, and, hence, this affects the overall management of epilepsy in this population. Governmental and nongovernmental organizations involved in epilepsy care in these countries have to recognize this fact and work toward (1) prevention of various causal factors for the disease, (2) reducing the treatment gap, (3) nurturing of epileptologists who can spearhead improvements in epilepsy care in the community, (4) imparting better education on epilepsy and epilepsy care in the community, and (5) development of epilepsy surgery centers.

REFERENCES

1. de Bittencourt PR, Adamolekum B, Bharucha N, et al. Epilepsy in the tropics: I. Epidemiology, socioeconomic risk factors, and etiology. Epilepsia 1996; 37:1121–7.
2. Carod-Artal FJ. Tropical causes of epilepsy. Rev Neurol 2009;49:475–82.
3. Placencia M, Shorvon SD, Paredes V, et al. Epileptic seizures in an Andean region of Ecuador. Incidence and prevalence and regional variation. Brain 1992; 115:771–82.
4. Wang W, Wu J, Wang D, et al. Epidemiological survey on epilepsy among rural populations in five provinces in China. Zhonghua Yi Xue Za Zhi 2002; 82:449–52.
5. Li SC, Schoenberg BS, Wang CC, et al. Epidemiology of epilepsy in urban areas of the People's Republic of China. Epilepsia 1985;26:391–4.
6. Sawhney IM, Singh A, Kaur P, et al. A case control study and one year follow-up of registered epilepsy cases in a resettlement colony of North India, a developing tropical country. J Neurol Sci 1999; 165:31–5.
7. Radhakrishnan K. Challenges in the management of epilepsy in resource poor countries. Nat Rev Neurol 2009;5:323–30.
8. Jallon P. Epilepsy and epileptic disorders, an epidemiological marker? Contribution of descriptive epidemiology. Epileptic Disord 2002;4:1–13.
9. Mac TL, Tran DS, Quet F, et al. Epidemiology, aetiology, and clinical management of epilepsy in Asia: a systematic review. Lancet Neurol 2007;6: 533–43.
10. Burneo JG, Tellez-Zenteno J, Wiebe S. Understanding the burden of epilepsy in Latin America: a systematic review of its prevalence and incidence. Epilepsy Res 2005;66:63–74.
11. Preux PM, Druet-Cabanac M. Epidemiology and etiology of epilepsy in sub-Saharan Africa. Lancet Neurol 2005;4:21–31.
12. Sridharan R, Murthy BM. Prevalence and pattern of epilepsy in India. Epilepsia 1999;40:631–6.
13. Aarli JA. Neurology and WHO: challenges and issues. A report. World Neurol 2002;17:10–1.

14. Dua T, de Boer HM, Prilipko LL, et al. Epilepsy care in the world: results of an ILAE/IBE/WHO global campaign against epilepsy survey. Epilepsia 2006; 47:1225–31.

15. Sylaja PN, Radhakrishnan K, Kesavadas C, et al. Seizure outcome after anterior temporal lobectomy and its predictors in patients with apparent temporal lobe epilepsy and normal MRI. Epilepsia 2004;45: 803–8.

16. Rathore C, Kesavadas C, Ajith J, et al. Cost-effective utilization of single photon emission computed tomography (SPECT) in decision making for epilepsy surgery. Seizure 2011;20:107–14.

17. Meinardi H, Scott RA, Reis R, et al. The treatment gap in epilepsy: the current situation and ways forward. Epilepsia 2001;42:136–49.

18. Mbuba CK, Ngugi AK, Newton CR, et al. The epilepsy treatment gap in developing countries: a systematic review of the magnitude, causes, and intervention strategies. Epilepsia 2008;49:1491–503.

19. Sylaja PN, Radhakrishnan K. Surgical management of epilepsy. Problems and pitfalls in developing countries. Epilepsia 2003;44:48–50.

20. Radhakrishnan K, Pandian JD, Santhoshkumar T, et al. Prevalence, knowledge, attitude and practice of epilepsy in Kerala, South India. Epilepsia 2000; 41:1027–35.

21. Lim KS, Tan LP, Lim KT, et al. Survey of public awareness, understanding and attitudes toward epilepsy among Chinese in Malaysia. Neurol J Southeast Asia 1999;4:31–6.

22. Rambe AS, Sjahrir H. Awareness, attitudes and understanding towards epilepsy among school teachers in Medan, Indonesia. Neurol J Southeast Asia 2002;7:77–80.

23. Commission on Epidemiology and Prognosis of the International League Against Epilepsy. Guidelines for epidemiological studies on epilepsy. Epilepsia 1993;34:592–6.

24. Arruda WO. Etiology of epilepsy. A prospective study of 210 cases. Arq Neuropsiquiatr 1991;49:251–4.

25. Hauser WA, Annerges JF, Kurland LT. Incidence of epilepsy and unprovoked seizures in Rochester, Minnesota: 1935–1984. Epilepsia 1993;34:453–68.

26. Guerreiro CA, Silveira DC, Costa EL, et al. Classification and etiology of newly diagnosed epilepsies in the southeast Brazil. Epilepsia 1993;34:14.

27. Rajshekhar V, Haran RP, Prakash GS, et al. Differentiating solitary small cysticercus granuloma and tuberculoma in patients with epilepsy. Clinical and computerized tomographic criteria. J Neurosurg 1993;78:402–7.

28. Rajshekhar V, Chandy MJ. Validation of diagnostic criteria for solitary cerebral cysticercal granuloma in patients presenting with seizures. Acta Neurol Scand 1997;96:76–81.

29. Garg RK. Diagnostic criteria for neurocysticercosis: some modifications are needed for Indian patients. Neurol India 2004;52:171–7.

30. Goulatia RK, Verma A, Mishra NK, et al. Disappearing CT lesions in epilepsy. Epilepsia 1987;28:523–7.

31. Garg RK. Single enhancing computerized tomography-detected lesion in immunocompetent patients. Neurosurg Focus 2002;12:e4.

32. Chandy MJ, Rajshekhar V, Ghosh S, et al. Single small enhancing CT lesions in Indian patients with epilepsy: clinical, radiological and pathological considerations. J Neurol Neurosurg Psychiatry 1991;54: 702–5.

33. Kathuria MK, Gupta RK, Roy R, et al. Measurement of magnetization transfer in different stages of neurocysticercosis. J Magn Reson Imaging 1998;8: 473–9.

34. Pradhan S, Kathuria MK, Gupta RK. Perilesional gliosis and seizure outcome: a study based on magnetization transfer magnetic resonance imaging in patients with neurocysticercosis. Ann Neurol 2000;48:181–7.

35. Pretell EJ, Martinot C, Garcia HH, et al. Differential diagnosis between cerebral tuberculosis and neurocysticercosis by magnetic resonance spectroscopy. J Comput Assist Tomogr 2005;29:112–4.

36. Trivedi R, Saksena S, Gupta RK. Magnetic resonance imaging in central nervous system tuberculosis. Indian J Radiol Imaging 2009;19:256–65.

37. Patro SN, Kesavadas C, Thomas B, et al. Uncommon presentation of intracranial cryptococcal infection mimicking tuberculous infection in two immunocompetent patients. Singapore Med J 2009;50:e133–7.

38. Aydin A, Ergor A, Ozkan H. Effects of sociodemographic factors on febrile convulsion prevalence. Pediatr Int 2008;50:216–20.

39. Cendes F, Andermann F, Dubeau F, et al. Early childhood prolonged febrile convulsions, atrophy and sclerosis of mesial structures, and temporal lobe epilepsy: an MRI volumetric study. Neurology 1993; 43(6):1083–7.

40. Rein AG. Temporal mesial sclerosis syndrome in epilepsy. Neurologia 1998;13:132–44.

41. Cendes F. Febrile seizures and mesial temporal sclerosis. Curr Opin Neurol 2004;17:161–4.

42. Chinchure S, Kesavadas C, Thomas B. Structural and functional neuroimaging in intractable epilepsy. Neurol India 2010;58:361–70.

43. Raymont V, Salazar AM, Lipsky R, et al. Correlates of posttraumatic epilepsy 35 years following combat brain injury. Neurology 2010;20(75):224–9.

44. Björkman ST, Miller SM, Rose SE, et al. Seizures are associated with brain injury severity in a neonatal model of hypoxia-ischemia. Neuroscience 2010; 166:157–67.

45. Huang BY, Castillo M. Hypoxic-ischemic brain injury: imaging findings from birth to adulthood. Radiographics 2008;28:417–39.

46. Kuchukhidze G, Unterberger I, Dobesberger J, et al. Electroclinical and imaging findings in ulegyria and epilepsy: a study on 25 patients. J Neurol Neurosurg Psychiatry 2008;79:547–52.

47. Crepin S, Houinato D, Nawana B, et al. Link between epilepsy and malnutrition in a rural area of Benin. Epilepsia 2007;48:1926–33.

48. Kumar S. Recurrent seizures: an unusual manifestation of vitamin B12 deficiency. Neurol India 2004;52:122–3.

49. Akaike A, Tamura Y, Sato Y, et al. Protective effects of a vitamin B12 analog, methylcobalamin, against glutamate cytotoxicity in cultured cortical neurons. Eur J Pharmacol 1993;241:1–6.

50. Sander JW, Perucca E. Epilepsy and comorbidity: infections and antimicrobials usage in relation to epilepsy management. Acta Neurol Scand Suppl 2003;180:16–22.

51. Bird TD. Major patterns of human inheritance: relevance to the epilepsies. Epilepsia 1994;35:2–6.

52. Sharma K. Genetic epidemiology of epilepsy: a twin study. Neurol India 2005;53:93–8.

Neuroimaging in Craniovertebral Anomalies as Seen in the Tropics

Shilpa S. Sankhe, MD[a,*], S.K. Susheel Kumar, MD[b]

KEYWORDS

• Neuroimaging • Tropics • Craniovertebral junction

The junction between the head and neck is called the occipitocervical or craniovertebral junction (CVJ). It provides a bony confine for the spinomedullary junction. It is a complex region that incorporates the occiput as well as the C1 and C2 vertebrae. This region is the most mobile part of the cervical spine and functions as a funnel that confers twin features of stability and motion. This combination of stability and flexibility is provided by the bony as well as ligamentous nature of atlantooccipital and atlantoaxial joints. These joints allow complex movements, with the ligamentous fastenings permitting these motions and the osseous elements providing stability without compromising the traversing neural elements as well as the vertebral artery.

CVJ anomaly is an important clinicopathologic condition among certain ethnic groups and is found more frequently in the Indian subcontinent than anywhere else in the world. Even in India, these anomalies are more frequently documented from northern and north-western states. However, the reason for this, and the incidence, remain elusive. In India, these are the one of the major causes of cervical cord compression. Hence, in every patient presenting with high cervical cord compression in India, CVJ anomalies must be excluded.

The craniovertebral complex is well visualized on midsagittal magnetic resonance (MR) imaging and reconstructed computed tomography (CT) images (**Fig. 1**).

This article discusses the normal anatomy of the CVJ and describes the common developmental anomalies affecting it. Relevant embryologic references are also discussed.

NORMAL BONY ANATOMY

The occipital bone has 3 parts. The basiocciput, which is located anteriorly in the midline, unites with the basisphenoid to form the sphenooccipital synchondrosis in the clivus. It has 2 parts on either side of the foramen magnum, comprising the exoccipital part of the occipital bone. The part of the occipital bone posterior to the foramen magnum is called the supraoccipital part.

The atlas is the first cervical vertebra that holds up the head. It is unique in that it does not have a body, the expected location of which is occupied by the dens. The atlas has 2 lateral masses that are connected by a short anterior, and a longer posterior, arch. The atlas ossifies from 3 ossification centers. The lateral masses of the atlas articulate with the occipital condyles. These articular facets are oval, with their long axes converging anteriorly. The atlantoarticular facets are concave and tilt medially. The transverse processes of the atlas are longer than those of all cervical vertebrae except C7.

The axis is the second cervical vertebra, and acts as a pivot for rotation of the atlas and head around the strong dens. The dens is conical and projects upward from the body of the axis. The

[a] Department of Radiology, King Edward Memorial Hospital, Parel, Mumbai 400012, Maharashtra, India
[b] Department of Radiology, Priyam Zhaveri PET-CT Centre, Dr Balabhai Nanavati Hospital, Mumbai 400056, Maharashtra, India
* Corresponding author.
E-mail address: drshilpas@hotmail.com

Neuroimag Clin N Am 21 (2011) 879–895
doi:10.1016/j.nic.2011.07.014
1052-5149/11/$ – see front matter © 2011 Elsevier Inc. All rights reserved.

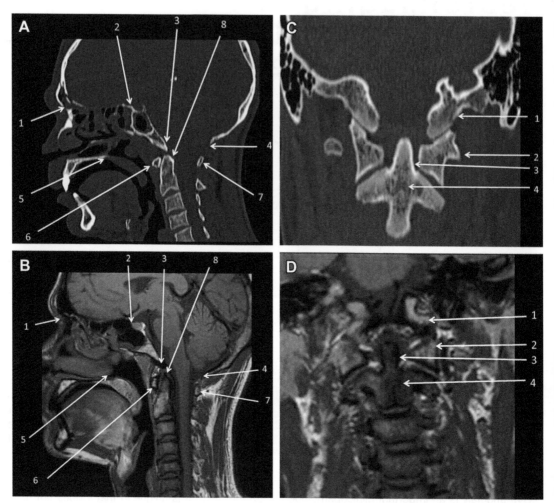

Fig. 1. Normal anatomy. Midsagittal CT (*A*) and MR imaging (*B*) show the appearance of normal CVJ and anatomic landmarks used for CVJ craniometry. 1, nasion; 2, tuberculum sella; 3, basion; 4, opisthion; 5, posterior margin of hard palate; 6, anterior arch of atlas; 7, posterior arch of atlas; 8, odontoid process. Coronal CT (*C*) and MR (*D*) images reveal occipitoatlantal and atlantoaxial articulation. 1, occipital condyles; 2, lateral mass of atlas; 3, odontoid process; 4, axis body.

posterior surface of the dens is held against the anterior arch of the atlas by the transverse ligament; in doing so, the transverse ligament divides the vertebral canal at the level of the atlas into 2 compartments. The anterior compartment is occupied by the dens, and the posterior two-thirds are occupied by the spinal cord and its covering. In the posterior part, about half is occupied by the cord itself. The axis ossifies from 5 primary and 2 secondary sides of ossification.

Craniovertebral Joints

The articulation between the cranium and the vertebral column is specialized in providing stability along with wide range of motion (**Fig. 2**).

It comprises articulations between the occipital condyles and the atlas and axis, which provides a universal joint permitting horizontal and vertical scanning movements of the head. The atlantooccipital joint articulates the occipital bone of the skull with a pair of synovial joints. The articulating surfaces consist of 2 reciprocally curved articular surfaces, with participation of the occipital condyle and the lateral masses of the atlas. This joint is stabilized by the anterior and the posterior occipital membrane. The atlantoaxial joint has 3 synovial joints; these are a pair of joints between the lateral masses and a median complex between the dens of the axis, which is held between the anterior arch and the transverse ligament of the atlas. The lateral articulating aspects of the

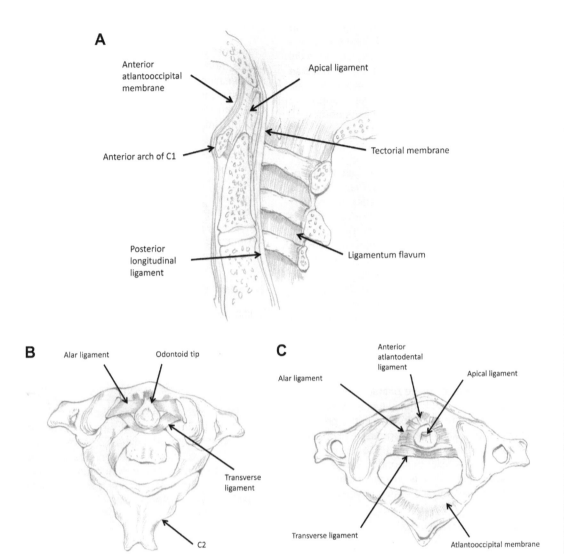

Fig. 2. Ligamentous anatomy of craniovertebral junction. (*A*) Midsagittal view. (*B, C*) Diagram showing axial view of C1 and C2 demonstrating the alar, apical and transverse ligaments.

atlantoaxial joints are planar. The transverse atlanto ligament is a broad, strong band that arches across the atlantal ring behind the dens. It is cruciate, with a horizontal component located behind the dens; from the median location of this horizontal part, fibers arise that pass upward and downward to insert into the basilar part of the occipital bone and the posterior surface of the axis, respectively.

The dens and the occipital bone are connected by the membrana tectoria, the paired alar ligaments, the median apical ligament, and the longitudinal components of the cruciform ligament. The membrana tectoria is the upward continuation of the posterior longitudinal ligament. The alar ligaments are a pair of ligaments that pass horizontally and laterally from the posterolateral aspect of the

apex of the dens to the occipital condyles. The apical ligament of the dens passes from the apex of the dens into the anterior margin of the foramen magnum between the alar ligaments. It represents the cranial continuation of the notochord and its sheath. The longitudinal component of the cruciform ligament also connects the axis to the occipital bone.

Movements of the CVJ

The CVJ represents a unique and complex interface responsible for more than half of the rotation and flexion-extension of the cervical spine.

The combination of the bony anatomy, joint articulations, and ligamentous fastenings of the CVJ allow a variety of movements. The atlantoaxial joint allows flexion, extension, axial rotation, and lateral bending. The atlantoaxial ligament allows flexion, extension, and lateral rotation. In axial rotation, as the head rotates in the transverse plane, the axis of motion is the odontoid process. The osseous articulations and their supporting ligaments must resist forces in all axes of motion.

PATHOGENESIS

Although most of the CVJ anomalies are developmental, trauma plays a role in unmasking these occult abnormalities. The type of trauma also varies; it may be a single episode of significant trauma or may be in the form of repetitive trauma.[1] This may also be in the form of repetitively carrying heavy loads on the head or the upper back.[2] In addition, recurrent viral throat infection, associated with fever, may cause ligamentous laxity caused by hyperemia; these, along with genetic predisposition, are believed to be the causative factors of CVJ anomalies.[3]

Kothari and Goel[4] speculated that basilar invagination is secondary to abnormally inclined alignment of the facets of the atlas and axis. The lateral atlantoaxial joints are planar, which permits slippage. The lack of obliquely locked facet joints also predisposes to this slippage in the presence of ligamentous laxity. The progressive slippage of the atlas over the axis secondary to this malalignment, a process similar to spondylolisthesis in the lumbosacral spine, results in invagination of the odontoid process into the craniocervical cord.

CLINICAL PRESENTATIONS

Although these anomalies are present at birth, the onset of clinical symptoms is usually observed between 11 and 40 years of age.[5] Male preponderance is seen, with gradual onset.

This condition may take the form of dysfunction of the brainstem, cervical spinal cord, cranial nerves, or the vascular supply to these structures. Myelopathy with pyramidal symptoms forms a dominant component. Spinothalamic dysfunction is less frequent.

Neck pain was a major presenting symptom in 77% of patients, whereas torticollis was present in 41% of patients.[6] Lower cranial nerve dysfunction has been found to be present in 20% of children with basilar invagination.[5] Neck pain, muscle spasms, and restriction of neck movements are frequently noted, suggesting instability of the region.

In addition, patients with atlantooccipital assimilation have a characteristic appearance with a short, broad neck, scapular elevation, low posterior hairline, and limitation of neck movements.[7]

CRANIOMETRY

Craniometry of the CVJ uses a series of lines, planes, and angles to define the normal anatomic relationships of the CVJ.[8,9] There has been renewed interest in the normal anatomy and pathology of the CVJ with the development of high-resolution CT and MR imaging. The anatomic landmarks described for plain radiographs and tomograms are well visualized on midsagittal MR and reformatted CT images (see **Fig. 1**A, B). Some of these lines (**Table 1**) have been recently reviewed[10] and are shown in **Fig. 3**. Another measurement of importance is the distance of the odontoid tip to the pontomedullary junction. This distance, as observed on MR imaging, is a useful index to define the reduction of the posterior cranial fossa bone size.

IMAGING CONSIDERATIONS

Multimodality imaging of the craniocervical junction is integral to the detection, classification, and surgical planning for the treatment of basilar invagination.

Conventional Radiography

Standard views of the cervical spine with minimal magnification are taken and these include lateral, open-mouth frontal, and dynamic flexion-extension views. Manipulation for flexion/extension views needs to be done gently and cautiously to minimize the risk of neurologic compression resulting from manipulating an unstable joint.

CT

High-resolution multidetector CT (MDCT) with isotropic reconstruction is an ideal modality for evaluation of complex osseous anatomy associated with CVJ anomalies. After axial images are obtained, these are isotropically reconstructed in multiple planes. In addition to multiplanar reconstructions (MPR), shaded surface displays (SSD) as well as volume-rendered techniques (VRT) are useful in the evaluation of bony anomalies. In the pediatric age group, rapid scanning with CT allows an examination to be performed even without sedation. The short scan time associated with CT is also beneficial in the evaluation of dynamic mobile atlantoaxial subluxation. The inherent risk of neurologic compression associated with manipulation of these unstable dislocations is reduced owing to the shorter scan time. In addition, CT angiography can also help in detecting the osseous abnormalities associated with an abnormal route of the vertebral artery, especially in patients with occipitalization of the atlas (**Figs. 4** and **5**).

Table 1
Craniometric lines and angles

	Synonyms	Definition	Normal Measurements	Implications
1.	Chamberlain line	Joins posterior margin of hard palate to opisthion	Tip of dens should not exceed 5 mm above the line	Odontoid process bisects the line in basilar invagination
2.	McGregor line	Joins posterior margin of hard plate to undersurface of occipital bone	Tip of dens should not exceed 7 mm above the line	Line position varies with flexion/extension hence has low significance
3.	McRae line	Joins anterior and posterior edges of foramen magnum (basion to opisthion)	Tip of dens does not exceed this line	When sagittal diameter is <20 mm, neurologic symptoms occur (foramen magnus stenosis)
4.	Wackenheim clivus line	Line drawn along clivus into cervical canal	Odontoid tip is ventral and tangential to this line	Odontoid process transects the line in basilar invagination or forward position of skull
5.	Height index of Klaus	Distance between tip of dens and tuberculum-torcular line	40–41 mm	<30 mm seen in basilar invagination
6.	Welcher basal angle	Angle between the lines drawn from nasion to tuberculum sellae and tuberculum sellae to basion	124°–142°	Widening is called platybasia
7.	Clivus canal angle	Angle formed at junction of Wackenheim line and posterior vertebral body line	180° in extension 150° in flexion <150° considered abnormal	
8.	Atlantooccipital joint axis angle (Schmidt)	Angle formed at the junction of lines traversing the atlantooccipital joints	125°–130°	Less than 124° is seen in condylar hypoplasia
9.	Fishgold digastric line	Joins the fossae for digastric muscles on undersurface of skull (just medial to mastoid process)	Dens tip should not project above this line. Central axis of dens should be perpendicular to the line	Corresponds to McRae line on lateral view; may be oblique in unilateral condylar hypoplasia; oblique odontoid suggests paramedian abnormality
10.	Fishgold bimastoid line	Line connecting tips of mastoid process	Runs across atlantooccipital joints, line is 10 mm below digastric line	Odontoid tip may be the line

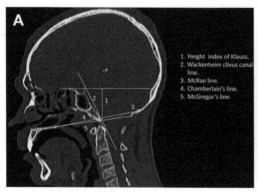
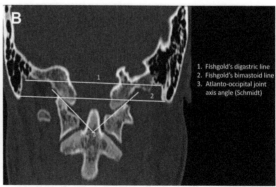

1. Height index of Klauss.
2. Wackenheim clivus canal line.
3. McRae line.
4. Chamberlain's line.
5. McGregor's line.

1. Fishgold's digastric line
2. Fishgold's bimastoid line
3. Atlanto-occipital joint axis angle (Schmidt)

Fig. 3. Sagittal and coronal CT showing various craniometric lines in lateral (*A*) and anteroposterior (*B*) views.

MR Imaging

MR imaging, with its multiplanar capabilities and high soft tissue contrast resolution, has become the mainstay in radiological evaluation of the CVJ. MR imaging has the advantage that it reveals cord, soft tissue, and ligamentous and vascular anatomy in detail. Dynamic MR imaging is useful for evaluating CVJ abnormalities and, in particular, spinal cord compression. MR imaging is able to detect cord compression that is not seen in the neutral position and is diagnostic for mobile atlantoaxial instability.[11] Assessment of the biomechanics of the joints assists in formulation of a rational surgical strategy.

CLASSIFICATION OF COMMON CVJ ANOMALIES IN THE TROPICS

In our experience, congenital atlantoaxial dislocation (AAD) is the commonest of these congenital anomalies and may occur with or without other

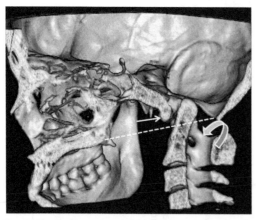

Fig. 4. Three-dimensional (3D) CT shows spatial relationships of complex skeletal disorders such as assimilation of atlas (*arrow*), fusion of C1 and C2 (*curved arrow*), and basilar invagination. Note violation of Chamberlain line demarcated by dotted line.

developmental anomalies (Table 2). Bony atlas anomalies, predominantly occipitalization of C1 along with basilar invagination with or without Chiari malformation, constitute the rest of the disorders. Os odontoideum is also seen in many patients. These findings are consistent with the literature.[12]

ANOMALIES OF THE OCCIPUT
Basilar Invagination

Basilar invagination is a developmental anomaly of the CVJ in which the odontoid abnormally moves up into the foramen magnum. It is often associated with other osseous anomalies of the CVJ, including atlantooccipital assimilation, incomplete ring of C1, hypoplasia of the basiocciput, occipital condyles, and atlas (see Fig. 5). Basilar invagination is also associated with neural axis abnormalities, including Chiari malformation, syringomyelia, syringobulbia, and hydrocephalus. The basiocciput may be short, such that the clivus is small and horizontally oriented (Fig. 6).[9,13–15]

Although congenital, basilar invagination may remain asymptomatic and unrecognized until adulthood, and it may ultimately require surgical treatment in a substantial subset of patients.

Goel and colleagues[16] classified basilar invagination into 2 types. Patients in group A have basilar invagination associated with an atlantodental subluxation; this type is more commonly encountered in the Indian subcontinent. In group B, basilar invagination exists with the maintained alignment of the odontoid and atlas; these patients do not have neurologic instability. Furthermore, patients having group A basilar invagination (ie, basilar invagination associated with atlantoaxial subluxation) are again subdivided into 2 groups. The basilar invagination may be reduced on extension, called vertically mobile AAD, or the basilar invagination may be fixed and not reduce on extension, which is

Table 2
Congenital anomalies affecting the CVJ

Anomalies of the Occiput	Anomalies of Atlas	Anomalies of Axis
Basilar invagination	Assimilation of the atlas	Os odontoideum
Platybasia	Posterior arch atlas agenesis	Hypoplastic odontoid
Basioccipital hypoplasia	Occipital vertebrae	Ossiculum terminale persistans
Occipital condyle hypoplasia	Ponticles of the atlas	
Chiari malformations		

called vertical fixed atlantoaxial dislocation. In addition, there is a subset of patients in the latter group in whom the basilar invagination may reduce on traction. Patients with basilar invagination with atlantoaxial dislocation, which is reducible in a certain posture, are treated only by posterior fixation in a reduced position, whereas vertical fixed atlantoaxial dislocation, which is not reducible even on traction, needs to be managed by atlantoaxial distraction, reduction, and fixation or by transoral decompression and posterior fixation.[17]

Literature related to CVJ often incorrectly uses the terms basilar invagination, basilar impression, cranial settling, and platybasia as if they were synonymous. However, these entities should be distinguished from true congenital basilar invagination.

Basilar impression is the acquired basilar invagination caused by the softening of bones, as occurs in hyperparathyroidism, rickets, osteomalacia, Paget disease, Hurler syndrome, osteogenesis imperfecta, and so forth. These conditions are not common in tropics and are not discussed further here.

Platybasia is commonly associated with basilar invagination and is diagnosed by an abnormally obtuse basal angle. The superior position of the odontoid process is associated with a more horizontal angulation and shortening of the clivus.[18] It is less commonly associated with basilar invagination in the tropics compared with the West. In addition, isolated platybasia is asymptomatic.

Basioccipital Hypoplasia

The basioccipital portion of the occipital bone is derived from fusion of 4 occipital sclerotomes. Hypoplasia may be mild or severe depending on

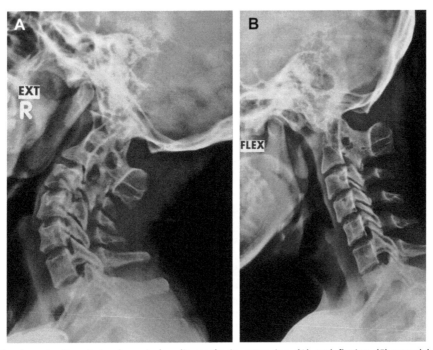

Fig. 5. Basilar invagination. Lateral cervical radiographs in extension *(A)* and flexion *(B)* reveal high placed odontoid with cervical 2 to 3 vertebral fusion.

how many of the 4 occipital sclerotomes have not formed. The hypoplasia decreases the length of the clivus, hence the term short clivus (Fig. 7). The Chamberlain line may be violated, and associated basilar invagination is common. The Wackenheim clivus canal angle is decreased along with bowstring deformity of the underlying cervicomedullary junction.[9,19]

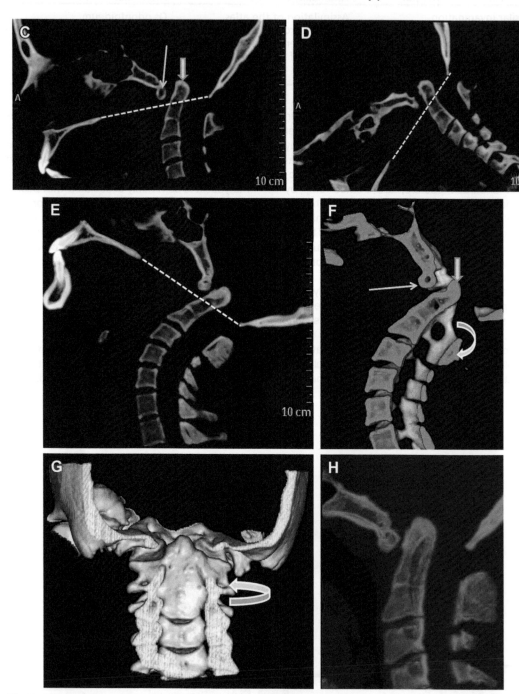

Fig. 5. (C) Sagittal reconstructed CT image in a neutral position shows high placed odontoid. The Chamberlain line is demarcated by a dotted line (C–E), the odontoid tip lies 9 mm above this line. Also note assimilation of atlas (arrow). Cervical vertebrae 2 to 3 are fused. (D) CT in flexion and (E) CT in extension showing persistence of vertical dislocation (basilar invagination). (F, G) Sagittal and coronal 3D CT images confirming assimilation of atlas (arrow) and fusion of C2 to C3 (curved arrow) and basilar invagination (block arrow). (H) Maximum intensity projection aids in showing all the abnormalities seen.

Occipital Condyle Hypoplasia

Occipital condylar hypoplasia may be unilateral or bilateral; it is more commonly the latter. The vertical height of the occipital condyles, which articulate with the lateral masses of the atlas, is reduced. The subsequent reduction in vertical height of the lateral articulations with preserved height of the median located dens, causes disruption of the Chamberlain line (basilar invagination)

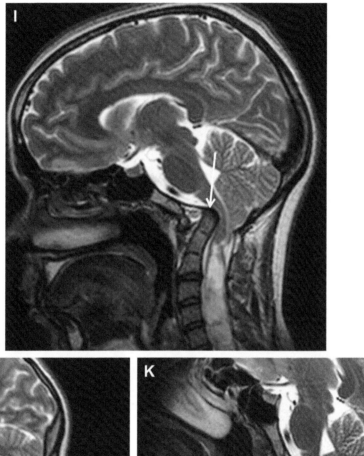

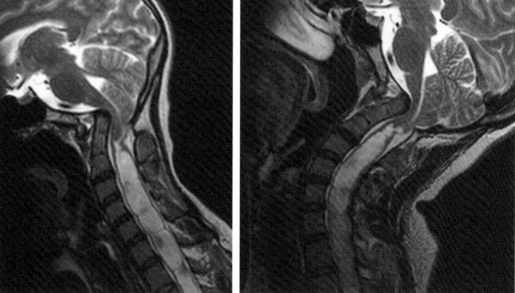

Fig. 5. (*I*) Sagittal T2-weighted images in neutral position show basilar invagination with retroflexed odontoid (*arrow*) causing compression of brainstem (medulla). A large syringohydromyelia is also seen. (*J, K*) Flexion and extension views depict the extent of ventral and dorsal cervicomedullary compression. There is an increase in cord compression in flexion with partial relief in extension.

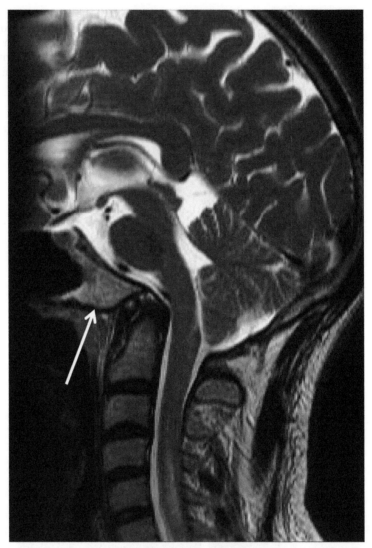

Fig. 6. T2-weighted midsagittal image showing basiocciput hypoplasia with horizontally oriented clivus (*arrow*).

and an associated increased atlantooccipital joint axis angle. In cases in which the occipital condylar hypoplasia is unilateral, the difference in the height is compensated for by a scoliosis of the cervical spine, the skull thus remaining in the midline. Clinically, condylar hypoplasia can reduce the range of movements, or even completely abolish movement, at the atlantooccipital joint, which can lead to compression of the vertebral artery as result of excessive movement of the occipital bone in relation to the atlas.[20]

ANOMALIES OF THE ATLAS

Isolated atlas anomalies do not disturb the occipitoatlantoaxial relationship and are not associated with basilar invagination (see **Fig. 6**).

Assimilation of the Atlas

Assimilation of the atlas is also called occipitocervical fusion, occipital cervical synostosis, or occipitalization of the atlas.[21] It refers to congenital fusion of the atlas to the occiput, a union that may be partial or complete. It may involve the anterior and posterior arch, or the lateral elements, either in a solitary fashion or in different subsets. The most common abnormality is fusion of the anterior of arch of the atlas to the basion (see **Fig. 5**). In this condition, the atlantooccipital joint is redundant, and flexion occurs at the atlantoaxial joint. This condition is often associated with agenesis of the posterior arch of the atlas (**Fig. 8**). In these conditions, a comma-shaped anterior margin of the foramen magnum is

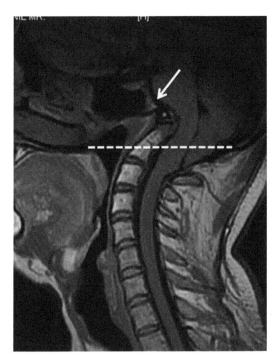

Fig. 7. Chiari I malformation with severe basioccipital hypoplasia with basion at the midpons level (*arrow*). The Chamberlain line is demarcated by the dotted line; the odontoid tip lies far above this line.

identified on sagittal MR images. This assimilation is a characteristic feature of basilar invagination. In addition, similar assimilation associated with C2 to C3 nonsegmentation is seen and is referred to as Klippel-Feil syndrome.[22] Other systemic congenital abnormalities associated with occipitalization of the atlas are incomplete clefting of the nasal cartilage, cleft palate, congenital external ear deformities, cervical rib and urinary tract abnormalities, and atlas arch abnormalities.[23]

Atlas Arch Anomalies

A defect may be seen in the anterior or posterior arch of the atlas. Defects of the posterior arch of the atlas are wrongly called spina bifida of the atlas, because the atlas lacks a true spinous process. Hence, the term posterior rachischisis is appropriate. The most common atlas arch anomaly is a midline posterior arch rachischisis, which may be associated with atlantoaxial instability.[23]

Anterior arch anomalies are less common; they are rarely identified in isolation and typically occur in association with posterior arch anomalies. This combined entity is called split atlas.[24] On an open-mouth odontoid view, a posterior arch defect may be superimposed on the axis and simulate a fracture. In this condition, thin-section CT with bone window reconstruction helps to differentiate these developmental abnormalities from a fracture. The margins of a developmental discontinuity are smooth and regular with contiguous cortical margins, and are not associated with adjacent hematoma. Fractures

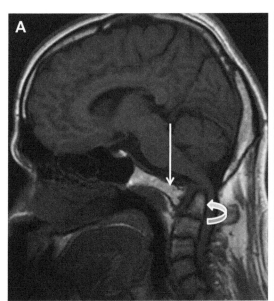

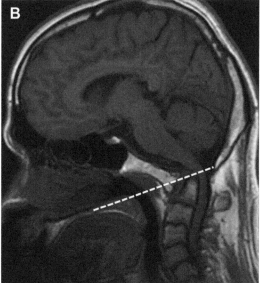

Fig. 8. (*A*) Midsagittal T1-weighted MR imaging shows assimilation of anterior arch of atlas (*arrow*) with agenesis of its posterior arch. There is associated odontoid hypoplasia (*curved arrow*). (*B*) The Chamberlain line demarcated by the dotted line shows that there is no basilar invagination.

are sharp, noncorticated, and are associated with adjacent hematoma.[25]

ANOMALIES OF THE AXIS

Most anomalies of the axis are confined to the odontoid process. These anomalies are usually not associated with basilar invagination. A brief understanding of the development of the dens is imperative before its anomalies are described.[26]

The fifth, sixth, and seventh occipital sclerotomes giving rise to the axis are designated as X, Y, Z. The X gives rise to the tip of the dens, the Y gives rise to the base of the dens, and the Z forms the centrum of the axis. An intervertebral

disc appears temporarily between the inferior part of the dens (Y) and the C2 body (Z) during development. No disc develops between the X and Y, which gives rise to the apical and basal parts of the dens, respectively, during development. Failure of fusion of the X with the YZ complex produces an ossiculum terminale (of Bergman), a disassociated apical odontoid epiphysis. Failure of the fusion between the XY complex and the Z at the dentocentral synchondrosis produces an os odontoideum. In addition, hypoplasia and aplasia of the X and Y centra and aplasia of the Z centrum lead to reduced height of the dens. In addition, hypoplasia of the dens is usually accompanied by the atlantooccipital assimilation and basilar invagination.

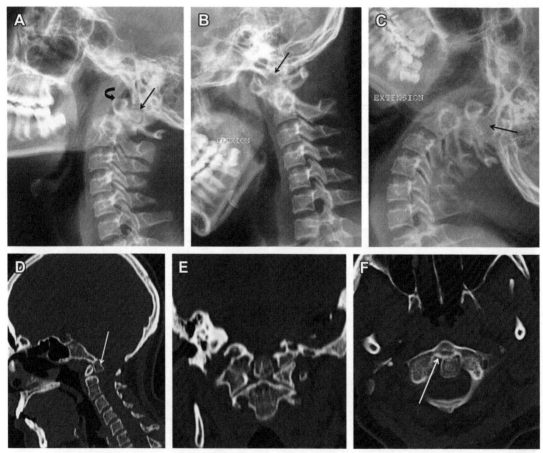

Fig. 9. Os odontoideum. (A–C) Neutral, flexion, and extension lateral radiographs of patient with os odontoideum. Note the presence of independent osseous structure (arrow), suggestive of os odontoideum posterior to the anterior arch of atlas (curved arrow). It is associated with hypoplastic odontoid process. The flexion and extension views exhibit movement of os odontoideum in unison with the clivus. (D) Sagittal reconstructed CT image shows Os odontoideum (arrow) in alignment with the basion (clivus). This is indicative of dystopic Os odontoideum. (E) Coronal reconstructed magnified CT image confirms the presence of well corticated margins of Os odontoideum. (F) Axial CT image shows marked hypertrophy of anterior arch of atlas with concave posterior margins (arrow).

Abnormalities of the dens can also be associated with atlantoaxial subluxation.

Os Odontoideum

This rare lesion of the second cervical vertebra was first described in 1886 by Giacomini. The name originates from the Latin *os* (bone) and *odontoideum* (tooth form). The term os odontoideum refers to an independent ossicle lying cephalad to the body of axis in the location of the odontoid process.[27] It has well-corticated margins with separation from the foreshortened odontoid peg.[28]

The cause of os odontoideum remains controversial, but there is now emerging consensus on a traumatic cause of os odontoideum rather than a congenital source.[29]

Two anatomic types of os odontoideum exist: orthotopic[30] and dystopic.[31] Orthotopic refers to an ossicle in a normal anatomic position that moves in unison with the anterior arch of C1 and therefore can be surgically reduced to be normally aligned with the dens. Dystopic defines an ossicle that has migrated toward the clivus and is functionally fused to the basion. It may also partially dislocate anterior to the C1 arch. The gap between the axis and the free ossicle usually extends above the level of the superior facets of the axis. This condition leads to incompetence of the cruciate ligament and to atlantoaxial instability. The degree of instability must be assessed by flexion and extension studies (**Fig. 9**).[32]

It is imperative to differentiate an os odontoideum from an acute D'Alonzo type II fracture of the dens. A D'Alonzo type II fracture of dens separates the dens at its base from the centrum of the axis vertebra. This differentiation is imperative, because treatment varies for each condition. Acute dens fractures are unstable and need to be immobilized immediately to prevent neurologic damage. Patients with os odontoideum may also be unstable; however, they do not need immediate treatment in the absence of neurologic signs. CT with bone window reconstruction is useful to differentiate these entities. An os odontoideum is associated with hypertrophy of the anterior arch of the atlas, with increased vertical dimensions, cortical thickening, and a convex posterior border.[33] This condition is likely to be a sympathetic compensatory reaction to chronic stress at an unstable joint. In addition, in a patient with os odontoideum, the axis body has a corticated convex upper margin, however, in an acute fracture, the upper margin of the axis body where it articulates with the dense is sharp, discontinuous, and uncorticated (**Fig. 10**).

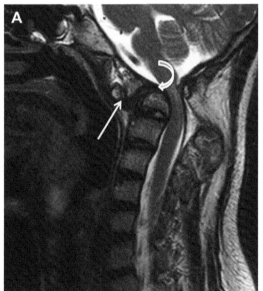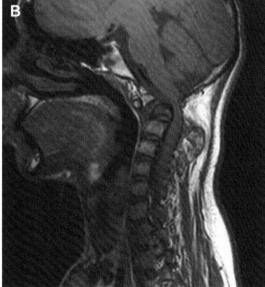

Fig. 10. Midsagittal T2-weighted (*A*) and T1-weighted (*B*) MR imaging showing presence of os odontoideum. There is hypoplastic odontoid process and presence of an independent ossicle (*arrow*) posterior to the anterior arch of atlas. Note that the body of axis has a well-corticated convex upper margin (*curved arrow*). Atlantodental interval is increased. Cord compression is seen, as shown by hyperintense signal suggestive of edema.

Odontoid Hypoplasia/Aplasia

Odontoid hypoplasia is more common than aplasia and is associated with various syndromes; of relevance here is Klippel-Feil syndrome. Both conditions may cause atlantoaxial instability bercause the ligamentous attachments are often missing, allowing excessive atlas rotation that may produce neurologic symptoms because of cervicomedullary compression.

Chiari Malformations

This group of malformations range from I to III and are characterized by increasing degrees of hindbrain dysgenesis.

Chiari I malformation

Chiari I malformation has been described as caudal protrusion of peg-shaped cerebellar tonsils below the foramen magnum. Tonsillar herniation of greater than 5 mm is essential for diagnosis. Posterior cranial fossa volume is typically small as measured by the Klaus height index.[34] The tentorium is clearly identified on MR imaging and the distance of the tip of the odontoid from the line of the tentorium indicates the height of the posterior cranial fossa (see **Fig. 8**). The incidence of syringomyelia is high, varying from 30% to 50%.[35,36] Osseous abnormalities include basiocciput hypoplasia with basilar invagination (see **Fig. 7**), and, less commonly, atlantooccipital assimilation (**Fig. 11**), nonsegmentation C2 to C3, and Klippel-Feil anomalies.

Chiari II malformation

Chiari II malformation is defined as dysgenesis and herniation of the hindbrain, which includes inferior portions of vermis, fourth ventricle, and medulla into the spinal canal. It is invariably associated with meningomyeloceles with or without syringohydromyelia. CVJ manifestations include thinning of the basiocciput with resultant concavity of the clivus and scalloping of the posterior aspect of the odontoid process (**Fig. 12**).[9]

Chiari III malformation

Chiari III malformation is a rare malformation with herniation of the hindbrain associated with occipital encephalocele in combination with features of Chiari II malformation.

Klippel-Feil Syndrome

Klippel-Feil syndrome is a classic triad of low posterior hairline, short neck, and limitation of neck movement, along with nonsegmentation of 2 or more cervical vertebrae.[28,37–39]

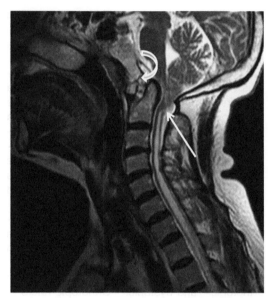

Fig. 11. Chiari I malformation. Midsagittal T2-weighted image reveals inferior displacement of the cerebellar tonsils (*arrow*) with mild basilar invagination. Compression of the cervicomedullary junction causes syringohydromyelia. In addition, there is associated AAD (*curved arrow*).

Associated CVJ anomalies are basilar invagination, odontoid hypoplasia, assimilation of the atlas, platybasia, and Chiari I malformation. Visceral congenital anomalies include Sprengel shoulder,

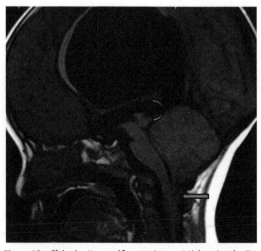

Fig. 12. Chiari II malformation. Midsagittal T1-weighted image shows tectal beaking (*curved arrow*) with concavity of the clivus (*arrow*). The posterior fossa is small with inferior tonsillar herniation causing obstruction to the outlet foramina (*block arrow*). Resultant obstructive hydrocephalus is seen.

syndactyly, and cardiovascular, genitourinary, ophthalmologic, and otolaryngologic anomalies.

These patients are predisposed to severe cervical cord injury following minor trauma. Accelerated degeneration of cervical spine occurs because of hypermobility at levels adjacent to the nonsegmented vertebrae (**Fig. 13**).

Atlantoaxial Instability

Congenital AAD is a common condition in tropical countries, with the highest incidence in India. Wadia[40] in 1960 first drew attention to its occurrence, whereas Pandya[41] published an excellent review article in 1972. The pattern of presentation is different from that found in the West.[42] Based on a large series of patients, pediatric congenital AADs were analyzed based on clinicoradiological findings and surgical outcome.[43] They were divided into congenital irreducible AAD (IAAD) (**Fig. 14**) and reducible AAD (RAAD). A significantly higher incidence of C1 assimilation, C2 to C3 fusion, asymmetrical occiput C2 facet joints, and basilar invagination were seen in patients with IAAD, whereas os odontoideum was observed in those with RAAD (see **Fig. 7**). Radiological differences in the anatomy of patients with IAAD and those with RAAD are likely to be caused by improper segmentation of the occipital and upper cervical sclerotomes in the former and dysfunction of the transverse ligament in the latter.[43] Dynamic flexion-extension studies are important for complete evaluation of the type of instability (ie, whether it is mobile or fixed) because this affects management.

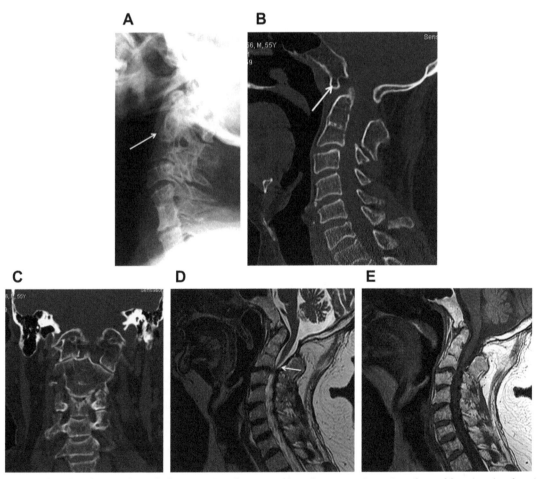

Fig. 13. Klippel-Feil anomaly with degenerative changes and cord compromise at interface of fused and unfused vertebrae. Lateral radiograph (*A*) showing fusion of C2 and C3 vertebrae (*arrow*). (*B*, *C*) Sagittal and coronal reconstructed CT confirms the findings. In addition, there is assimilation of atlas (*arrow*). No canal compromise is seen at the CVJ. Midsagittal T2-weighted (*D*) and T1-weighted (*E*) images showing cord compression at the interface of fused and unfused vertebrae (*arrow*).

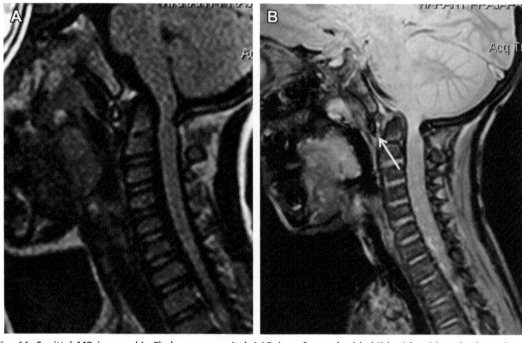

Fig. 14. Sagittal MR images (*A, B*) show congenital AAD in a 6-month-old child with widened atlantodental interval (*arrow*).

SUMMARY

CVJ disorders in the Occident are usually associated with systemic disorders. In contrast, in the Orient, a greater incidence of isolated CVJ anomalies is seen. More importantly, although these are developmental anomalies, they manifest late in life, with trauma and/or infection playing a promotive role. The most significant and common of these anomalies are basilar invagination and atlantodental dislocation, which also occur together. Accurate diagnosis of these anomalies is now feasible by using state-of-the-art high spatial resolution imaging using CT and MR imaging. This technique allows not only precise diagnosis but also permits detailed pretreatment selection as well as preoperative planning. Greater awareness of this subset of patients is essential for greater understanding and effective management of these ailments.

ACKNOWLEDGMENTS

I would like to acknowledge my colleagues Dr S. Jaggi from Bombay Hospital, and B. Yeragi from Nair hospital for **Figs. 13** and **14** respectively, and A. Ihare from KEM Hospital for photographic assistance.

REFERENCES

1. Menezes AH. Primary craniovertebral anomalies and hindbrain herniation syndrome (Chiari I): data base analysis. Pediatr Neurosurg 1995;23: 260–9.
2. Bharucha EP, Dasyur HM. Craniovertebral anomalies: a report on 40 cases. Brain 1964;87:469–80.
3. Pradhan M, Behari S, Kalra SK, et al. Association of methylenetetrahydrofolate reductase genetic polymorphisms with atlantoaxial dislocations. J Neurosurg Spine 2007;7:623–30.
4. Kothari M, Goel A. Transatlantic odonto-occipital listhesis: the so-called basilar invagination. Neurol India 2007;55:6–7.
5. Sambasivan M. Anatomy of the craniovertebra anomalies. Prog Clin Neurosci 1988;1:81–100.
6. Goel A. Treatment of basilar invagination by atlantoaxial joint distraction and direct lateral mass fixation. J Neurosurg Spine 2004;1:281–6.
7. Van gilder JC, Menezes AH, Dolan KD. The craniovertebral junction and its abnormalities. New York: Futura; 1987.
8. Dolan KD. Cervicobasilar relationships. Radiol Clin North Am 1977;15:155–66.
9. Smoker WR. MR imaging of the craniovertebral junction. Magn Reson Imaging Clin N Am 2000;8(3):636, 637, 640.

10. Smoker WR. Craniovertebral junction: normal anatomy, craniometry and congenital anomalies. Radiographics 1994;14:225–7.

11. Gupta V, Khandelwal N, Mathuria SN. Dynamic magnetic resonance imaging evaluation of craniovertebral junction abnormalities. J Comput Assist Tomogr 2007;31(3):354–9.

12. Chopra JS, Sawhey IM, Kak VK, et al. Analysis of 82 cases of craniovertebra anomalies. Br J Neurosurg 1988;2:455–63.

13. Menezes AH. Congenital and acquired abnormalities of the craniovertebral junction. In: Youmans Neurological Surgery, 4. Philadelphia: WB Saunders; 1996. p. 1035–89.

14. Von Torklus D, Ghele W. The upper cervical spine. New York: Grune & Statton; 1972.

15. Wackenheim A. Cervico-occipital Joint. Berlin: Springer-Verlag; 1985.

16. Goel A, Bhatjiwale M, Desai K. Basilar invagination: a study based on 190 surgically treated cases. J Neurosurg 1998;88:962–8.

17. Goel A, Shah A, Rajan S. Vertical mobile and reducible atlantoaxial dislocation. J Neurosurg Spine 2009;11: 9–14.

18. Malis LI, Cohen I, Gross SW. Arnold-Chiari malformation. Arch Surg 1951;63:783–98.

19. Penning L. Normal movements of the cervical spine. AJR Am J Roentgenol 1978;130:317–26.

20. Bernini FP, Elefante R, Smaltino F, et al. Angiographic study on the vertebral artery in cases of deformities of the occipitocervical joint. Am J Roentgenol 1969;107:526–9.

21. Dubonsett J. Torticollis in children caused by congenital anomalies of the atlas. J Bone Joint Surg Am 1986; 68:178.

22. McRae DL, Barnum AS. Occipitalization of the atlas. AJR Am J Roentgenol 1953;70:23–46.

23. Smoker WR. Congenital anomalies of the cervical spine. Neuroimaging Clin N Am 1995;5:427–49.

24. Wackenheim A. Roentgen diagnosis of the craniovertebral region. New York: Springer-Verlag; 1974.

25. Gehweiler JA, Daffner RH, Robert SL. Malformation of the atlas simulating the Jefferson fractures. AJR Am J Roentgenol 1983;4:187–90.

26. Gray H, Standring S. Gray's anatomy. 39th edition. London: Elsevier, Churchill Livingstone; 2005. p. 729, 744–5, 793–5.

27. Giacomini C, Sull'Esistenza D. "Os Odontoideum" nell'uomo, Gior. Acad Med 1886;49:24–38.

28. Smoker WR, Khanna G. Imaging the craniocervical junction. Childs Nerv Syst 2008;24(10):1123–45.

29. Babak A, Gosselin MP, Fehlings MJ. Os odontoideum: etiology and surgical management. Neurosurgery 2010;66:A22–31.

30. Vargas TM, Rybicki FJ, Ledbetter SM, et al. Atlantoaxial instability associated with as orthotopic os odontoideum: a multimodality imaging assessment. Emerg Radiol 2005;11(4):223–5.

31. Egashira T, Nose T, Ono Y, et al. A case with dystopic os odontoideum. No Shinkei Geka 1980;8(5): 489–93 [in Japanese].

32. Thomasan M, Young JW. Os odontoideum. Skeletal Radiol 1984;11:144–6.

33. Holt R, Helms C, Munk P, et al. Hypertrophy of the C1 anterior arch: useful sign to distinguish os odontoideum from acute dens fracture. Radiology 1989; 173:207–9.

34. Klaus E. Rontgendiagnostik der platybasic und basilaren impression. Fortscher Rontgenstr 1957; 86:460–9.

35. Elster AD, Chen MY. Chiari I malformations: clinical and radiological reappraisal. Radiology 1992;183: 347–53.

36. Seaz RJ, Onofrio BM, Yanagihara T. Experience with Arnold-Chiari malformations, 1960-1970. J Neurosurg 1976;45:416–22.

37. Ulmer JL, Elster AD, Ginsberg LE, et al. Klippel Feil Syndrome: CT and MR of acquired and congenital abnormalities of cervical spine and cord. J Comput Assist Tomogr 1993;17:215–24.

38. Elster AD. Quadriplegia after minor trauma in Klippel Feil Syndrome. A case report and review of literature. J Bone Joint Surg Am 1984;66:1473–4.

39. Nagib MG, Maxwell RE, Chou SN. Identification and management of high risk patients with Klippel Feil Syndrome. J Neurosurg 1984;61:523–30.

40. Wadia NH. Myelopathy complicating congenital atlanto-axial dislocation (A study of 28 case). Brain 1967;90:449–72.

41. Pandya SK. Atlantoaxial dislocation (Review). Neurol India 1972;20(1):13–48.

42. Jawalkar S, Chopra JS, Kak VK, et al. Craniovertebral anomalies in north-western India. Neurol India 1983;31(9):15–26.

43. Salunke P, Behari S, Kirankumar MV, et al. Pediatric congenital atlantoaxial dislocation: differences between the irreducible and reducible varieties. J Neurosurg 2006;104(2):115–22.

Vascular Brain Pathologies

Ajay Garg, MD

KEYWORDS

- Brain lesions • Vascular brain pathology
- Vasculitis • Vasculopathy • Takayasu arteriitis
- Moyamoya disease

Vascular pathologies of brain comprise a heterogeneous group of abnormalities such as vasculitis, dural arteriovenous malformations, carotid-cavernous fistulas, cerebral venous thrombosis (CVT), and intracerebral hemorrhage (ICH). Modern imaging techniques are increasingly unraveling these vascular lesions of the brain at a stage when many of them are still asymptomatic. This article focuses on acquired vascular pathologies prevalent in the tropical countries. Some of the common vascular pathologies of brain lesions encountered in clinical practice are enumerated here (**Box 1**).

VASCULITIS AND VASCULOPATHY

Cerebral vasculitis is heterogeneous group of multisystem disorders characterized pathologically by inflammation with or without necrosis of the blood vessel wall. Vasculitis, like inflammation in other tissues, may be caused by many different agents and pathogenic mechanisms; however, these different causes produce only a limited number of histologic expressions of injury—ischemia following vessel lumen compromise and hemorrhage following vessel wall disruption. Therefore, the same clinical manifestations can result from etiologically and pathogenetically different vasculitic diseases.

Important clinical factors that merit consideration include age, sex, and ethnic origin of the patient, presence of skin lesions (ulcers, palpable purpura), size of vessel involvement (small, medium, and large), involvement of other organs (in particular kidneys, lungs, and paranasal sinuses), use of medications, drug abuse, and neurologic signs including cognitive deterioration, focal deficit, transient ischemic attack, stroke, and thunderclap headache (TCH).[1] Relevant laboratory tests should include erythrocyte sedimentation rate (ESR), rheumatoid factor, C-reactive protein, complement level, immune status and antibodies in blood and cerebrospinal fluid (CSF), protein and cell count in CSF, and assessment of coagulation factors. Chest radiographs may reveal asymptomatic pulmonary involvement.[1]

Computed tomography (CT) of the brain is less useful for the diagnosis of acute central nervous system (CNS) vasculitis because of limited spatial resolution, and thus can demonstrate only large ischemic infarctions well, although it can show parenchymal brain calcifications found within old ischemic lesions. Magnetic resonance (MR) imaging plays a crucial role in the workup of patients of suspected vasculitis, even though the abnormalities found on MR imaging are not diagnostic. Involvement of small perforating arteries results in ischemic lesions localized in the deep or subcortical white matter and the basal ganglia. When larger arteries are occluded, the resulting infarctions are found in the cortical gray and white matter. During the acute stage of the infarction, diffusion-weighted MR imaging can distinguish acute from chronic ischemic abnormalities. Within a few days, acute infarctions progress to a subacute stage with neoangiogenesis, and may enhance following contrast administration. In addition, wall thickening and intramural contrast uptake are frequent findings in patients with active cerebral vasculitis affecting large brain arteries.[2]

Important clinical features and literature on different forms of vasculitis are briefly reviewed here.

Department of Neuroradiology, Neurosciences Centre, All India Institute of Medical Sciences, Ansari Nagar, New Delhi 110029, India
E-mail address: drajaygarg@gmail.com

Neuroimag Clin N Am 21 (2011) 897–926
doi:10.1016/j.nic.2011.07.007
1052-5149/11/$ – see front matter © 2011 Elsevier Inc. All rights reserved.

Classification of vascular pathologies of brain

- Vasculitis and Vasculopathy
  - Primary vasculitis
    - Primary central nervous system angiitis
    - Giant cell arteritis
  - Secondary Vasculitis
    - Systemic vessel wall disease
      - Takayasu arteritis
      - Moyamoya disease
      - Polyarteritis nodosa
    - Autoimmune Vasculitis
    - Infectious Vasculitis
      - Bacterial infection—acute septic meningitis, tubercular meningitis
      - Fungal infection—*Candida*, aspergillosis, coccidiomycosis, mucormycosis
      - Viral infection—varicella zoster infection, human immunodeficiency virus vasculopathy
      - Parasitic infection—neurocysticercosis
      - Mycotic aneurysms
    - Drug-induced vasculitis
    - Radiation vasculopathy
  - Reversible cerebral vasoconstriction syndrome
  - Arterial dissections
- Dural Arteriovenous Malformations
- Cerebral Venous Thrombosis
- Nontraumatic hemorrhage
  - Intracerebral hemorrhage
  - Subarachnoid hemorrhage
- Caroticocavernous Fistula
- Posterior reversible Encephalopathy Syndrome

Primary Vasculitis

Primary CNS angiitis (granulomatous angiitis)

Primary angiitis of the central nervous system (PACNS), also called primary CNS vasculitis, is an idiopathic inflammatory condition affecting medium-sized to small arteries, arterioles, and venules of brain parenchyma and meninges. Rarely, PACNS affects the spinal cord. PACNS is most often observed in the fifth to sixth decade; however, several pediatric cases have also been reported. Acute or subacute onset confusion, headache,

change of personality, paresis, cranial neuropathy, hallucinations, or loss of consciousness are often presenting signs but, as such, nonspecific. Laboratory findings include elevated inflammatory markers, particularly the ESR, and CSF analysis may reveal elevated opening pressure, raised protein levels, and/or lymphocytic pleocytosis.

Pathologically, transmural involvement of the vessel wall is commonly seen with dense infiltration of inflammatory cells, primarily lymphocytes and large mononuclear cells,[3] with or without the presence of granulomas. There may be fibrinoid necrosis in the vessel wall, and inflammation in the leptomeningeal and/or parenchymal vessels may be patchy, leading to false-negative biopsies.[4–6]

On imaging, findings in PACNS are highly variable and nonspecific. CT scan is abnormal in up to 67% of cases, and may reveal areas of low-density suggestive of ischemic events and, rarely, intraparenchymal or subarachnoid hemorrhage.[7] MR imaging shows discrete or diffuse supratentorial and infratentorial lesions involving the deep and superficial white matter (Fig. 1).[8–10] In addition, areas of infarcts and hemorrhage may be seen (see Fig. 1; Fig. 2). On diffusion-weighted imaging (DWI), some acute/subacute lesions show restricted diffusion, suggesting an ischemic mechanism, whereas other acute/subacute lesions have higher apparent diffusion coefficient values, implicating a nonischemic mechanism.[11] Post gadolinium, the lesions usually enhance in up to 90% of cases (see Figs. 1 and 2). In addition, enhancements can be seen in the Virchow-Robin spaces, leptomeninges, and spinal cord lesions (see Fig. 2). Patients with normal MR examination are unlikely to have abnormalities suggestive of angiitis on catheter angiography or brain biopsy. MR angiography is usually not informative, but may show vascular irregularities. Catheter angiography has a sensitivity and positive predictive value of less than 30%. It may show focal and/or multifocal segmental narrowing occlusion or irregularity of both small and medium-sized parenchymal and leptomeningeal blood vessels; collateral vessel formations, and prolonged circulation time (see Fig. 2; Fig. 3).[12] Angiographically, PACNS cannot be differentiated from secondary causes of angiitis of CNS.

Histopathological confirmation by leptomeningeal and brain parenchymal biopsy remains the gold standard for the diagnosis of PACNS. This method is invasive, and findings may be negative in some patients with primary angiitis of the CNS because of sampling error.[13,14] A negative biopsy does not rule out the condition. PACNS is managed with high-dose steroids and cytotoxic agents

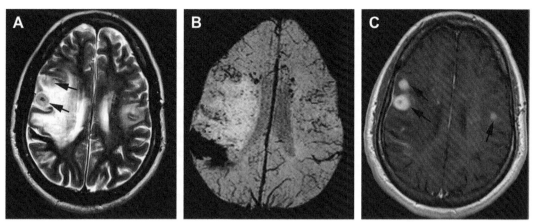

Fig. 1. Primary central nervous system (CNS) angiitis. Axial T2-weighted image (*A*) shows hyperintense lesions in bilateral frontoparietal white matter along with isointense nodules (*arrows*). Susceptibility-weighted image (SWI) (*B*) demonstrates tiny hypointense foci suggestive of petechial hemorrhages or possibly microthrombi throughout the white matter. Site of previous negative biopsy can be identified as area of hemorrhage in the right parietal region. Postgadolinium T1-weighted image (*C*) shows multiple enhancing nodular (*arrows*) and punctate lesions in both cerebral hemispheres.

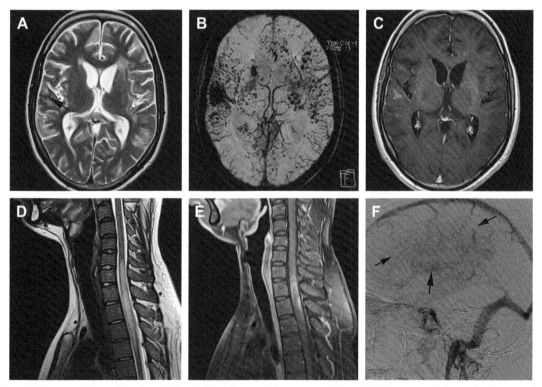

Fig. 2. Primary CNS angiitis. Axial T2-weighted image (*A*) shows multifocal white matter lesion in both cerebral hemispheres and area of old hemorrhage in right temporal lobe (*arrow*). SWI (*B*) demonstrates numerous tiny microhemorrhages throughout the white matter. Postgadolinium T1-weighted image (*C*) shows multiple linear and punctate enhancing foci in both cerebral hemispheres. Sagittal T2-weighted image (*D*) of cervicodorsal spine shows long-segment hyperintense lesion in cervicodorsal spinal cord that enhances following gadolinium administration (*E*). Early venous phase of right internal artery angiogram (*F*) shows irregularity of draining veins (*arrows*; flea-bitten appearance, pseudophlebitic pattern).

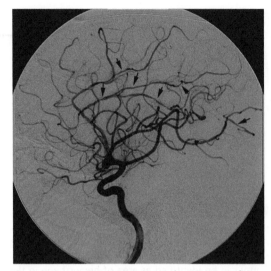

Fig. 3. Primary CNS angiitis. Lateral projection of arterial phase of left internal carotid artery angiogram shows multifocal irregularities (*arrows*) of pericallosal, callosomarginal, and branches of middle cerebral arteries.

such as cyclophosphamide and azathioprine. Without treatment, the disease is usually fatal.

Giant cell arteritis

Giant cell arteritis (GCA) is a chronic, granulomatous vasculitis of large and medium-sized arteries. It involves the superficial temporal artery, but may also include other cranial arteries, for example, the occipital arteries.[15] It usually occurs in patients older than 55 years. There are two common constellations of findings in GCA: temporal arteritis and polymyalgia rheumatica. Symptoms of temporal arteritis include unilateral headache, facial pain, jaw claudication, or loss of vision. Temporal arteritis is a common manifestation of GCA and may be confirmed by using temporal artery biopsy.[16] Histologic analysis may reveal granulomatous inflammatory changes. In many patients, the clinical manifestation and laboratory values are suggestive of a diagnosis of temporal arteritis, and a biopsy is unnecessary. However, in cases of clinical uncertainty, biopsy may be required for a definitive diagnosis.

A characteristic gray-scale ultrasound finding of GCA involvement of the temporal artery is a diffusely thickened hypoechoic arterial wall or halo. Color and spectral Doppler ultrasonography may depict turbulent flow and stenosis of the affected vessel.[17] Contrast-enhanced, high-resolution MR imaging may depict mural thickening and enhancement of vessel wall, thereby suggesting the diagnosis.[18]

Secondary Vasculitis

Systemic vessel wall disease

Takayasu arteritis Takayasu arteritis (TA) is an idiopathic chronic inflammatory disease affecting the aorta, its main branches, and the pulmonary arteries.[19] TA leads to inflammation and fibrosis in the involved vessel walls resulting in luminal stenosis, occlusion, dilation, and aneurysm formation.[20] This disease is also known as aortitis syndrome, nonspecific aortoarteritis, pulseless disease, atypical coarctation of aorta, and aortic syndrome, among others.[20] Although reported worldwide, it is more frequently seen in Asia, the Mediterranean basin, South Africa, and Latin America.[21] The annual incidence of TA in North America was previously estimated to be 2.6 per million. TA has overall female preponderance, although the female to male ratio seems to decline from eastern Asia toward the West.[22,23] TA commonly occurs in the second and third decades of life.

The exact etiopathology remains unknown. The pathologic basis for this disease is a vasa vasoritis in the adventitia of large and medium-sized arteries.[22] TA involves a continuous length of the vessel, producing mural and luminal changes in some areas, and only mural changes in the intervening segments.[24,25] Even the angiographically normal areas have extensive wall changes on cross-sectional imaging.

The clinical manifestations of TA are usually divided into early and late phases. First there is an early or prepulseless phase characterized by nonspecific systemic features such as low-grade fever, night sweats, weight loss, arthralgia, and fatigue. The initial "inflammatory phase" is often followed by a secondary "pulseless phase"[26] characterized by vascular insufficiency from intimal narrowing of the vessels manifesting as arm or leg claudication, renal artery stenosis causing hypertension, and neurologic symptoms secondary to renovascular hypertension or ischemia (postural dizziness, seizures, amaurosis, hemiparesis, aphasia, cranial nerve palsies, and vertigo).

Imaging features of acute phase Significant findings of the acute phase of TA are wall thickening of the aorta and pulmonary artery.[26–30] High-resolution B-mode ultrasonography can detect increased intimal-medial thickness (IMT),[31] which is a reliable marker of active disease, especially in the absence of angiographically visible disease.[31] Similarly, unenhanced CT scans may show a high-density wall of variable thickness in the aorta or its branches along with calcification, and enhanced CT scan may show enhancement of the thickened wall in patients with an active inflammation (Fig. 4).[32,33] MR imaging can show subtle wall thickening in early cases, and may show a bright signal due to edema in and around the inflamed vessel on T2-weighted images (Fig. 5). During the acute phase, enhancement of the vessel wall and periadventitious soft tissues can also be observed (see Fig. 5).[34] Delayed contrast-enhanced MR imaging may also be a useful technique to identify inflammation in the arterial wall.[35] Overall these MR criteria are not highly sensitive, but are highly specific of disease activity.[34] Sometimes occlusion of the aortic branches or pulmonary artery, or both, is seen in the acute phase. Rarely, pseudoaneurysm formation occurs in the acute phase.[28] ^{18}F-Fluorodeoxyglucose positron emission tomography images coregistered with enhanced CT images have also demonstrated the distribution and inflammatory activity in the aorta, its branches, and the pulmonary artery in patients with active disease. The intensity of accumulation has been shown to decrease in response to therapy.[36]

Imaging features of late phase Significant findings of the late phase of TA include diffuse narrowing of the descending thoracic and abdominal aorta. Dilatation occurs most commonly in the ascending aorta.[26,28,30] Stenosis, the most common finding, involves all arteries arising from the aorta, most commonly the common carotid and subclavian arteries (see Fig. 5; Fig. 6). Occlusion is the second most common finding. Abrupt occlusion, abrupt transition to collateral vessels, and flame-shaped termination are characteristic. Among branches of abdominal aorta, the renal artery is the most frequently involved.[26,28] Pulmonary artery involvement is relatively high, with an estimated occurrence rate of 50% to 80%.[26,28] TA is also associated with aortic dissection and pseudoaneurysm formation in the late phase. MR angiography depicts these findings well, and is also useful for evaluation of bypass graft. Cine MR imaging can depict aortic regurgitation caused by dilatation of the ascending aorta.[28] Angiographic findings considered diagnostic of TA include a spectrum of changes ranging from minimal intimal irregularity to typical rat-tail narrowing, complete obstruction, or aneurysm formation in the involved vessels. Involvement of the aorta and/or at least 2 medium-sized branches is considered essential for diagnosis.

The diagnosis requires correlation of clinical, radiologic, and biochemical findings. The criteria for diagnosis include the presence of (1) symptoms caused by ischemia of the CNS, upper extremities, or kidneys; (2) fever, absent or decreased pulses, bruits, and fundoscopic findings; and (3) increased ESR and presence of C-reactive protein.

The goals of therapy in TA include the control of clinical activity by pharmacologic treatment using steroids and/or immunosuppressive therapy, restoration of blood flow to the stenosed vessel by surgical or endovascular techniques, pharmacologic control of blood pressure, and supportive

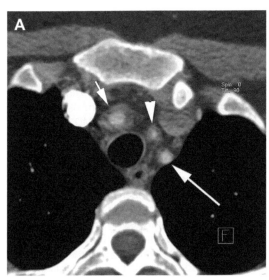
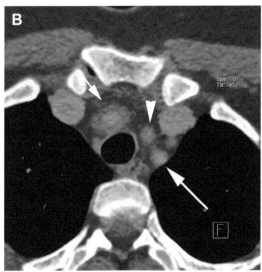

Fig. 4. Computed tomography (CT) findings in Takayasu arteritis. CT angiogram in early arterial phase (*A*) at level of root of great vessels shows increased thickness of brachiocephalic (*short arrow*), left common carotid (*arrowhead*), and left subclavian arteries (*long arrow*). CT angiogram in delayed phase (*B*) shows enhancement of thickened wall, suggesting active disease.

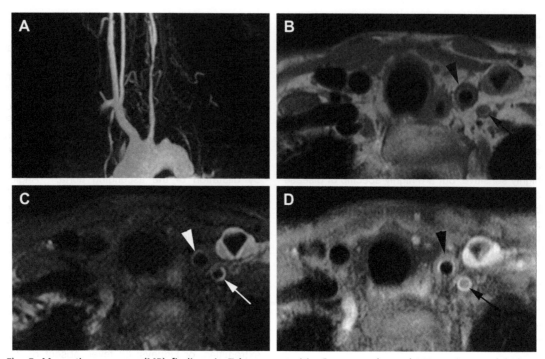

Fig. 5. Magnetic resonance (MR) findings in Takayasu arteritis. Contrast-enhanced MR angiogram (*A*) shows occlusion of left subclavian artery and long-segment irregularity and stenosis of left common carotid artery from its origin up to carotid bifurcation. Fat-saturated T1-weighted image (*B*) and T2-weighted image (*C*) show mural thickening and T2-hyperintensity of left common carotid (*arrowhead*) and left subclavian artery (*arrow*). Postgadolinium fat-saturated T1-weighted image (*D*) shows enhancement of the vessel wall. (*Courtesy of* Gurpreet Gulati, MD, Department of Cardiac-Radiology, All India Institute of Medical Sciences, New Delhi.)

management. Supra-aortic angioplasty is often not feasible in patients with TA because of involvement of the long segment of arteries.[37] Surgical treatment can be offered in the form of a bypass graft (ascending aorta to carotid/subclavian).[38,39] This repair is recommended in the "burnt-out" phase of the disease when further progression is unlikely.[40]

Moyamoya disease Moyamoya disease (MMD; *moyamoya* translates from Japanese as "puff of smoke") represents a rare cerebral steno-occlusive disease characterized by progressive occlusion of the terminal segments of the internal carotid arteries (ICAs)[41] and compensatory development of tortuous, dilated collateral networks. The result of these steno-occlusions is a severe impairment of the cerebrovascular reserve capacity. MMD is a progressive disease, as reflected by the MMD classification proposed by Suzuki and colleagues.[42] The term moyamoya syndrome is used in cases in which an underlying cause (sickle cell anemia, Down syndrome, Marfan syndrome, tuberous sclerosis, Turner syndrome, von Recklinghausen disease, atherosclerotic disease, coarctation of the aorta, fibromuscular dysplasia, and tuberculosis) can be identified.

In MMD, vascular occlusion results from a combination of hyperplasia of smooth muscle cells and luminal thrombosis. The media is often attenuated with irregular elastic lamina.[43] By definition, the pathognomic arteriographic findings are bilateral in MMD, although they can be asymmetric in degree and extent.[44] Patients with unilateral findings have the moyamoya syndrome and eventually up to 40% develop contralateral disease during follow-up.[45] Proximal posterior cerebral arteries may show stenosis or occlusion in up to 25% of patients with MMD.[46]

The exact etiology of MMD is unknown. The disease may be hereditary and multifactorial and may occur in a previously healthy individual. Whereas most cases have been reported in East Asia thus far, the number of pediatric as well as adult cases of MMD reported within the Caucasian population is growing steadily, due to an increasing awareness of the disease.[47] MMD has a bimodal age presentation, with the first peak occurring in the first decade of life and second peak in the fourth decade. Among pediatric patients, ischemic symptoms are the most common presentation, whereas adults may present with either ischemic or a hemorrhagic stroke, or both. In the United States, the rate

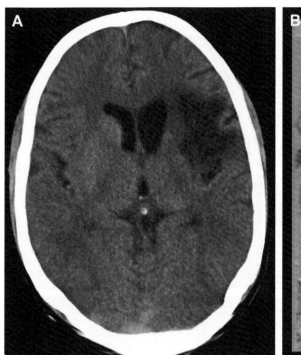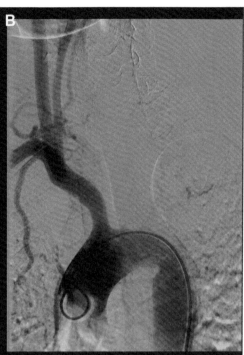

Fig. 6. Takayasu arteritis. Noncontrast computed tomography (NCCT) of head (A) shows a chronic infarct in left middle cerebral artery territory. Arch aortogram (B) shows complete occlusion of left common carotid and left subclavian artery from the arch. Mild stenosis of proximal branchiocephalic artery is also seen. (*Courtesy of* Gurpreet Gulati, MD, Department of Cardiac-Radiology, All India Institute of Medical Sciences, New Delhi.)

of hemorrhage among adults is approximately 7 times as high as the rate among children (20% vs 2.8%).[48,49] Compared with adults in the United States, adults in the Asian population have a much higher (42%) rate of hemorrhage in MMD.[50,51]

Depending on presentation, imaging may show evidence of ischemia (acute, subacute, or chronic) or hemorrhage (parenchymal, intraventricular or, rarely, subarachnoid). MR imaging can reveal stenosis or occlusion of distal ICA, decrease in size of flow voids of middle cerebral arteries (MCAs) and anterior cerebral arteries, presence of moyamoya vessels with signal voids within the basal ganglion and thalami, as well as ischemia, infarction, atrophy, and ventriculomegaly (Fig. 7).[52] T2*-weighted MR images may detect asymptomatic microbleeds in about 15% to 44% of adult patients.[53] On fluid-attenuated inversion recovery (FLAIR) images, diffuse leptomeningeal collaterals may appear as sulcal hyperintensity, referred to as the ivy sign (see Fig. 7). This ivy sign is seen in hemisphere with decreased cerebrovascular reserve. Diffusion-weighted and perfusion imaging are useful for evaluating cerebral ischemia in MMD. Regional cerebral perfusion in patients with MMD is decreased and delayed with posterior cerebral artery (PCA) stenosis, with a greater decrease and delay with PCA occlusion. If the PCA is occluded, the number of leptomeningeal collateral vessels to the anterior circulation presumably decreases; thereby causing severe cerebral ischemia that results in an infarction. Contrast-enhanced T1-weighted images show marked leptomeningeal enhancement along the cortical sulci, as well as enhancement of moyamoya vessels in cases with advanced MMD.[54]

MR angiography is also useful for the diagnosis of MMD in a noninvasive way. MR angiography shows terminal ICA stenosis or occlusion, and the presence of moyamoya collaterals (see Fig. 7). Conventional arteriography, the ultimate gold standard in the evaluation of patients suspected to have MMD, is reserved for presurgical evaluation before vascular anastomosis and is also useful in assessing the development of collateral pathways following surgical revascularization (Fig. 8). Incidental major artery aneurysms can be found in 3.6% of adult patients with nonhemorrhagic MMD, an observed frequency that increases with age. About half of these aneurysms are located in the posterior circulation, particularly in older patients with bilateral MMD (Fig. 9).[55]

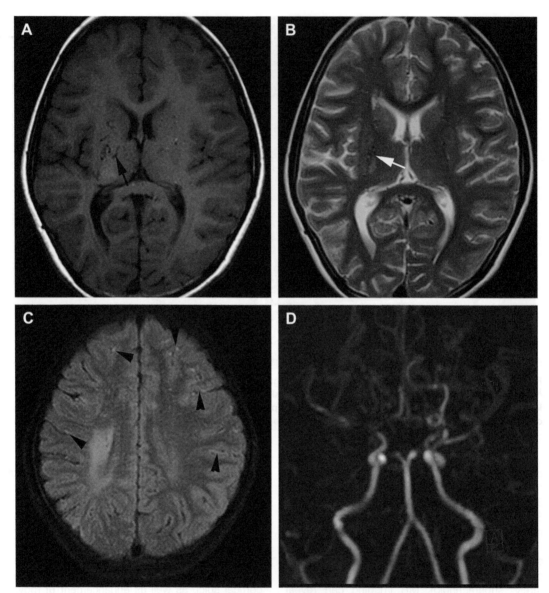

Fig. 7. MR imaging findings in moyamoya disease. Axial T1-weighted image (*A*) and T2-weighted image (*B*) show flow-void signals resulting from basal collaterals (*arrow*). Axial unenhanced fluid-attenuated inversion recovery (FLAIR) image (*C*) shows multiple areas of high signal intensity (*arrowheads*) in leptomeninges "ivy sign." MR angiography (*D*) shows stenosis of bilateral terminal internal carotid arteries (ICAs), and proximal anterior cerebral arteries and middle cerebral arteries (MCAs), typical of moyamoya.

Patients with MMD seem to progress with time, even if they are asymptomatic. Surgical treatment has been advocated as the treatment of choice to improve cerebral hemodynamics and to reduce the risk of subsequent strokes.[56] Three types of surgical revascularization procedures can be done: direct (superficial temporal artery-MCA anastomosis), indirect (encephaloduroarteriosynangiosis, encephalomyosynangiosis, and so forth), or combined.

Polyarteritis nodosa Polyarteritis nodosa (PAN) is a focal panmural necrotizing vasculitis in small and medium-sized arteries (and sometimes small veins) that can involve any organ and in varying degrees.[57] The kidneys may be involved in 70% to 80% of cases; the gastrointestinal tract, peripheral nerves, and skin in 50%; skeletal muscles and mesentery in 30%; and the CNS in 10%.[58] The characteristic pathologic findings are fibrinoid necrotizing inflammatory foci in the walls of small

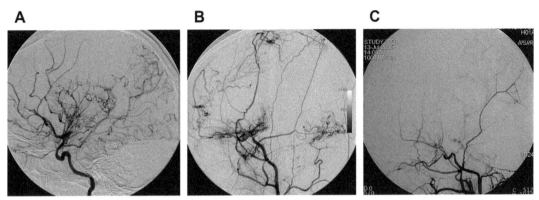

Fig. 8. Angiographic findings in different stages of moyamoya. (*A*) Suzuki grades I to II, with stenosis of terminal ICA with development of basal and pial collaterals. (*B*) Suzuki grades III to IV, with significant narrowing of the internal carotid artery and characteristic "puff-of-smoke" collaterals. There is diminished cortical perfusion. (*C*) shows Suzuki grades V to VI, with obliteration of the ICA distal to the origin of ophthalmic artery with concomitant disappearance of the puff-of-smoke collaterals.

and medium-sized arteries, with multiple small aneurysms (**Fig. 10**). In the reparative and chronic stages, fibroblast proliferation causes wall thickening and may produce areas of stenosis or occlusion, which may lead to ischemia or infarction. This pathophysiology produces the two angiographic findings of polyarteritis nodosa, aneurysms on the one hand and stenoses or occlusions on the other. If left untreated, polyarteritis nodosa is usually fatal. However, treatment with corticosteroids and cyclophosphamide improves the chance for survival.

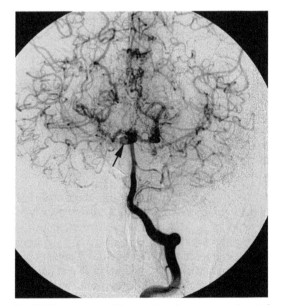

Fig. 9. Moyamoya with associated aneurysm. Frontal projection of left vertebral artery angiogram shows dysplastic basilar top aneurysm (*arrow*) and diffuse leptomeningeal collaterals.

Autoimmune vasculitis

Systemic lupus erythematosus, Behçet disease, Wegener granulomatosis, and Sjögren syndrome comprise the majority of autoimmune conditions associated with CNS vasculitis. In all of these disorders, the precise pathogenesis remains obscure; in all, however, the immune system seems to play a central role, and immunosuppressive agents are the cornerstones of treatment.

On MR imaging of brain the typical appearance of CNS vasculitis includes multiple subcortical infarctions, although substantial variation in the number, size, and location of the lesions may occur in this condition. MR imaging may not reveal all abnormal brain regions in such patients. MR studies reveal abnormalities in the vast majority of patients with CNS autoimmune vasculitis, and in this sense the sensitivity of MR imaging is quite high. However, findings on MR imaging are not specific for vasculitis, and similar MR findings may occur in patients suffering from multiple sclerosis, low-grade gliomas, mitochondrial disorders, substance abuse, and other conditions.

Table 1 contains a brief summary of clinical findings and imaging features in various autoimmune vasculitides.

Infectious vasculitis

Infection is a well-recognized cause of secondary vasculitis; many different agents have been implicated. It is important to have a high index of suspicion for infection as the cause of vasculitis, because treatment can be directed at the underlying organism. General clues to infectious vasculitis are associated fever, abnormality of the peripheral leukocyte count, and recent or current extraneural infection.

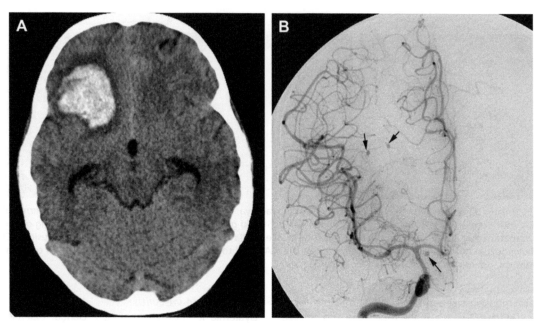

Fig. 10. Polyarteritis nodosa. NCCT (*A*) shows right frontal acute hematoma. Anteroposterior projection of arterial phase of right ICA angiogram (*B*) shows microaneurysms (*arrows*) in smaller MCA branches.

Bacteria Acute septic meningitis, attributable to several bacterial agents, may cause vasculitis and cerebral infarcts in 5% to 15% of adults with bacterial meningitis and in up to 30% of neonates.

Mycobacterium tuberculosis is the commonest cause of chronic meningitis, and typically follows rupture of an old tubercle with the release of myco-bacteria in the subarachnoid space. The thick gelatinous inflammatory exudate that typically contains organisms, mononuclear cells, tubercles, and caseation necrosis settles at the base of the brain along cisterns, particularly in the Sylvian fissure, where arteritis can form along traversing blood vessels. Resultant ischemic infarction occurs in up to 41% of patients.[59] The infection may include vasculitis of the smaller and middle-sized cerebral arteries, often the lenticulostriate arteries or the posterior cerebral branches and the thalamoperforating arteries, leading to small infarctions in the basal ganglion and deep white matter (**Fig. 11**).

Fungi Four fungal agents, *Aspergillus*,[60] *Candida*, *Coccidioides*,[61] and *Mucormycetes*, are important CNS pathogens, particularly in the setting of leukopenia, sepsis, drug-induced or human immu-nodeficiency virus (HIV)-related immunosuppres-sion, and severe debilitation. All have the capacity to invade arteries of the CNS in the course of disseminated infection and meningitis. Vasculitis may be acute, subacute, or a late complication of CNS infection. Cerebral infarction results from direct vascular injury leading to aneu-rysm formation, vascular thrombosis, endarteritis, and cerebral hemorrhage, or results from microab-scesses, or extension along contiguous sites of infection. Mucormycosis may be particularly ag-gressive in poorly controlled diabetes. There may be associated spread from sites of nasopharyngi-tis, oropharyngitis, and sinusitis to the cavernous sinus and ICA, leading to focal thrombosis and cerebral infarction, detectable by imaging studies (**Fig. 12**).

Viral agents CNS vasculitis can occur in the course of infection by varicella zoster virus (VZV) and retroviral infection. Hepatitis virus types A and C are also associated with CNS vasculitis, but preferably affect the peripheral nervous system. Cytomegalovirus causes retinitis, menin-goencephalitis, myelitis, and CNS vasculitis in association with HIV infection.

VZV vasculopathy VZV vasculopathies can com-plicate zoster (secondary VZV infection) or vari-cella (primary VZV infection). The spectrum of VZV vasculopathy is widening and includes ischemic infarction of the brain and spinal cord, aneurysm formation,[62] subarachnoid and cerebral hemorrhage, carotid dissection and, rarely, pe-ripheral arterial disease.[63] VZV vasculopathy in immunocompetent or immunocompromised indi-viduals can be unifocal or multifocal with both deep-seated and superficial infarctions. Lesions at the gray-white matter junction on brain imaging are a clue to diagnosis.[63] Angiography reveals segmental narrowing, thrombosis, and beading along proximal branches of the anterior and MCAs.

HIV vasculopathy HIV-infected children have an increased incidence of cerebrovascular disease that is associated with severe immune suppression[64] and with vertically acquired HIV infection or exposure to the virus in the neonatal period. Both medium-sized arteries and veins are involved, with the development of aneurysms, vessel occlusion, embolic disease, and venous thrombosis. The aneurysms tend to be fusiform in shape and involve both major arteries of the circle of Willis and second- and third-order branches, which differentiates these aneurysms from berry aneurysms (**Fig. 13**).[65,66] Vasculopathy often remains asymptomatic until a complication, such as the rupture of an aneurysm or a stroke, occurs. Vasculopathy can be identified both on MR and digital angiography as caliber variation and irregularity of vessels (see **Fig. 13**). Early diagnosis is important because treatment with highly active antiretroviral therapy and corticosteroids may stop disease progression or even induce regression of the vasculopathy.[67]

Parasites—cysticercosis Cerebrovascular complications of neurocysticercosis include lacunar infarction or large-vessel disease, progressive midbrain syndrome, transient ischemic attacks, and brain hemorrhage.[68,69] Mechanisms of cerebrovascular complications include luminal narrowing due to subintimal cushions, vasospasm due to arteritis in midsized and small perforating vessels of the brain, and fresh thrombi.[69] Vasculitis must be suspected when segmental narrowing, a beaded appearance, or an abrupt or tapered area of vascular obstruction is noted at angiography.[70] Based on angiographic criteria, arteritis is seen in up to 53% of patients with subarachnoid neurocysticercosis, including asymptomatic patients, with the middle and posterior cerebral arteries being most commonly affected (**Fig. 14**).[70] Multivessel involvement is noted in nearly 50% of cases, and infarction associated with arteritis is seen in 2% to 12%.[70] Neuroimaging studies reveal cysts, mural nodules, basilar meningitis, hydrocephalus, and vascular lesions (see **Fig. 14**).

Mycotic aneurysms It is estimated that mycotic aneurysms (MAs) develop in approximately 2% to 5% of patients with infective endocarditis.[71] Common bacterial pathogens associated with MA are *Streptococcus viridans* (approximately 50%) and *Staphylococcus aureus* (approximately

10%).[72] Mechanisms of aneurysm formation include direct bacterial infection, septic or bland embolic occlusion of the vasa vasorum,[71] and immune complex deposition injuring the arterial wall. MAs tend to develop at arterial branch points, which are the common sites of embolic impaction, particularly in the distal middle cerebral artery branches at bifurcations (**Fig. 15**).

Drug-induced vasculopathy

Some antibiotics (sulfonamide), chemotherapeutic agents (thiouracil), and illicit drugs (cocaine, heroin, amphetamine) can cause vasculitis or vasculopathy.[73] Cocaine usually affects medium-sized arteries, resulting in infarction. The diagnosis of vasculitis is based on the pathologic findings and not on the aforementioned angiographic findings.

Radiation vasculopathy

Radiation-induced injuries to large cerebral arteries that result in stenotic and/or occlusive vasculopathy are an important delayed complication of radiation therapy. These injuries usually evolve slowly to produce ischemic effects, years or even decades after irradiation.[74] MR images of wall thickening and prominent ring enhancement of the wall of affected large cerebral arteries[75,76] may be a diagnostic clue in differentiating radiation-induced arteritis from MMD.[77]

Reversible Cerebral Vasoconstriction Syndrome

Reversible cerebral vasoconstriction syndrome (RCVS) describes a group of disorders characterized by reversible segmental cerebral vasoconstriction. These disorders include TCH with vasoconstriction, benign angiopathy of the CNS, Call-Fleming syndrome, postpartum angiopathy, and drug-induced vasospasm.[78–80] Patients can present with isolated TCH or TCH in conjunction with altered cognition, motor and sensory deficits, seizures, visual disturbances, ataxia, speech abnormalities, nausea, and vomiting. Patients with RCVS may have a normal MR examination, or MR imaging may show abnormalities consistent with posterior reversible leukoencephalopathy or watershed infarctions in the distal vascular territory of cerebral vessels, with severe spasm.[81] Angiography shows reversible alternating segments of vasoconstriction and dilation in the proximal and distal branches of the circle of Willis. RCVS cannot be differentiated from PACNS by a single vascular imaging study. However, in patients with RCVS, substantial improvement in vasospasm, even in the absence of specific treatment, is expected within 4 weeks of symptom onset. Several months might be needed

Table 1
Clinical, laboratory, and imaging findings in various autoimmune disorders with vasculitis

	Disease Name	Systemic Diagnosis	Neurologic Symptoms	Laboratory Findings	Imaging
1	Rheumatic Disease	Severe constitutional symptoms Prominent extra-articular manifestations of vasculitis affecting the skin, eyes, heart, and/or lungs	Nonspecific multitude of neurologic signs and symptoms	Rheumatic factor Elevated ESR	Scattered WM lesions
2	Systemic Lupus Erythematosus (SLE)		Often presents with neuropsychiatric symptoms	Antinuclear antibodies Antibodies against dsDNA	Cortical infarctions mimicking MELAS Scattered WM lesions mimicking multiple sclerosis Severe basal ganglion changes mimicking deep venous thrombosis Extensive calcification of the basal ganglion, dendrate nucleus, centrum semiovale, and corticosubcortical region Normal MR imaging
3	Sneddon syndrome	Generalized livedo recemosa	Large and small arterial infarcts with severe neurologic consequences and often cognitive deterioration	Elevated ESR Anticardiolipin antibodies	Multiple smaller and large infarcts with prominent cortical involvement Multiple hemosiderin deposits with extensive superficial hemosiderosis
4	Antiphospholipid antibody syndrome (1° or 2° to SLE, postinfections drug induced)	Hypercoagulative state, which leads to thrombotic complications, stroke, myocardial infarctions, dementia, and fetal loss. Cardiac value vegetations, mitral regurgitation	Infarcts Early-onset dementia		Multiple WM lesions, lesion usually extends into the cortical layers

5	Sjögren syndrome	Involvement of salivary and lachrymal glands; constitutional symptoms: fatigue, malaise, low-grade fever; Reynaud syndrome; lymphadenopathy	Trigeminal neuropathy Recurrent aseptic meningoencephalitis Transverse myelitis Chronic progressive myelitis Neuropsychiatric symptoms		Nonspecific extensive gray and white matter lesions Microhemorrhages
6	Scleroderma	CREST (Calcinosis, Reynaud syndrome, Esophageal problems, Sclerodactylia, and Telangiectasia syndrome)	Pain and parethesias from nerve entrapment; territorial strokes, epileptics seizures, recurrent loss of consciousness, multiple spontaneous intracerebral hemorrhages	Anticentromere antibiotics	Nonspecific Middle-sized artery infarcts Macrohemorrhages and microhemorrhages Extensive calcifications
7	Neurosarcoidosis (5% of patients with systemic sarcoidosis)	Systemic granulamatous disease, affecting lungs with lung fibrosis, hilar lymph nodes skin, liver, spleen	Facial nerve paralysis (most common manifestation)	Not very helpful Positive angiotensin-converting enzyme test in CSF pleocytosis	Suprasellar leptomeningeal disease WM lesions
8	Wegener granulomatosis	Recurrent epistaxis or sinusitis, pulmonary infiltrates and/or nodules, glomerulonephritis, ocular involvement Dyspnea, hoarseness, cough, wheezing, and other symptoms of tracheal or parenchymal lung diseases	Cranial neuropathy Seizure Peripheral neuropathy, stroke, or TIAs Headache	Cytoplasmic antineutrophil antibodies in 90%	Sinusitis Destruction of petrous part of temporal lobe Erosion of lamina papyracea Enhancement of cranial nerves Pachymeningeal thickening and enhancement Infarct
9	Churg-Strauss syndrome, granulamatous inflammation, and necrotizing vasculitis involving small to medium-sized vessels	Allergic rhinitis, asthma, eosinophilia, pulmonary infiltrates, coronary arteritis, intestinal ischemia	Commonly involves the peripheral nervous system and presents as a mononeuritis multiplex CNS involvement is seen in 10% of patients	Perinuclear antineutrophil antibodies (pANCA)	Macroinfarctions or microinfarctions Macrohemorrhages or microhemorrhages

(continued on next page)

Table 1
(continued)

	Disease Name	Systemic Diagnosis	Neurologic Symptoms	Laboratory Findings	Imaging
10	Microscopic polyarteritis (polyangiopathy), necrotizing vasculitis of small vessels, arterioles, capillaries, or veins without granulomas	Pulmonary hemorrhage, glomerulonephritis	Peripheral and cranial nerve involvement Stroke	pANCA (+vein 50%–80%)	Macroinfarcts or microinfarcts
11	Behçet disease (multisystem recurrent vasculitis of supposedly autoimmune origin); blood vessels of all sizes are involved, arteries as well as veins	Clinical triad: recurrent oral ulcers, genital ulcers, and anterior or posterior uveitis	CNS involvement in 5%–10% of cases Headache Meningoencephalitis Cranial nerve palsies Cerebellar ataxia Spastic paraparesis or tetraparesis Raised intracranial pressure Dementia	CSF pleocytosis, elevated protein, and elevated pressure	Asymmetric mesodiencephalic junction lesion with edema extending along certain long tracts in the brainstem, sparing red nucleus and involving diencephalon, pontobulbar region lesions; brainstem lesions are more frequent, larger, and more extensive than in multiple sclerosis Hemispheric WM lesions: focal or confluent, more likely to be subcortical than periventricular Spinal cord lesion: posterolateral, mainly cervical cord Cranial nerve enhancement, enhancement of intracranial and spinal cord lesions Cerebral venous thrombosis

Abbreviations: CNS, central nervous system; CSF, cerebrospinal fluid; ESR, erythrocyte sedimentation rate; MELAS, Mitochondrial Encephalopathy, Lactic Acidosis, and Stroke-like episodes; TIA, transient ischemic attack; WM, white matter.

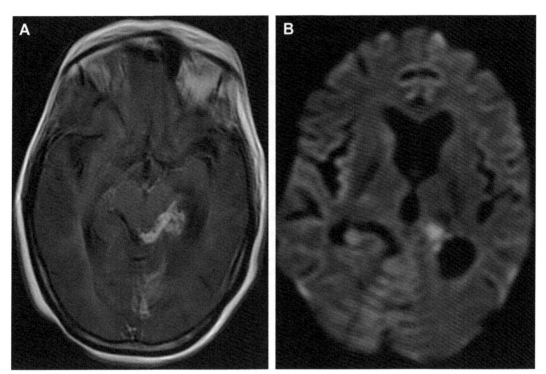

Fig. 11. Tuberculous vasculitis with infarct. Contrast-enhanced axial T1-weighted image (*A*) shows enhancing exudates in left perimesencephalic cistern. Axial diffusion-weighted MR image (*B*) shows an acute infarct in left posterior thalamus.

for complete normalization of vascular imaging. On the other hand, vascular imaging abnormalities in patients with PACNS rarely normalize completely.

Arterial Dissection

Dissections are defined as mural hemorrhage with formation of a hematoma between the tunica media and the tunica intima of involved artery, or

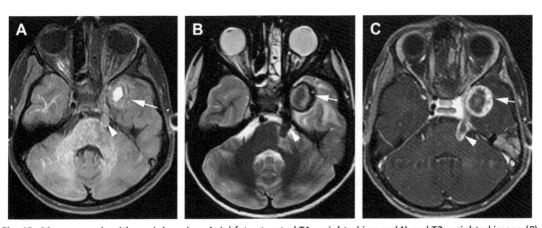

Fig. 12. Mucormycosis with angioinvasion. Axial fat-saturated T1-weighted image (*A*) and T2-weighted image (*B*) show T2-hypointense and T1-hyperintense lesions in sphenoid sinus, left cavernous sinus (CS), and extending posteriorly along the left trigeminal nerve, suggestive of fungal sinusitis with involvement of left CS and left trigeminal nerve (*arrowhead*). The left cavernous ICA flow void is not seen. In addition, a globular lesion (*arrow*) with T2-hypointense rim and core of T1-and T2-hypointensity is present in left CS, suggestive of thrombosed aneurysm. The wall of the aneurysm, sphenoid sinusitis, left CS, and left trigeminal nerve enhance following intravenous gadolinium administration (*C*).

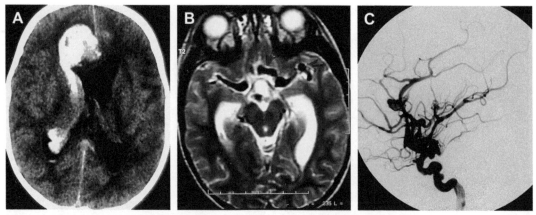

Fig. 13. Human immunodeficiency virus (HIV) vasculopathy. A 14-year-old boy (seropositive for HIV) presented with sudden onset severe headache. Contrast-enhanced CT (*A*) shows acute right frontal hematoma with intraventricular extension. Axial T2-weighted image (*B*) reveals multiple aneurysms involving circle of Willis. Brain parenchyma appears normal. Lateral view of left ICA angiogram (*C*) shows multiple dysplastic aneurysms involving ICA and its branches.

rarely subadventitial. Dissection may cause a variety of clinical presentations, including stroke, headache, neck pain, tinnitus, Horner syndrome, and cranial neuropathies.[82] Trauma is the most common cause of arterial dissection. Nontraumatic causes of dissection include fibromuscular dysplasia, hypertension, collagen vascular disorders, migraines, and oral contraceptive use. Nontraumatic dissections most often affect the cervical ICA at the bifurcation or at the proximal supraclinoid segment. Vertebral artery dissection is predominantly located in the pars transversaria (V2) or the atlas loop (V3).

On unenhanced CT, arterial dissection may appear as increased external diameter and a crescent-shaped hyperdense area corresponding to a wall hematoma.[83] On CT angiography, fairly reliable signs of arterial dissection are an intimal flap, a dissecting aneurysm, and a narrowed lumen with crescent-shaped mural thickening.

On MR imaging, diagnosis of arterial dissection depends on the characteristics of the intramural hematoma (size, shape, intensity), surrounding structures (fat, venous plexus, skull base, CSF), and MR imaging sequences (matrix, section thickness, pulse sequence).[84,85] The hematoma follows

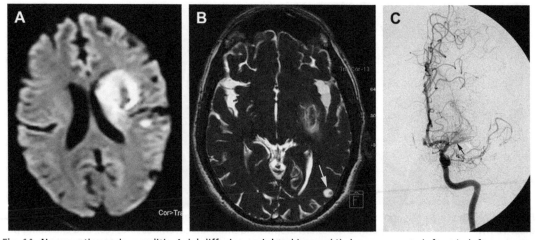

Fig. 14. Neurocysticercosis vasculitis. Axial diffusion-weighted image (*A*) shows an acute infarct in left corona radiata. Axial constructive interference in steady state image (*B*) shows racemose neurocysticercosis in left sylvian fissure. Another cysticercus with scolex is present in the left occipital lobe (*arrow*). Anteroposterior projection of left ICA angiogram (*C*) shows stenosis and irregularity of proximal left MCA (*arrow*) and nonvisualization of distal left MCA branches.

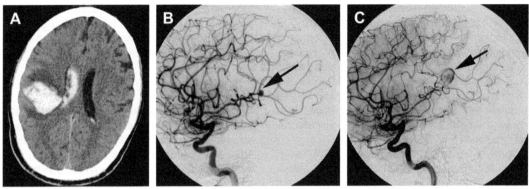

Fig. 15. Mycotic aneurysm. A 12-year-old boy with infective endocarditis presented with sudden-onset left hemiparesis. NCCT (*A*) shows right frontal hematoma. Lateral view of right ICA angiogram (*B*) reveals a small aneurysm (*arrow*) in distal branches of the right MCA. This patient was managed conservatively. Repeat angiogram (*C*) after 6 weeks shows increase in size of the aneurysm (*arrow*).

a typical evolution of signal intensity depending on the state of products of hemoglobin breakdown.[84,85] In the early and chronic stage, the hematoma is usually isointense to surrounding structures and may be obscured on T1-weighted images.[84] Subacute hematoma appears characteristically on T1-weighted image as a crescent-shaped hyperintense area around an eccentric flow void corresponding to the vessel lumen (Fig. 16). The hematoma usually becomes isointense within 6 months or disappears.[84]

MR angiography with 3-dimensional time-of-flight (3D TOF) imaging demonstrated excellent sensitivity and specificity of 95% and 99%, respectively, in diagnosis of carotid dissection, but poor sensitivity (20%) in diagnosis of vertebral artery dissection compared with conventional angiography.[86] Accurate evaluation of dissection

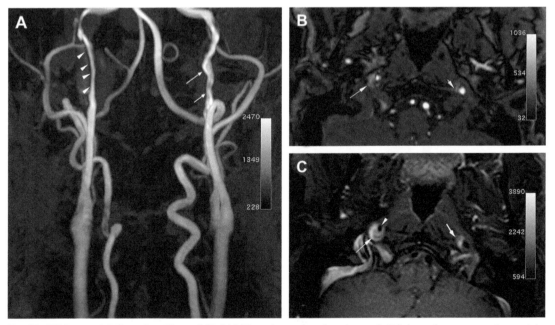

Fig. 16. MR in arterial dissection. Time-of-flight MR angiography of neck vessels (*A*) shows long segment eccentric stenosis of right ICA (*arrowheads*) and double lumen in cervical segment of left ICA (*arrows*). Base image of TOF angiography (*B*) shows flow-related enhancement with eccentric hyperintense thrombus with false lumen (*arrows*). Fat-saturated T1-weighted image (*C*) clearly demonstrates flow void of patient vessel (*arrowheads*) and eccentric subacute thrombi within vessel wall (*arrows*).

relies on a combined reading of axial MR images and MR angiogram source images.[86] On TOF MR angiography, subacute dissection appears as pseudoenlargement of the lumen corresponding to flow associated with the intramural hematoma, simulating blood flow.[86] Contrast-enhanced MR angiography is able to demonstrate luminal irregularities and stenosis with an increased field of view, from the aortic arch through the intracranial circulation.[87,88]

Digital subtraction angiography (DSA), even though regarded as gold standard, is not always definitive in the diagnosis of dissection because the thickness and configuration of the arterial wall are not appreciable. DSA may reveal long, tapered, usually eccentric, and irregular stenosis that begins distal to the carotid bulb ("string" sign),[89] focal narrowing with a distal site of dilatation ("string and pearl" sign), a tapered occlusion that spares the carotid bulb ("flame" sign),[90]

tapered stenosis with concomitant dissecting aneurysm, occlusion, and only dissecting aneurysm (Fig. 17). Pathognomonic signs, such as a double lumen or intimal flap, are rarely observed.[89,91]

DURAL ARTERIOVENOUS FISTULAS

Dural arteriovenous fistulas (DAVFs), also called dural arteriovenous malformations, are acquired lesions in the dura mater and represent 10% to 15% of all intracranial vascular malformations.[92] Although DAVFs can occur anywhere in the dura mater covering the brain, they occur most frequently in the cavernous and transverse-sigmoid sinuses. Venous outflow obstruction, sometimes associated with sinus thrombosis, can precede formation of some DAVFs.

Typically, DAVFs are acquired. Patients may be asymptomatic or may experience symptoms ranging from mild symptoms to fatal hemorrhage.

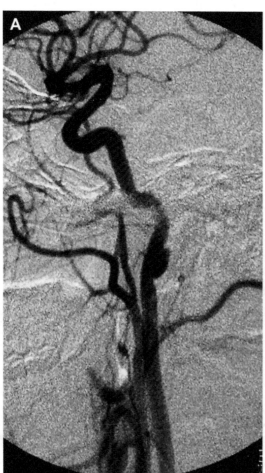 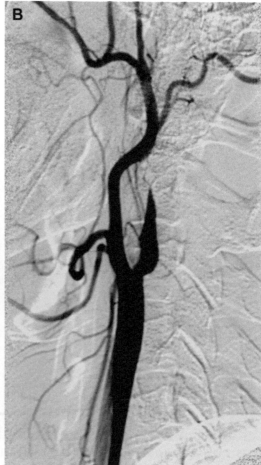

Fig. 17. Digital subtraction angiography (DSA) in arterial dissection. Lateral left ICA angiogram (A) shows a dissecting aneurysm in distal cervical segment of ICA. Lateral view of ICA angiogram (B) demonstrates tapered occlusion of ICA distal to carotid bulb, suggesting occlusion secondary to dissection.

Furthermore, these symptoms may be characterized as either nonaggressive (benign) (eg, tinnitus) or aggressive (eg, intracranial hemorrhage, neurologic deficits). DAVFs with direct or indirect cortical venous drainage are considered to carry a high risk for hemorrhage that mandates prompt diagnosis and treatment.

Head CT typically does not detect DAVFs, although dilated veins may suggest their presence. The spectrum of MR imaging findings is very variable. Fistulas may be seen as a flow void cluster around the dural venous sinus on MR imaging or as flow-related enhancement along the involved sinus on MR angiography. Other MR imaging findings may include engorged ophthalmic vein/proptosis, white matter hyperintensity, intracranial hemorrhage, dilated leptomeningeal or medullary vessels, venous pouch, and leptomeningeal or medullary vascular enhancements (Fig. 18).[93–95] DAVFs may be better appreciated on susceptibility-weighted images (SWI) where venous vasculature appears prominent because of venous engorgement and slow flow, allowing increased oxygen extraction.[96] MR angiography is a complementary tool for the identification of DAVF and may show identifiable fistulas, venous flow–related enhancement, and prominent extracranial vessels. It has been reported that an MR imaging demonstration of leptomeningeal or medullary vascular dilation and enhancements predicts poor outcome and indicates a need for emergent therapy.[93] Four-dimensional contrast-enhanced MR angiography on a 3-T scanner with parallel imaging is a reliable diagnostic tool for the characterization of intracranial DAVFs, especially with respect to the fistula site and the route of venous drainage.[97]

Intra-arterial DSA remains the criterion standard for the assessment of intracranial DAVFs. Its inherent high spatial and temporal resolution facilitates the accurate analysis of the fistula site and the discernment of the feeding arteries and draining veins. General approaches for the treatment of DAVFs include conservative treatment, radiation therapy, endovascular intervention, and surgery.

CEREBRAL VENOUS THROMBOSIS

CVT is a relatively uncommon but serious neurologic disorder. Tissue damage and stasis (eg, trauma, surgery, and immobilization), hematologic disorders (eg, protein C and protein S deficiencies), malignancies, collagen vascular diseases, pregnancy, and some medications (eg, oral contraceptives) have been reported to be predisposing factors for CVT. Nearly 20% of cases of CVT are idiopathic.[98]

On unenhanced CT, acute blood clot or thrombus within the dural sinus (dense triangle sign) (Fig. 19) or cortical vein (cord sign) may be identified as an elongated high-attenuation lesion in 20% of patients.[98,99] An ischemic infarction, sometimes with a hemorrhagic component, may be seen. An ischemic lesion that crosses the usual arterial boundaries (particularly with a hemorrhagic component) or in close proximity to a venous sinus is suggestive of CVT.[100–102] In 10% to 30% of cases of CVT, the findings on either unenhanced or contrast-enhanced CT are negative.

MR imaging is more sensitive than CT in early detection of thrombosis and is more accurate in depicting the extent and complications of CVT.[103] The principal early signs of CVT on

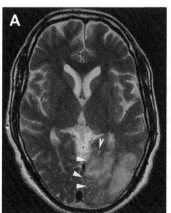 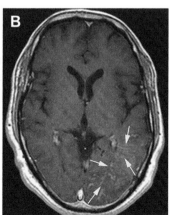 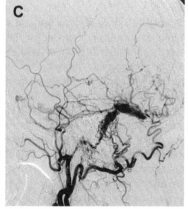

Fig. 18. Dural arteriovenous malformation. (A) Axial T2-weighted image shows hyperintensity with effacement of cortical sulci in left occipital lobe. In addition, multiple tiny tortuous flow voids (arrowheads) are seen. Postgadolinium axial T1-weighted image (B) shows enhancement of medullary veins (arrows) in left occipital lobe. Early arterial phase left vertebral artery angiogram (C) shows left sigmoid transverse sinus dural arteriovenous malformation.

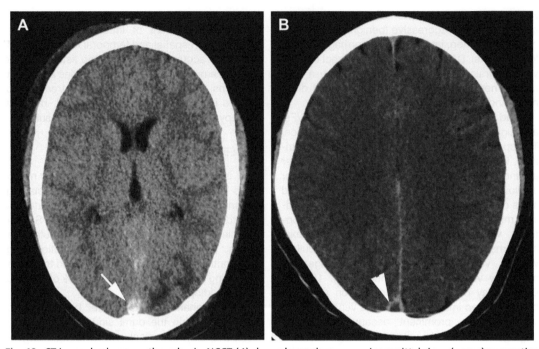

Fig. 19. CT in cerebral venous thrombosis. NCCT (*A*) shows hyperdense superior sagittal sinus (*arrow*) suggesting thrombosis. Contrast-enhanced CT (*B*) shows filling defect (*arrowhead*) within posterior superior sagittal sinus (empty delta sign).

unenhanced MR imaging are the combination of absence of a flow void with alteration of signal intensity in the dural sinus due to thrombus (**Fig. 20**). Because the signal intensity of venous thrombi on MR images changes over time according to the biochemical status of hemoglobin, the signal intensity of dural sinuses in different MR sequences also changes with time. The secondary signs of MR imaging may show similar patterns to CT, including cerebral swelling, edema, and/or hemorrhage.[104,105] On MR imaging, FLAIR and T2-weighted images show cortical and subcortical high-signal-intensity lesions.[106] DWI may reveal mixed signal intensity, which relates to both cytotoxic and vasogenic edema.[106,107] SWI may show a prominent hypointense signal in the veins due to increased concentration of deoxyhemoglobin in the involved veins. If treated successfully, this effect disappears.[108] An infarction not conforming to a major arterial vascular territory, such as the presence of multiple isolated lesions, involvement of a subcortical region with sparing of the cortex, and extension over more than one arterial distribution are highly suspicious of a venous origin.[109] Bilateral parasagittal hemispheric lesions are suggestive of superior sagittal sinus thrombosis. Ipsilateral temporo-occipital and cerebellar lobe lesions can be found in transverse sinus thrombosis. Bilateral or unilateral infarction in the

thalami, basal ganglia, and internal capsule is typically seen in deep venous thrombosis (**Fig. 21**).

MR venography can add to the diagnostic value of routine MR imaging, and better demonstrates the layout of the major cerebral veins and dural venous sinuses. In MR venography, thrombosis is suggested by absence of normal flow signal in a sinus or a vein, or frayed appearance of the venous sinus. CT venography can provide a rapid and reliable modality for detecting CVT.[110,111] CT venography is much more useful in subacute or chronic situations because of the varied density in thrombosed sinus. CT venography is at least equivalent to MR venography in the diagnosis of CVT.[109,112] Invasive cerebral angiographic procedures are less commonly needed to establish the diagnosis of CVT given the availability of MR venography and CT venography.[105,113] These techniques are reserved for situations in which the MR venography or CT venography results are inconclusive or if an endovascular procedure is being considered.

NONTRAUMATIC HEMORRHAGE
Intracerebral Hemorrhage

Neuroimaging studies are not only required for diagnosis but also provide important insights into the type of hemorrhage, the underlying etiology,

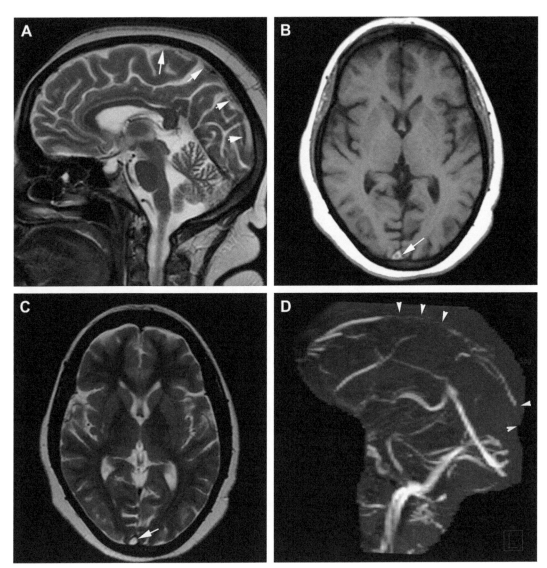

Fig. 20. Superior sagittal sinus thrombosis. Sagittal T2-weighted (*A*), axial T1-weighted (*B*), and axial T2-weighted (*C*) images show loss of flow void in superior sagittal sinus (*small arrows* in *A, B* and *C*). TOF MR angiography (*D*) shows nonvisualization of posterior superior sagittal sinus (*arrowheads* in *D*), confirming thrombosis.

and the accompanying pathophysiology. Unenhanced CT is still the modality of choice for the assessment of ICH, owing to its widespread availability and rapid acquisition time.

On unenhanced CT, acute intracerebral hematoma typically appears hyperdense, with associated mass effect depending on size and location of hematoma (**Fig. 22**). Rapidly accumulating hematoma and unretracted semiliquid clot may result in hypodense areas within generally hyperdense acute hematomas, the so-called swirl sign. Sometimes acute hematoma may be isodense if there is severe anemia, impaired clot formation due to coagulopathy, or volume averaging with

adjacent hematoma. Fluid-fluid levels within the clot can also occur, and are more common in hematomas caused by anticoagulation, but this is not specific and has also been described in hematomas due to hypertension, trauma, tumor, or arteriovenous malformation. More than 33% of patients with ICH have substantial hematoma expansion when imaged within 3 hours of onset, and expansion is associated with poorer outcome.[114] It has been found that contrast extravasation on CTA is an early predictor of hematoma expansion.[115]

On MR imaging, the appearance of ICH is more complicated and time dependent. The MR signal

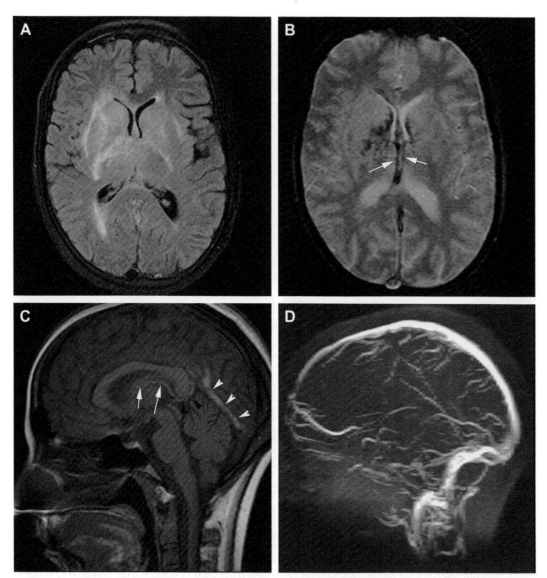

Fig. 21. Deep venous sinus thrombosis. Axial unenhanced FLAIR MR image (*A*) shows hyperintensity in bilateral corpus striatum and thalami. Axial T2-weighted MR imaging (*B*) demonstrates hemorrhages in bilateral basal ganglia. Both internal cerebral veins are hypointense (*arrows*). Sagittal T1-weighted MR image (*C*) shows hyperintensity in region of internal cerebral veins (*arrows*), veins of Galen (*black arrowheads*), and straight sinus (*white arrowheads*), suggestive of subacute thrombosis. MR venography (*D*) shows nonvisualization of deep venous system.

intensity of hemorrhage is mainly dependent on both the chemical state of the iron atoms within the hemoglobin molecule and the integrity of the red blood cell membrane. In practice, there is considerable variability in the orderly progression of hematoma signal change over time. It is common to see different stages appear simultaneously. For these reasons, "dating" of bleed onset using MR imaging data alone is intrinsically imprecise.

Pattern recognition clues to the etiology of ICH
It may be possible to predict the cause of ICH based on the age of the patient, and distribution and imaging characteristics of hematoma (**Table 2**).

Subarachnoid Hemorrhage

Subarachnoid hemorrhage (SAH) is a serious condition that accounts for 5% of all strokes.[116]

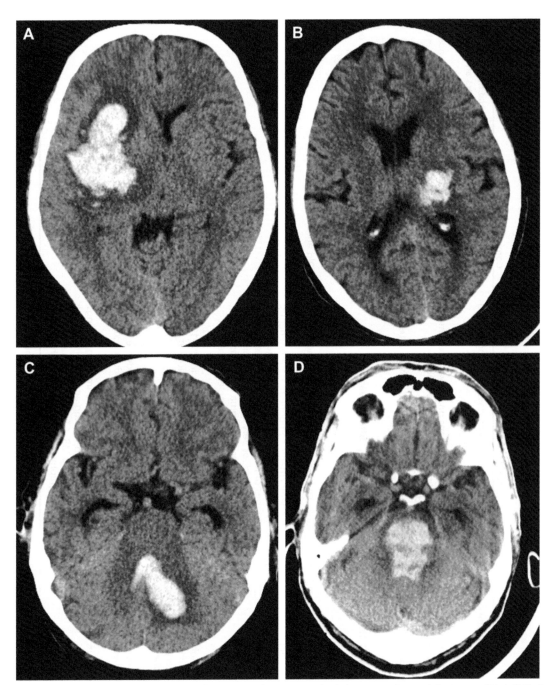

Fig. 22. Hypertensive hematoma. NCCT shows acute hematomas in right external capsule/putamen (*A*), left thalamus (*B*), left cerebellum (*C*), and pons (*D*).

The clinical hallmark of SAH is a history of a TCH or an unusually severe headache that started suddenly in a previously healthy patient, especially when associated with meningism and/or loss of consciousness. The most common cause of a nontraumatic SAH is an aneurysm rupture. The differential diagnosis of nonaneurysmal SAH is broad, including perimesencephalic nonaneurysmal SAH, arteriovenous malformations, tumors, pituitary apoplexy, CVT, vasculitis, hematological conditions (including leukemia and coagulopathies), and drugs (including cocaine, ephedrine, and amphetamine).

If SAH is suspected, unenhanced CT scan is the first line of investigation in confirming its presence. Acute SAH appears as hyperdensity in the CSF

Table 2
Pattern recognition in intracerebral hemorrhage (ICH)

	Location	Imaging Findings	Comments
Hypertension (see Fig. 22)	External capsule/putamina, thalamus, pons, cerebellum	Acute hematoma with classic imaging findings	Suggest angiography for putaminal hemorrhage unless patient is older than 55 years and is hypertensive[128]
Cavernoma (see Fig. 23)	Pons is favorite location; abuts pal or ventricular surface	"Popcorn"-like lesions on T2-weighted image with hypointense rim, rim booms on gradient sequences	May be associated with developmental venous anomaly, scan best after intravenous contrast
Hemorrhagic transformation of infarct	Hemorrhage localized to cortex	Nonhemorrhagic component within arterial territory	
Venous infarct	Hematoma in WM or WM-gray matter junction	Evidence of CVT, Diffusion variable	Parasagittal region if thrombosis is superficial or bithalamic if thrombosis is in deep venous system; posterior temporal lobe if vein of Labbe occlusion
Cerebral amyloid angiopathy	Lobar bleed, spares basal ganglion	Multiple hemorrhages of different ages	Old age
Neoplasm	Anywhere in brain	Nonhemorrhagic component; heterogeneous; delayed evolution of signal changes; multiple stages of hematoma in the same lesion; absent, diminished, or very irregular hypointense rim; persistent perihematoma edema and mass effect; inappropriate enhancement in acute lesion	
Aneurysm	Medial frontal lobe (ruptured anterior communicating artery or anterior cerebral artery aneurysm) and temporal lobe (ruptured MCA aneurysm)	Parenchymal hematoma is seen in 4%–19% of patients with SAH due to saccular aneurysm	When ICH is immediately adjacent to the subarachnoid space at the base of the brain or basal interhemispheric fissure, vascular imaging should be strongly considered to exclude saccular aneurysm
Trauma	Orbitofrontal regions, anterior temporal lobes	Presence of fluid-blood level; evidence of head trauma: scalp hematoma, subdural/extradural hematomas	
Arteriovenous malformations (AVMs)	Anywhere in brain	Suggestive but not sensitive imaging findings include dilated feeding and draining vessels on T2-weighted MR, CT angiography, or MR angiography, as well as patchy enhancement	Young age

Abbreviations: CVT, cerebral venous thrombosis; MCA, middle cerebral artery; SAH, subarachnoid hemorrhage.
Adapted from Garg A, Vibha D, Singh MB, et al. Neuroimaging, CSF and EEG in the neurology emergency. In: Singh MB, Bhatia R, editors. Emergencies in neurology. Manipal: Byword Books Private Limited; 2011. p. 15; with permission.

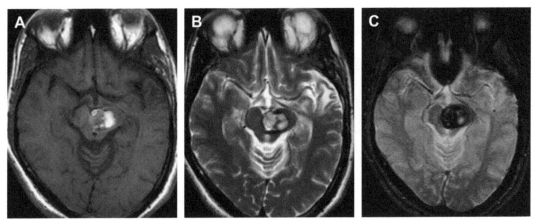

Fig. 23. Midbrain cavernoma. The lesion has mixed signal intensity core with hypointense hemosiderin rim on T2-weighted (*A*) and T1-weighted (*B*) images, and blooms in gradient-echo T2-weighted image (*C*).

spaces. In the first 12 hours after SAH, the sensitivity of CT for SAH is 98% to 100%, declining to 93% at 24 hours[117,118] and to 57% to 85% 6 days after SAH.[119,120] When the CT scan is negative in a patient with suspected SAH, diagnostic lumbar puncture for analysis of CSF is strongly recommended.[120] In addition, CT scan can provide important information about the potential complications of SAH, which include hydrocephalus, infarcts secondary to vasospasm, and so forth.

MR imaging techniques using FLAIR images have improved the diagnosis of acute SAH.[121] However, MR imaging will not quickly replace CT in the routine investigation of patients suspected of having SAH because of the practical limitations of MR imaging in the emergency setting (availability, logistics [including difficulty in scanning acutely ill patients], sensitivity to motion artifact, patient compliance, longer study time, and cost). It does, however, have a role to play in subacute or chronic cases, where CT may have returned to normal.[122]

Selective catheter cerebral angiography is currently the standard for diagnosing cerebral aneurysms as the cause of SAH. DSA provides accurate assessment of the aneurysm's location, size, geometry, relationship to adjacent vessels, and potential multiplicity. Approximately 20% to 25% of DSA performed for SAH will not indicate a source of bleeding.[123] MR angiography and multisection CTA may be considered when conventional angiography cannot be performed in a timely fashion. The sensitivity of 3D TOF MR angiography for cerebral aneurysms is between 85% and 100% for detecting aneurysms larger than 5 mm, and drops to 56% for detecting aneurysms smaller than 5 mm.[124,125] Multisection CTA

is a rapid, readily available, less invasive alternative to catheter angiography. CTA is better able to define aneurysmal wall calcification, intraluminal aneurysm thrombosis, orientation of aneurysm with respect to intraparenchymal hemorrhage, and the relationship of the aneurysm with bony landmarks. Recent literature has demonstrated a high accuracy of detecting aneurysms more than 3 to 4 mm in size using 4-section and 16-section CTA in the range of 92% to 100%, but with a much lower sensitivity in detecting smaller aneurysms (<3–4 mm), in the range of 74% to 84%.[126–128]

CAROTID-CAVERNOUS FISTULA

Carotid-cavernous fistulas (CCFs) are abnormal communications between the carotid arterial system and the venous cavernous sinus (CS). CCFs may be divided into spontaneous or traumatic in relation to cause, and direct or indirect (dural) in relation to angiographic findings.

On imaging studies such as CT scan and MR imaging, CCF may present with enlarged superior ophthalmic vein, proptosis, thick extraocular muscles, and evidence of enlarged CS with a convexity of the lateral wall (Fig. 24).[129] These changes can only make one suspect a fistula. The presence of flow-related enhancement in the CS on MR angiography suggests the diagnosis in the right clinical setting. DSA, currently the standard of reference for the diagnosis of dural and direct CCFs, characterize the blood supply and venous drainage of CCFs (see Fig. 24B). With direct or dural CCFs, the venous drainage may be multidirectional. At present, the treatment modality of choice is endovascular intervention.

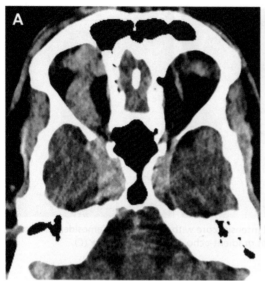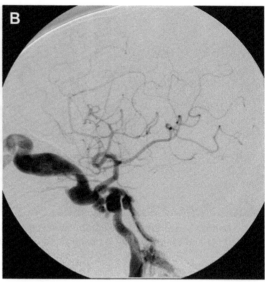

Fig. 24. Caroticocavernous fistula. Contrast-enhanced CT scan of brain (*A*) shows prominent bilateral cavernous sinuses and dilated right superior ophthalmic vein. Lateral view of right ICA angiogram (*B*) shows a direct caroticocavernous fistula, with anterior drainage into ophthalmic venous system and posterior drainage into inferior petrosal sinus.

POSTERIOR REVERSIBLE ENCEPHALOPATHY SYNDROME

In the posterior reversible encephalopathy syndrome (PRES), catheter angiography, MR angiography, and MR perfusion demonstrate evidence of vasculopathy with focal and diffuse vasoconstriction, focal vasodilation, and a string-of-bead pattern along with reduced relative cerebral blood volume, suggesting a state of brain hypoperfusion.[130–132] When performed, repeat MR angiography often demonstrates reversal of the vasculopathy.

SUMMARY

Vascular disease of brain is a heterogeneous group of disorders with diverse clinical presentation. To establish a differential diagnosis clinical features, disease progression, age of onset, blood results, and CSF examinations have to be taken into consideration. Neuroimaging techniques, such as MR imaging and DSA, play a central role in the diagnosis and monitoring of disease. Imaging plays an important role in narrowing down the differential diagnosis. The imaging protocol for suspected cases of vascular disorder should include DWI and SWI.

REFERENCES

1. Knaap MS, Valk J, Barkhof F. Vasculitis. In: Heilmann U, editor. Magnetic resonance of myelination and myelin disorders. 3rd edition. Berlin: Birkhäuser; 2005. p. 773–800.

2. Küker W, Gaertner S, Nagele T, et al. Vessel wall contrast enhancement: a diagnostic sign of cerebral vasculitis. Cerebrovasc Dis 2008;26(1):23–9.

3. Vanderzant C, Bromberg M, MacGuire A, et al. Isolated small-vessel angiitis of the central nervous system. Arch Neurol 1988;45(6):683–7.

4. Nabika S, Kiya K, Satoh H, et al. Primary angiitis of the central nervous system mimicking dissemination from brainstem neoplasm: a case report. Surg Neurol 2008;70(2):182–5.

5. Chu CT, Gray L, Goldstein LB, et al. Diagnosis of intracranial vasculitis: a multi-disciplinary approach. J Neuropathol Exp Neurol 1998;57(1):30–8.

6. Duna GF, Calabrese LH. Limitations of invasive modalities in the diagnosis of primary angiitis of the central nervous system. J Rheumatol 1995; 22(4):662–7.

7. Siva A. Vasculitis of the nervous system. J Neurol 2001;248(6):451–68.

8. Campi A, Benndorf G, Martinelli V, et al. Spinal cord involvement in primary angiitis of the central nervous system: a report of two cases. AJNR Am J Neuroradiol 2001;22(3):577–82.

9. Campi A, Benndorf G, Filippi M, et al. Primary angiitis of the central nervous system: serial MRI of brain and spinal cord. Neuroradiology 2001;43(8):599–607.

10. Greenan TJ, Grossman RI, Goldberg HI. Cerebral vasculitis: MR imaging and angiographic correlation. Radiology 1992;182(1):65–72.

11. White ML, Zhang Y. Primary angiitis of the central nervous system: apparent diffusion coefficient lesion analysis. Clin Imaging 2010;34(1):1–6.

12. Alhalabi M, Moore PM. Serial angiography in isolated angiitis of the central nervous system. Neurology 1994;44(7):1221–6.

13. Younger DS, Calabrese LH, Hays AP. Granulomatous angiitis of the nervous system. Neurol Clin 1997;15(4):821–34.

14. Lie JT. Primary (granulomatous) angiitis of the central nervous system: a clinicopathologic analysis of 15 new cases and a review of the literature. Hum Pathol 1992;23(2):164–71.

15. Pfadenhauer K, Weber H. Giant cell arteritis of the occipital arteries—a prospective color coded duplex sonography study in 78 patients. J Neurol 2003;250(7):844–9.

16. Savage CO, Harper L, Cockwell P, et al. ABC of arterial and vascular disease: vasculitis. BMJ 2000;320(7245):1325–8.

17. Schmidt WA. Doppler ultrasonography in the diagnosis of giant cell arteritis. Clin Exp Rheumatol 2000;18(4 Suppl 20):S40–2.

18. Bley TA, Uhl M, Carew J, et al. Diagnostic value of high-resolution MR imaging in giant cell arteritis. AJNR Am J Neuroradiol 2007;28(9):1722–7.

19. Numano F, Okawara M, Inomata H, et al. Takayasu's arteritis. Lancet 2000;356(9234):1023–5.

20. Liu YQ. Radiology of aortoarteritis. Radiol Clin North Am 1985;23(4):671–88.

21. Lande A, Bard R, Rossi P, et al. Takayasu's arteritis. A worldwide entity. N Y State J Med 1976;76(9):1477–82.

22. Johnston SL, Lock RJ, Gompels MM. Takayasu arteritis: a review. J Clin Pathol 2002;55(7):481–6.

23. Mwipatayi BP, Jeffery PC, Beningfield SJ, et al. Takayasu arteritis: clinical features and management: report of 272 cases. ANZ J Surg 2005;75(3):110–7.

24. Sharma S, Sharma S, Taneja K, et al. Morphologic mural changes in the aorta revealed by CT in patients with nonspecific aortoarteritis (Takayasu's arteritis). AJR Am J Roentgenol 1996;167(5):1321–5.

25. Sharma S, Sharma S, Taneja K, et al. Morphological mural changes in the aorta in non-specific aortoarteritis (Takayasu's arteritis): assessment by intravascular ultrasound imaging. Clin Radiol 1998;53(1):37–43.

26. Nastri MV, Baptista LP, Baroni RH, et al. Gadolinium-enhanced three-dimensional MR angiography of Takayasu arteritis. Radiographics 2004;24(3):773–86.

27. Gotway MB, Araoz PA, Macedo TA, et al. Imaging findings in Takayasu's arteritis. AJR Am J Roentgenol 2005;184(6):1945–50.

28. Matsunaga N, Hayashi K, Sakamoto I, et al. Takayasu arteritis: MR manifestations and diagnosis of acute and chronic phase. J Magn Reson Imaging 1998;8(2):406–14.

29. Yamada I, Nakagawa T, Himeno Y, et al. Takayasu arteritis: diagnosis with breath-hold contrast-enhanced three-dimensional MR angiography. J Magn Reson Imaging 2000;11(5):481–7.

30. Matsunaga N, Hayashi K, Sakamoto I, et al. Takayasu arteritis: protean radiologic manifestations and diagnosis. Radiographics 1997;17(3):579–94.

31. Seth S, Goyal NK, Jagia P, et al. Carotid intima-medial thickness as a marker of disease activity in Takayasu's arteritis. Int J Cardiol 2006;108(3):385–90.

32. Park JH. Conventional and CT angiographic diagnosis of Takayasu arteritis. Int J Cardiol 1996;54(Suppl):S165–71.

33. Park JH, Chung JW, Im JG, et al. Takayasu arteritis: evaluation of mural changes in the aorta and pulmonary artery with CT angiography. Radiology 1995;196(1):89–93.

34. Choe YH, Han BK, Koh EM, et al. Takayasu's arteritis: assessment of disease activity with contrast-enhanced MR imaging. AJR Am J Roentgenol 2000;175(2):505–11.

35. Desai MY, Stone JH, Foo TK, et al. Delayed contrast-enhanced MRI of the aortic wall in Takayasu's arteritis: initial experience. AJR Am J Roentgenol 2005;184(5):1427–31.

36. Kobayashi Y, Ishii K, Oda K, et al. Aortic wall inflammation due to Takayasu arteritis imaged with ^{18}F-FDG PET coregistered with enhanced CT. J Nucl Med 2005;46(6):917–22.

37. El Mesnaoui A, Sedki N, Bouarhroum A, et al. [Cerebral revascularisation in Takayasu's arteritis]. Ann Cardiol Angeiol (Paris) 2007;56(3):130–6 [in French].

38. Stoodley MA, Thompson RC, Mitchell RS, et al. Neurosurgical and neuroendovascular management of Takayasu's arteritis. Neurosurgery 2000;46(4):841–51 [discussion: 851–2].

39. Gu YQ, Wang ZG. Surgical treatment of cerebral ischaemia caused by cervical arterial lesions due to Takayasu's arteritis: preliminary results of 49 cases. ANZ J Surg 2001;71(2):89–92.

40. Scott D, Awang H, Sulieman B, et al. Surgical repair of visceral artery occlusions in Takayasu's disease. J Vasc Surg 1986;3(6):904–10.

41. Suzuki J, Kodama N. Moyamoya disease—a review. Stroke 1983;14(1):104–9.

42. Suzuki J, Takaku A, Kodama N, et al. An attempt to treat cerebrovascular 'Moyamoya' disease in children. Childs Brain 1975;1(4):193–206.

43. Takagi Y, Kikuta K, Nozaki K, et al. Histological features of middle cerebral arteries from patients treated for Moyamoya disease. Neurol Med Chir (Tokyo) 2007;47(1):1–4.

44. Suzuki J, Takaku A. Cerebrovascular "moyamoya" disease. Disease showing abnormal net-like vessels in base of brain. Arch Neurol 1969;20(3):288–99.

45. Fukui M. Guidelines for the diagnosis and treatment of spontaneous occlusion of the circle of Willis ('moyamoya' disease). Research Committee on

Spontaneous Occlusion of the Circle of Willis (Moyamoya Disease) of the Ministry of Health and Welfare, Japan. Clin Neurol Neurosurg 1997; 99(Suppl 2):S238–40.

46. Miyamoto S, Kikuchi H, Karasawa J, et al. Study of the posterior circulation in moyamoya disease. Part 2: visual disturbances and surgical treatment. J Neurosurg 1986;65(4):454–60.

47. Vajkoczy P. Moyamoya disease: collateralization is everything. Cerebrovasc Dis 2009;28(3):258.

48. Hallemeier CL, Rich KM, Grubb RL, et al. Clinical features and outcome in North American adults with moyamoya phenomenon. Stroke 2006;37(6): 1490–6.

49. Scott RM, Smith JL, Robertson RL, et al. Long-term outcome in children with moyamoya syndrome after cranial revascularization by pial synangiosis. J Neurosurg 2004;100(2 Suppl Pediatrics):142–9.

50. Ikezaki K, Han DH, Kawano T, et al. A clinical comparison of definite moyamoya disease between South Korea and Japan. Stroke 1997; 28(12):2513–7.

51. Yilmaz EY, Pritz MB, Bruno A, et al. Moyamoya: Indiana University Medical Center experience. Arch Neurol 2001;58(8):1274–8.

52. Yoon HK, Shin HJ, Lee M, et al. MR angiography of moyamoya disease before and after encephaloduroarteriosynangiosis. AJR Am J Roentgenol 2000; 174(1):195–200.

53. Kikuta K, Takagi Y, Nozaki K, et al. Asymptomatic microbleeds in moyamoya disease: T2*-weighted gradient-echo magnetic resonance imaging study. J Neurosurg 2005;102(3):470–5.

54. Yoon HK, Shin HJ, Chang YW. "Ivy sign" in childhood moyamoya disease: depiction on FLAIR and contrast-enhanced T1-weighted MR images. Radiology 2002;223(2):384–9.

55. Yeon JY, Kim JS, Hong SC. Incidental major artery aneurysms in patients with non-hemorrhagic moyamoya disease. Acta Neurochir (Wien) 2011;153(6): 1263–70.

56. Mesiwala AH, Sviri G, Fatemi N, et al. Long-term outcome of superficial temporal artery-middle cerebral artery bypass for patients with moyamoya disease in the US. Neurosurg Focus 2008;24(2):E15.

57. Stone JH. Polyarteritis nodosa. JAMA 2002; 288(13):1632–9.

58. Wold LE, Baggenstoss AH. Gastrointestinal lesions of periarteritis nodosa. Mayo Clin Proc 1949;24(2): 28–35.

59. Leiguarda R, Berthier M, Starkstein S, et al. Ischemic infarction in 25 children with tuberculous meningitis. Stroke 1988;19(2):200–4.

60. Martins HS, da Silva TR, Scalabrini-Neto A, et al. Cerebral vasculitis caused by *Aspergillus* simulating ischemic stroke in an immunocompetent patient. J Emerg Med 2010;38(5):597–600.

61. Blair JE. Coccidioidal meningitis: update on epidemiology, clinical features, diagnosis, and management. Curr Infect Dis Rep 2009;11(4):289–95.

62. Gürsoy G, Aktin E, Bahar S, et al. Post-herpetic aneurysm in the intrapetrosal portion of the internal carotid artery. Neuroradiology 1980;19(5):279–82.

63. Gilden D, Cohrs RJ, Mahalingam R, et al. Varicella zoster virus vasculopathies: diverse clinical manifestations, laboratory features, pathogenesis, and treatment. Lancet Neurol 2009;8(8):731–40.

64. Patsalides AD, Wood LV, Atac GK, et al. Cerebrovascular disease in HIV-infected pediatric patients: neuroimaging findings. AJR Am J Roentgenol 2002;179(4):999–1003.

65. Dubrovsky T, Curless R, Scott G, et al. Cerebral aneurysmal arteriopathy in childhood AIDS. Neurology 1998;51(2):560–5.

66. Shah SS, Zimmerman RA, Rorke LB, et al. Cerebrovascular complications of HIV in children. AJNR Am J Neuroradiol 1996;17(10):1913–7.

67. Berkefeld J, Enzensberger W, Lanfermann H. MRI in human immunodeficiency virus-associated cerebral vasculitis. Neuroradiology 2000;42(7):526–8.

68. terPenning B, Litchman CD, Heier L. Bilateral middle cerebral artery occlusions in neurocysticercosis. Stroke 1992;23(2):280–3.

69. Rodriguez-Carbajal J, Del Brutto OH, Penagos P, et al. Occlusion of the middle cerebral artery due to cysticercotic angiitis. Stroke 1989;20(8):1095–9.

70. Barinagarrementeria F, Cantú C. Frequency of cerebral arteritis in subarachnoid cysticercosis: an angiographic study. Stroke 1998;29(1):123–5.

71. Phuong LK, Link M, Wijdicks E. Management of intracranial infectious aneurysms: a series of 16 cases. Neurosurgery 2002;51(5):1145–51 [discussion: 1151–2].

72. Bayer AS, Bolger AF, Taubert KA, et al. Diagnosis and management of infective endocarditis and its complications. Circulation 1998;98(25):2936–48.

73. Ferro JM. Vasculitis of the central nervous system. J Neurol 1998;245(12):766–76.

74. Zidar N, Ferluga D, Hvala A, et al. Contribution to the pathogenesis of radiation-induced injury to large arteries. J Laryngol Otol 1997;111(10):988–90.

75. Haltia M, Iivainainen M, Majuri H, et al. Spontaneous occlusion of the circle of Willis (moyamoya syndrome). Clin Neuropathol 1982;1(1):11–22.

76. Hosoda Y. Pathology of so-called "spontaneous occlusion of the circle of Willis". Pathol Annu 1984;(19 Pt 2):221–44.

77. Aoki S, Hayashi N, Abe O, et al. Radiation-induced arteritis: thickened wall with prominent enhancement on cranial MR images report of five cases and comparison with 18 cases of moyamoya disease. Radiology 2002;223(3):683–8.

78. Call GK, Fleming MC, Sealfon S, et al. Reversible cerebral segmental vasoconstriction. Stroke 1988; 19(9):1159–70.

79. Hajj-Ali RA, Furlan A, Abou-Chebel A, et al. Benign angiopathy of the central nervous system: cohort of 16 patients with clinical course and long-term followup. Arthritis Rheum 2002;47(6):662–9.

80. Calabrese LH, Gragg LA, Furlan AJ. Benign angiopathy: a distinct subset of angiographically defined primary angiitis of the central nervous system. J Rheumatol 1993;20(12):2046–50.

81. Lu SR, Liao YC, Fuh JL, et al. Nimodipine for treatment of primary thunderclap headache. Neurology 2004;62(8):1414–6.

82. Schievink WI. Spontaneous dissection of the carotid and vertebral arteries. N Engl J Med 2001;344(12):898–906.

83. Chen CJ, Tseng YC, Lee TH, et al. Multisection CT angiography compared with catheter angiography in diagnosing vertebral artery dissection. AJNR Am J Neuroradiol 2004;25(5):769–74.

84. Kitanaka C, Tanaka J, Kuwahara M, et al. Magnetic resonance imaging study of intracranial vertebrobasilar artery dissections. Stroke 1994;25(3):571–5.

85. Mascalchi M, Bianchi MC, Mangiafico S, et al. MRI and MR angiography of vertebral artery dissection. Neuroradiology 1997;39(5):329–40.

86. Lévy C, Laissy JP, Raveau V, et al. Carotid and vertebral artery dissections: three-dimensional time-of-flight MR angiography and MR imaging versus conventional angiography. Radiology 1994;190(1):97–103.

87. Huston J, Bernstein MA, Riederer SJ. Feathering: vertebral artery pseudostenosis with elliptical centric contrast-enhanced MR angiography. AJNR Am J Neuroradiol 2006;27(4):850–2.

88. Leclerc X, Lucas C, Godefroy O, et al. Preliminary experience using contrast-enhanced MR angiography to assess vertebral artery structure for the follow-up of suspected dissection. AJNR Am J Neuroradiol 1999;20(8):1482–90.

89. Houser OW, Mokri B, Sundt TM, et al. Spontaneous cervical cephalic arterial dissection and its residuum: angiographic spectrum. AJNR Am J Neuroradiol 1984;5(1):27–34.

90. Ozdoba C, Sturzenegger M, Schroth G. Internal carotid artery dissection: MR imaging features and clinical-radiologic correlation. Radiology 1996;199(1):191–8.

91. Provenzale JM, Morgenlander JC, Gress D. Spontaneous vertebral dissection: clinical, conventional angiographic, CT, and MR findings. J Comput Assist Tomogr 1996;20(2):185–93.

92. Newton TH, Cronqvist S. Involvement of dural arteries in intracranial arteriovenous malformations. Radiology 1969;93(5):1071–8.

93. Kwon BJ, Han MH, Kang HS, et al. MR imaging findings of intracranial dural arteriovenous fistulas: relations with venous drainage patterns. AJNR Am J Neuroradiol 2005;26(10):2500–7.

94. Chen JC, Tsuruda JS, Halbach VV. Suspected dural arteriovenous fistula: results with screening MR angiography in seven patients. Radiology 1992;183(1):265–71.

95. De Marco JK, Dillon WP, Halback VV, et al. Dural arteriovenous fistulas: evaluation with MR imaging. Radiology 1990;175(1):193–9.

96. Saini J, Thomas B, Bodhey NK, et al. Susceptibility-weighted imaging in cranial dural arteriovenous fistulas. AJNR Am J Neuroradiol 2009;30(1):E6.

97. Nishimura S, Hirai T, Sasao A, et al. Evaluation of dural arteriovenous fistulas with 4D contrast-enhanced MR angiography at 3T. AJNR Am J Neuroradiol 2010;31(1):80–5.

98. Ameri A, Bousser MG. Cerebral venous thrombosis. Neurol Clin 1992;10(1):87–111.

99. Shinohara Y, Yoshitoshi M, Yoshii F. Appearance and disappearance of empty delta sign in superior sagittal sinus thrombosis. Stroke 1986;17(6):1282–4.

100. Ford K, Sarwar M. Computed tomography of dural sinus thrombosis. AJNR Am J Neuroradiol 1981;2(6):539–43.

101. Keiper MD, Ng SE, Atlas SW, et al. Subcortical hemorrhage: marker for radiographically occult cerebral vein thrombosis on CT. J Comput Assist Tomogr 1995;19(4):527–31.

102. Lee SK, terBrugge KG. Cerebral venous thrombosis in adults: the role of imaging evaluation and management. Neuroimaging Clin N Am 2003;13(1):139–52.

103. Tsai FY, Wang AM, Matovich VB, et al. MR staging of acute dural sinus thrombosis: correlation with venous pressure measurements and implications for treatment and prognosis. AJNR Am J Neuroradiol 1995;16(5):1021–9.

104. Liauw L, van Buchem MA, Spilt A, et al. MR angiography of the intracranial venous system. Radiology 2000;214(3):678–82.

105. Yoshikawa T, Abe O, Tsuchiya K, et al. Diffusion-weighted magnetic resonance imaging of dural sinus thrombosis. Neuroradiology 2002;44(6):481–8.

106. Forbes KP, Pipe JG, Heiserman JE. Evidence for cytotoxic edema in the pathogenesis of cerebral venous infarction. AJNR Am J Neuroradiol 2001;22(3):450–5.

107. Ducreux D, Oppenheim C, Vandamme X, et al. Diffusion-weighted imaging patterns of brain damage associated with cerebral venous thrombosis. AJNR Am J Neuroradiol 2001;22(2):261–8.

108. Barnes SR, Haacke EM. Susceptibility-weighted imaging: clinical angiographic applications. Magn Reson Imaging Clin N Am 2009;17(1):47–61.

109. Poon CS, Chang JK, Swarnkar A, et al. Radiologic diagnosis of cerebral venous thrombosis: pictorial review. AJR Am J Roentgenol 2007;189(Suppl 6):S64–75.

110. Casey SO, Alberico RA, Patel M, et al. Cerebral CT venography. Radiology 1996;198(1):163–70.

111. Ozsvath RR, Casey SO, Lustrin ES, et al. Cerebral venography: comparison of CT and MR projection venography. AJR Am J Roentgenol 1997;169(6): 1699–707.

112. Rodallec MH, Krainik A, Feydy A, et al. Cerebral venous thrombosis and multidetector CT angiography: tips and tricks. Radiographics 2006; 26(Suppl 1):S5–18 [discussion: S42–3].

113. Lafitte F, Boukobza M, Guichard JP, et al. MRI and MRA for diagnosis and follow-up of cerebral venous thrombosis (CVT). Clin Radiol 1997;52(9): 672–9.

114. Brott T, Broderick J, Kothari R, et al. Early hemorrhage growth in patients with intracerebral hemorrhage. Stroke 1997;28(1):1–5.

115. Kim J, Smith A, Hemphill JC, et al. Contrast extravasation on CT predicts mortality in primary intracerebral hemorrhage. AJNR Am J Neuroradiol 2008; 29(3):520–5.

116. King JT. Epidemiology of aneurysmal subarachnoid hemorrhage. Neuroimaging Clin N Am 1997; 7(4):659–68.

117. Sames TA, Storrow AB, Finkelstein JA, et al. Sensitivity of new-generation computed tomography in subarachnoid hemorrhage. Acad Emerg Med 1996;3(1):16–20.

118. van der Wee N, Rinkel GJ, Hasan D, et al. Detection of subarachnoid haemorrhage on early CT: is lumbar puncture still needed after a negative scan? J Neurol Neurosurg Psychiatry 1995;58(3):357–9.

119. van Gijn J, van Dongen KJ. The time course of aneurysmal haemorrhage on computed tomograms. Neuroradiology 1982;23(3):153–6.

120. Bederson JB, Connolly ES, Batjer HH, et al. Guidelines for the management of aneurysmal subarachnoid hemorrhage: a statement for healthcare professionals from a special writing group of the Stroke Council, American Heart Association. Stroke 2009;40(3):994–1025.

121. Wiesmann M, Mayer TE, Yousry I, et al. Detection of hyperacute subarachnoid hemorrhage of the brain by using magnetic resonance imaging. J Neurosurg 2002;96(4):684–9.

122. Noguchi K, Ogawa T, Seto H, et al. Subacute and chronic subarachnoid hemorrhage: diagnosis with fluid-attenuated inversion-recovery MR imaging. Radiology 1997;203(1):257–62.

123. Cioffi F, Pasqualin A, Cavazzani P, et al. Subarachnoid haemorrhage of unknown origin: clinical and tomographical aspects. Acta Neurochir (Wien) 1989;97(1–2):31–9.

124. Atlas SW. Magnetic resonance imaging of intracranial aneurysms. Neuroimaging Clin N Am 1997; 7(4):709–20.

125. Huston J, Nichols DA, Luetmer PH, et al. Blinded prospective evaluation of sensitivity of MR angiography to known intracranial aneurysms: importance of aneurysm size. AJNR Am J Neuroradiol 1994; 15(9):1607–14.

126. Tipper G, U-King-Im JM, Price SJ, et al. Detection and evaluation of intracranial aneurysms with 16-row multislice CT angiography. Clin Radiol 2005; 60(5):565–72.

127. Yoon DY, Lim KJ, Choi CS, et al. Detection and characterization of intracranial aneurysms with 16-channel multidetector row CT angiography: a prospective comparison of volume-rendered images and digital subtraction angiography. AJNR Am J Neuroradiol 2007;28(1):60–7.

128. Wintermark M, Uske A, Chalaron M, et al. Multislice computerized tomography angiography in the evaluation of intracranial aneurysms: a comparison with intraarterial digital subtraction angiography. J Neurosurg 2003;98(4):828–36.

129. Viñuela F, Fox AJ, Debrun GM, et al. Spontaneous carotid-cavernous fistulas: clinical, radiological, and therapeutic considerations. Experience with 20 cases. J Neurosurg 1984;60(5):976–84.

130. Sengar AR, Gupta RK, Dhanuka AK, et al. MR imaging, MR angiography, and MR spectroscopy of the brain in eclampsia. AJNR Am J Neuroradiol 1997;18(8):1485–90.

131. Lin JT, Wang SJ, Fuh JL, et al. Prolonged reversible vasospasm in cyclosporin A-induced encephalopathy. AJNR Am J Neuroradiol 2003;24(1):102–4.

132. Ito T, Sakai T, Inagawa S, et al. MR angiography of cerebral vasospasm in preeclampsia. AJNR Am J Neuroradiol 1995;16(6):1344–6.

Neurobrucellosis

Osman Kizilkilic, MD[a],*, Cem Calli, MD[b]

KEYWORDS

• Neurobrucellosis • Brucellosis • Neuropathology

Brucellosis is a multisystem infection that can involve any organ system and may present with a broad spectrum of clinical presentations. Nervous system involvement of brucellosis is known as neurobrucellosis (NB). The nervous system may be one of several systems involved in chronic diffuse brucellosis[1] or, rarely, neurologic findings may be the only signs of brucellosis.[1–4]

NB has neither a typical clinical picture nor specific CSF findings. In endemic areas, NB must be considered in the differential diagnosis of patients presented with neurologic symptoms and concomitant fever.

PHYSIOPATHOLOGY OF NEUROBRUCELLOSIS

The exact mechanism by which the organism reaches nervous system is uncertain but, after gaining entry into the body, it invades the reticuloendothelial system from where it reaches the blood stream,causing bacteremia, and later reaches the meninges. When host immunity declines, the organism proliferates and invades other nervous system structures.[5,6]

The occurrence of NB during the acute phase of illness may be due to direct deleterious effects of organisms invading nervous tissues, to the release of circulating endotoxins, or to the immunologic and inflammatory reactions of the host to the presence of these organisms within the nervous system or within other tissues of the body.[1]

Brucella bacteria may affect the nervous system directly or indirectly as a result of cytokine or endotoxin on the neural tissue. Cytotoxic lymphocytes and microglia activation play an immunopathologic role in this disease. A depressed immune status is believed to be a risk factor for developing NB.[1]

Nervous system involvement in brucellosis might be due to the persisting intracellular microorganisms or, perhaps, the infection triggers an immune mechanism leading to neuropathology.[7,8] In an experimental animal model, the ganglioside-like molecules expressed on the surface of *Brucella melitensis* were found to induce anti-ganglioside membrane 1 (GM1) ganglioside antibodies, resulting in flaccid limb weakness and ataxia-like symptoms.[7,9]

Involvement of the CNS in brucellosis has been reported with the incidence varying between 0.5% and 25% in different series.[10–16] Neurologic complications of *Brucella* are rarely seen in children[17–22]; the rate of neurologic complications is 0.8% of children affected with systemic brucellosis.[22] NB is categorized according to the clinical manifestation, which is CNS or peripheral nervous system involvement, or a combination.[23] Some immunologic mechanisms operate to produce the demyelinating lesions in the cerebral and spinal cord white matter.[13,20,24]

Although the NB is not very common, it has marked clinical importance for its severity and morbidity.

CLINICAL PRESENTATION OF NEUROBRUCELLOSIS

Clinical presentations of NB vary widely because *Brucella* exhibits a great affinity for the meninges. *Brucella* enters the CNS during the first stage of the disease by hematogenous spread; then, latent or clinical meningitis occur, from which microorganisms may eventually invade the neighboring nervous structures.[17] The early manifestations appear during the course of the septicemia or

[a] Department of Radiology, Cerrahpasa Medical Faculty, University of Istanbul, 34300 Kocamustafapasa, Istanbul
[b] Department of Radiology, Medical Faculty, Ege University, 35100 Bornova, Izmir, Turkey
* Corresponding author.
E-mail address: ebos90@hotmail.com

Neuroimag Clin N Am 21 (2011) 927–937
doi:10.1016/j.nic.2011.07.008

shortly after its termination, whereas the late ones, which are more frequent, may last months or years after having occurred in the septicemic period, which many times are subclinical.[17]

NB can present at any stage of systemic brucellosis and several clinical forms, such as meningitis, meningoencephalitis, brain abscess, epidural abscess, myelitis, radiculoneuritis, cranial nerve involvement, or demyelinating or vascular disease, may be seen.[10,13,15,25] The clinical manifestation in this group included fever, headache, sweating, weight loss, and neurologic manifestations, such as papilledema, seizures, confusion, polyradiculopathy, and lymphocytic meningitis.[7,26] Headache and psychiatric symptoms may develop owing to the toxic effect of NB.[20]

The most common clinical form is meningitis or meningoencephalitis, occurring in 50% of the cases (Figs. 1 and 2). Development of basal meningitis may lead to lymphocytic pleocytosis, cranial nerve enhancement, and intracranial hypertension. It is characterized by CSF pleocytosis and high protein levels.[1,12,27] In cases with brucellosis, other possible causes of infection of inflammatory disease such as tuberculosis, fungal infection, or sarcoidosis can be ruled out by the negative culture of CSF or granuloma, and the high index of suspicion of brucellosis with positive Brucella titers and marked improvement with adequate treatment.

Various chronic manifestations are perhaps best divided into those presenting with peripheral neuropathy or radiculopathy and those presenting with more diffuse CNS involvement including myelitis with cranial nerve involvement and a syndrome of parenchymatous dysfunction.[1,2,15]

Symptoms of peripheral neuropathy and radiculopathy include back pain, areflexia, and paraparesis with involvement of the proximal nerve radicals. In patients with diffuse CNS involvement, myelitis is evidenced by back pain, spastic paraparesis, and demyelination and can also occur with cerebellar dysfunction.

The syndrome of parenchymatous dysfunction can occur at any point in the CNS but it most commonly affects the cerebellum, spinal cord and cerebral white matter. Meningovascular complications, in particular mycotic aneurysms, ischemic strokes, and subarachnoid hemorrhage are relatively common.[1–3] NB can present with other rare neurologic manifestations including isolated intracranial hypertension, Guillain-Barre syndrome, solitary extraaxial posterior fossa abscess, cerebral venous thrombosis, and subdural hemorrhage.[1,28–31]

Both pseudotumor cerebri and papillitis (optic neuritis) have been implicated in the pathophysiology of papilledema.[11,32,33] Pseudotumor cerebri is characterized by increased CSF pressure,

papilledema, but with generally preserved vision, and pupillary reflexes. Papillitis (optic neuritis) presents as pain on movement of the eyes, papilledema, rapidly occurring visual loss and relative afferent pupillary defect.[32]

Spinal granuloma or abscess because of brucellosis may cause an upper motor neuron-type lesion, whereas brucellar spinal root involvement may cause a lower motor neuron-type lesion.[34]

All these manifestations can lead to confusion and delay in diagnosis. It may also lead to difficulty in differentiating NB from other chronic infections, especially tuberculosis and syphilis.[35]

DIAGNOSIS OF NEUROBRUCELLOSIS

NB has neither a typical clinical picture nor specific CSF findings.[36] The diagnosis of NB is based on the existence of a neurologic picture not explained by any other neurologic disease, evidenced by systemic brucellar infection, and the presence of inflammatory alteration in CSF.[37]

Examination of CSF typically reveals an elevated protein concentration, a depressed glucose concentration, and a moderate leukocytosis composed mainly of lymphocytes.[2,15,38] The exception is the cerebellar syndrome, in which the protein concentration is elevated but there is no leukocytosis.[1,39]

Blood culture is not an ideal test for diagnosis of NB because of low yield and long time it requires.[1,40] As a result of low rate of Brucella isolation from CSF (<20%), the diagnosis of NB mainly depends on the detection of specific antibodies in CSF.[1,15,41] Although the positive culture is the gold standard for diagnosis, it has been thought to be suboptimal.[37,42]

Neuroimaging and neurophysiologic evaluation combined with the microbiological diagnostic tools is useful for both diagnosis and detection of complications. Accurate diagnosis and proper management of central nervous system brucellosis appears to be fundamental since it is a very subtle disease.[7]

IMAGING OF NEUROBRUCELLOSIS

Magnetic resonance imaging (MRI) is the imaging modality with capability to show both parenchymal lesions, and cranial nerve involvement; contrast administration is mandatory for the evaluation of leptomeningeal involvement.

Although the imaging methods are important for the diagnosis of neurobrucellosis, the test results must be in accordance with the patient's clinical condition to have diagnostic value. A focal cortical cerebral lesion with nodular enhancement and surrounding edema, increase in perivascular

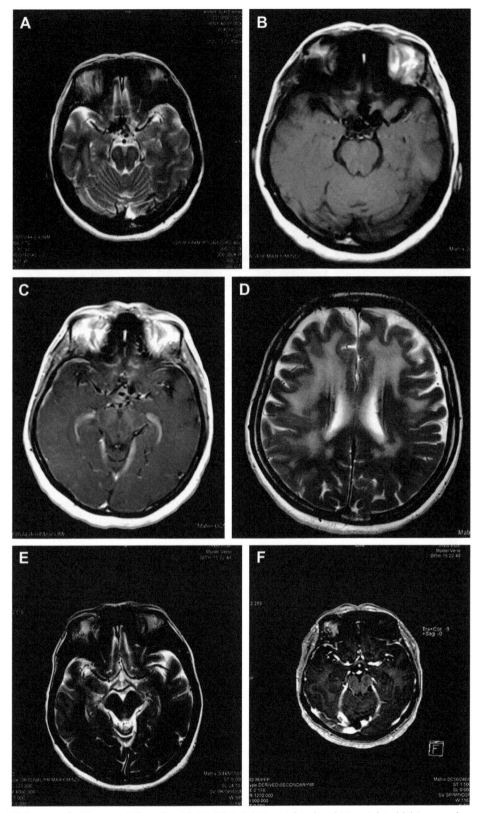

Fig. 1. MR images of a 51-year-old female with NB (A) Axial T2 weighted and T1 weighted (B) images show supra-sellar cistern located extraaxial lesion, hypointense on both sequences. Contrast enhanced T1 weighted image (C) shows slight leptomeningeal contrast enhancement consistent with inflammation. Axial T2 weighted superior section image (D) shows diffuse increased white matter intensity, secondary to white matter involvement 3 months post medication MR images obtained show: (E) Axial T2 weighted image, contrast enhanced T1 weighted image (F) show resolution of suprasellar cistern lesion and leptomeningeal contrast enhancement.

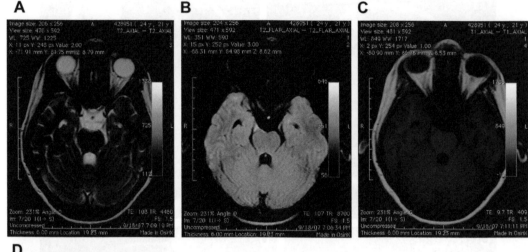

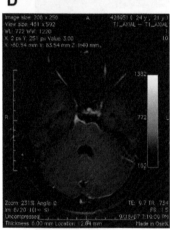

Fig. 2. MR images of 24-year-old female presented with headache and fever, CSF examination revealed neurobrucellosis. (A) Axial T2 weighted, (B) FLAIR, and (C) T1 weighted images, show leptomeningeal thickening in the right half of prepontine cistern that shows leptomeningeal thickening and contrast enhancement in the same location on postcontrast T1 weighted image (D).

vascularization and generalized inflammation of the white matter can be seen on CT and MRI.[17]

Imaging abnormalities in NB are variable and may mimic other infectious or inflammatory conditions. Imaging appearance reflects inflammatory or demyelinating processes or vascular insult and does not always correlate with clinical situation.[1,26] According to the Al Sous and colleagues[26] imaging findings of NB are divided into 4 categories: normal, inflammation (recognized by granulomas, abnormal enhancement of the meninges, perivascular space, or lumbar nerve roots), white matter changes and vascular changes.

INFLAMMATION AND IMAGING FEATURES

Involvement of one or more cranial nerves is seen in more than 50% of the cases with NB, this is mostly a result of basal meningitis. In cases with Brucellosis the causes of cranial nerve involvement include extension of meningeal infection, possible vasculitic processes, pseudotumor cerebri and side effect of tetracycline which is commonly used for the treatment of Brucellosis (see Figs. 1 and 2; Fig. 3). Cranial nerve paralyses are seen more frequently during the acute/subacute disease course associated with CNS involvement.[2,20,22] The vestibulocochlear nerve is the most common affected cranial nerve in NB. On the other hand isolated involvement of cranial nerve is a very rare.[23,27,33,43] Brucellar cranial nerve palsies usually resolve completely with the administration of antibiotics, whereas those with chronic CNS infections often have permanent neurologic deficits.[7,8,20,44]

The abducens nerve has the longest intracranial course and is therefore susceptible to direct and indirect insults like microvascular infarction or direct compression.[7,45]

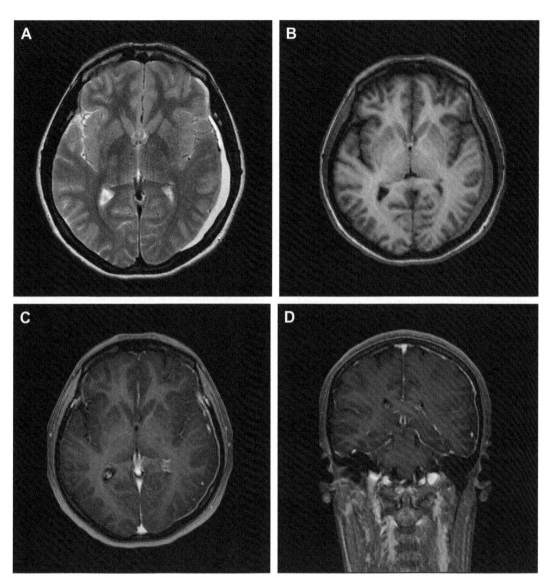

Fig. 3. MR images of a 18-year-old female presented with malasia, fever and headcahe. Physical examination revealed nuchal rigidity, microbiological examinations were consistent with NB and meningitis. (*A*) Axial T2 weighted, (*B*) T1 weighted images, show subdural collection on the left side and leptomeningeal thickening. Post contrast Axial (*C*) and Coronal (*D*) T1 weighted image shows diffuse leptomeningeal thickening, contrast enhancement and subdural effusion (empyema).

The pathogenesis of optic neuritis and abducens nerve palsy is speculative. Possible mechanisms include extension of meningeal infection secondary to an inflammation of the meninges in the subarachnoid cistern and microorganism reaching the neuroaxis via the bloodstream or lymphatic system. It attacks the Schwann cells and leads to demyelination. Another theory is a vasculitic process. The bacterial antigen, antibody, and complement complex are deposited in the vasa nervosum with vascular and perivascular infiltrates.[23,46,47]

Although formation of the granulomas results from inflammation that is relevant to infection, it is a rare manifestation in NB.

Brucella meningitis may behave as an exclusively neurologic disease mimicking vascular accidents that are frequently paroxysmal and recurrent.[3]

Computed tomography and MR studies in uncomplicated meningitis are usually normal or some enhancement of the meninges is seen on post contrast images. In granulomatous meningitis, enhancement is typically seen in basal meninges, whereas bacterial meningitis typically shows enhancement over the cerebral convexities. In all types of meningitis contrast MR is more sensitive than CT. Contrast enhanced FLAIR sequence may be even more sensitive in detecting enhancement. Extension of enhancing subarachnoid exudates deep into the sulci can be seen in severe cases.

Imaging of the affected patients is not performed routinely other than to ensure the absence of hydrocephalus or abscess before a lumbar puncture is performed. Neuroimaging is indicated if the clinical diagnosis is unclear, if neurologic deterioration occurs secondary to increased intracranial pressure or if patients' recovery from the disease is slow.

Cortical lesions with surrounding edema show a characteristic enhancement consisting of a central nodular intense enhancement and a faint peripheral enhancement (target sign) that might reflect diverse stages of brain inflammation, similar to those reported in chronic brain abscess, such as tuberculosis.[17,47] Early stage of the parenchymal infection is the cerebritis stage. In the cerebritis stage, an ill-defined subcortical hyperintense lesion can be seen in T2W images. During the late stage the central necrotic area is hyperintense on T2W images and show restricted diffusion on diffusion weighted imaging. The thick, somewhat irregularly marginated rim appears iso to mildly hyperintense on T1W images and enhances after administration of contrast media. Peripheral vasogenic edema is always present.

Despite its rareness, brucellosis should be considered in the differential diagnosis of focal brain lesions or leptomeningeal enhancing lesions, especially in the patients with a history of contact with domestic animals, consumption of non-pasteurized lactic products or previous brucellosis.[17]

WHITE MATTER INVOLVEMENT

Three patterns of white matter involvement that manifests as hyperintense lesions on T2 weighted images have been noted. The first pattern is a diffuse appearance affecting the arcuate fibers region, the second pattern is periventricular, and the third pattern is a focal demyelinating appearance.

Brain MRI shows extensive bilateral high signal abnormalities in the periventricular white matter on T2-weighted and FLAIR images. MR angiography could be normal (see Fig. 1; Fig. 4). Imaging of multifocal white matter hyperintensities on T2W and FLAIR MR Images are nonspecific, and the differential diagnosis of these lesions is very broad.

The nature and cause of white matter abnormalities are not known, but they may be due to an autoimmune reaction. The white matter involvement may mimic other inflammatory or infectious disease, such as multiple sclerosis, acute disseminated encephalomyelitis, or Lyme disease.[11,26,36,48–51] In contrast multiple sclerosis these white matter lesions do no tend to locate in the callosomarginal region and they do not enhance.

MRI features consisting of high-intensity confluent areas in the white matter of the brain around the lateral ventricles are in favor of a demyelinating process. In the presence of any posterior fossa or brain stem lesion highly probable diagnosis will be multiple sclerosis.

VASCULAR INVOLVEMENT

Brucella infection by itself triggers the immune mechanism leading to a demyelinating state. As the disease gets more chronic, the immune

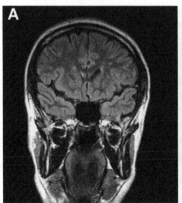
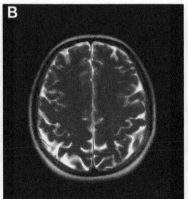
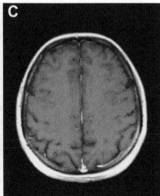

Fig. 4. MR images of a 37-year-old female. (A) Coronal FLAIR, Axial T2 (B) weighted images show millimetric hyperintense lesion in the periventricular white matter in both cerebral hemispheres. Axial post contrast T1 weighted image (C) shows lack of enhancement of periventricular lesions.

mechanism processes increase.[20,24] This disease does not show predilection of size or location of vascular structure.[20]

The vascular insult is likely due to one of the following two mechanisms. In the first, an inflammatory process of the small vessels or venous system causes lacunar infarcts, small hemorrhages, or venous thrombosis.[2,26,52–55] Brucella can cause vasculitis; it has no predilection of size or location of vascular structure. Arterial and/or venous structures may be affected.[56,57] Vascular involvement may result in lacunar infarcts, small hemorrhages or venous thrombosis.[10] The second possible mechanism is hemorrhagic stroke caused by rupture of a mycotic aneurysm, a likely sequel of embolic stroke from brucellar endocarditis.[2,26,58,59]

The pathogenesis of TIA and ischemic stroke in brucellosis still remains uncertain. Transient cerebral ischemic attacks can be seen secondary to the vascular-perivascular inflammatory reaction or vascular spasm. Large vessel involvement is rare in NB.[1,7,10] Most likely, ischemic stroke in NB is a consequence of an accompanying vasculitis.[2,25] Various degrees of vascular inflammation ranging from acute to chronic with the possibility of necrosis and aneurysmal formation have been described in NB.[25,60] It has been proposed that TIA in brucellosis may be related to infectious vasculitis, cerebral vasospasm or cardioembolism.[11,60,61] Vessel involvement in Brucella may also develop secondary to cardiac embolization leading to necrosis of the occluded vessel and formation of mycotic aneurysm that may rupture and lead to subarachnoid or cerebral hemorrhage.[55]

Carotid angiograms may disclose diffuse vascular spasm in the territory of the affected artery. Most of the patients with ischemic cerebral symptoms in the literature have normal cerebral angiograms.[61] Normal appearance of cerebral vessels in DSA is considered consistent with vasculitis of deep penetrating arteries.[11]

Diffusion weighted imaging is useful in the setting of acute ischemia, as it will detect infarctions earlier than conventional MR sequences or FLAIR sequence. Frequently multiple lacunar type infarcts are seen in the distribution of perforating vessels in the brainstem, basal ganglia, and white matter as a result of involvement of basal cisterns and vessels contained therein.

Myelitis is generally evidenced by back pain, ataxia, paresthesia, paraplegia and sphincter abnormalities.[7] Since NB mimics peripheral and central nervous system pathologies, differential diagnosis is important in probable patients. MR examination shows thickening of the spinal roots and diffuse enhancement along the distal cord and cauda equina.

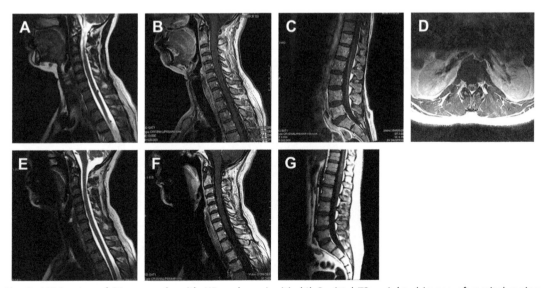

Fig. 5. MR images of 21-year-male with NB and meningitis (A) Sagittal T2 weighted image of cervical region shows intradural-extramedullary hypointense nodular lesions (consistent with granuloma formation). Sagittal postcontrast T1 weighted (B) cervical region image shows peripheral enhancement of the spinal cord, and lack of contrast enhancement of intradural-extramedullary lesions. (C) Sagittal and axial (D) postcontrast T1 weighted lumbar images show contrast enhancement of the cauda equina and thickening of the filum terminale roots. Imaging following medical treatment show: (E) Sagittal T2 weighted cervical MR image shows resolution of intradural-extramedullary lesions. Sagittal contrast enhanced T1 weighted image (F) shows resolution of same lesions and lack of contrast enhancement of cervical spinal cord. Sagittal T1 weighted postcontrast MR image (G) of lumbar region shows absence of contrast enhancement of the cauda equina.

MR imaging of focal brain involvement by NB is scant, and no specific reports in pediatric patients has been made to date.

MYELOPATY AND SPINAL DISEASE

Myelopathy may result from different mechanisms. Acute transvers myelitis, spinal cord infarction, adhesive arachnoiditis, compression from epidural abscess or from brucellar spondylitis

may occur. Brucella spondylitis affects the lumbosacral and lower thoracic region most frequently, causing erosion and vertebral collapse leading to cord or cauda equina compression.[35]

The major role of neuroimaging is to identify treatable conditions that can mimic myelopathy. These include acute disk herniation, hematoma, epidural abscess, or compressive myelopathy.

During the acute phase of the myelopathy, MR images are normal in half of the patients and

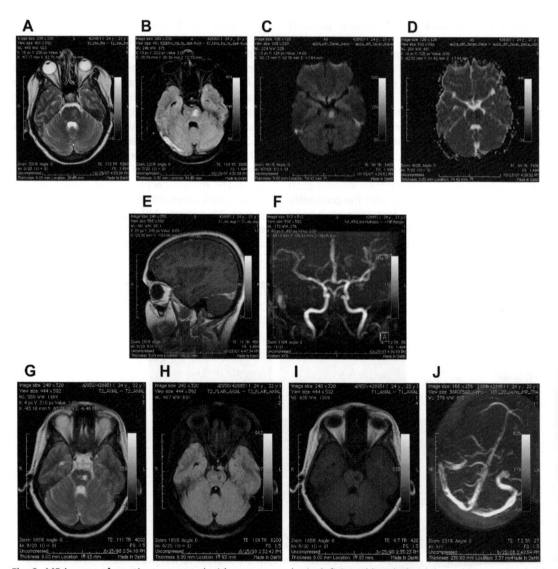

Fig. 6. MR images of a patient presented with acute neurologic deficit and headache. (*A*) Axial T2 weighted, (*B*) FLAIR images shows hyperintens lesion in the left half of pons. Diffusion weighted image (*C*) with b = 1000 sec/mm^2 with corresponding ADC map (*D*) shows restricted diffusion of the same lesion consistent with acute ischemic lesion. Sagittal T1 weighted postcontrast image (*E*) shows thrombosis of the right transvers sinus (filling defect-empty delta sign). MR angiography, MIP image (*F*) shows normal intracranial arteries. Imaging of the patient after success full medical treatment clinical recovery shows: (*G*) Axial T2 weighted, (*H*) FLAIR and (*I*) T1 weighted images show lesion on the left side of the pons with CSF-like signal intensity on all images, consistent with chronic lacune. MR venography MIP image (*J*) shows patency and recanalizationof the right transvers sinus.

nonspecific in the other half. Focal cord expansion, poorly delineated increased signal in the spinal cord on T2W images may seen. Varying degree of contrast enhancement occurs in some of the cases (Fig. 5).

CEREBRAL VENOUS THROMBOSIS AND VENOUS INFARCT

Cerebral venous thrombosis may occur as a complication of certain infections during pregnancy or postpartum, with contraceptives, in Behcet's disease or systemic lupus erythematosus, and in several coagulopathies including protein C and S antithrombin III deficiency, and in antiphospholipid antibody syndrome.[62]

In the acute phase (when the clot is dense), thrombus can be seen on CT as hyperdense in the sinus on non contrast CT. In the subacute phase of the thrombosis, contrast enhanced images show filling defect within the sinus.

MR imaging is very helpful for the diagnosis and is the best method of noninvasive investigation. The acutely thrombosed sinus is isointense to the brain parenchyma on T1W images and hypointense to brain on T2W images. This appearance cannot be distinguished from slow flow. When the thrombus is subacute and hyperintens on T1W images it is very easy to recognize (Fig. 6).

Advances in MR venography have greatly aided the diagnosis of venous sinus thrombosis by MR imaging. Two-dimensional time-of-flight MR venography or phase contrast MR venography can be used to make the diagnosis. Since time-of-flight MR angiography is acquired using T1W images, both moving blood and subacute thrombus may be seen equivocal. CT venography is also a fast and reliable way of making the diagnosis.

The MR differential diagnosis of dural sinus thrombosis is primarily imaging artifacts that can mimic intravascular clot. These include contrast enhanced scans with flow compensation methods, unenhanced scans with inflow of fully unsaturated spins into the imaged slice (entry phenomena), incorrect pulse sequence selection or misplaced saturation bands, incorporation of hyperintense clot.

On CT, venous infarcts are usually poorly delimited, hypodense or mixed attenuation areas involving the subcortical white matter and causing a slight mass effect on ventricles. On MR, early venous infarcts may be identified by prolongation of T1 and T2W images. Reduced diffusion is not an early sign of venous infarction; diffusion appears to be heterogenous with areas of increased, normal and decreased diffusion. Some of the venous infarct may be hemorrhagic or may cause hematoma.

SUMMARY

NB has neither a typical clinical picture nor specific CSF findings and its diagnosis is based on the existence of a neurologic picture not explained by any other neurologic disease, evidenced by systemic brucellar infection, and the presence of inflammatory alteration in CSF, especially in patients living in endemic areas for the infection. Neuroimaging and neurophysiologic evaluation combined with the microbiological diagnostic tools is useful for both diagnosis and detection of complications. Magnetic resonance imaging is the imaging modality, which may show both parenchymal lesions, and cranial nerve involvement; contrast administration is mandatory for the evaluation of leptomeningeal involvement.

REFERENCES

1. Abdolbagi MH, Rasooli-Nejad M, Jafari S, et al. Clinical and laboratory findings in neurobrucellosis: review of 31 cases. Arch Iran Med 2008;11(1):21–5.
2. McLean DR, Russell N, Khan MY. Neurobrucellosis: clinical and therapeutic features. Clin Infect Dis 1992;15(4):582–90.
3. Bouza E, Garcia de la Torre M, Parras F, et al. Brucellar meningitis. Rev Infect Dis 1987;9(4):810–22.
4. Bucher A, Gaustad P, Pape E. Chronic neurobrucellosis due to Brucella melitensis. Scand J Infect Dis 1990;22(2):223–6.
5. Vinod P, Singh MK, Garg RK, et al. Extensive meningoencephalitis, retrobulbar neuritis and pulmonary involvement in a patient of neurobrucellosis. Neurol India 2007;55(2):157–9.
6. Billard E, Cazevieille C, Dornand J, et al. High susceptibility of human dendritic cells to invasion by the intracellular pathogens Brucella suis, B.abortus, and B.melitensis. Infect Immun 2005;73(12):8418–24.
7. Gul HC, Erdem H, Bek S. Overview of neurobrucellosis: a pooled analysis of 187 cases. Int J Infect Dis 2009;13(6):339–43.
8. Akdeniz H, Irmak H, Anlar O, et al. Central nervous system brucellosis: presentation, diagnosis and treatment. J Infect 1998;36(3):297–301.
9. Watanabe K, Kim S, Nishiguchi M, et al. Brucella melitensis infection associated with Guillain-Barre syndrome through molecular mimicry of host structures. FEMS Immunol Med Microbiol 2005;45(2):121–7.
10. Adaletli I, Albayram S, Gurses B, et al. Vasculopathic changes in the cerebral arterial system with neurobrucellosis. AJNR Am J Neuroradiol 2006;27(2):384–6.

11. AlDeeb SM, Yaqub BA, Sharif HS, et al. Neurobru-cellosis:clinical characteristics, diagnosis, and out-come. Neurology 1989;39(4):498–501.

12. Nas K, Tasdemir N, Cakmak E, et al. Cervical intrame-dullary granuloma of Brucella: a case report and review of the literature. Eur Spine J 2007;16(3):255–9.

13. Bashir R, Zuheir Al-Kawi M, Harder EJ, et al. Nervous system brucellosis: diagnosis and treat-ment. Neurology 1985;35(11):1576–81.

14. Bingol A, Yucemen N, Meco O. Medically treated in-traspinal "Brucella" granuloma. Surg Neurol 1999; 52(6):570–6.

15. Shakir RA, Al-Din AS, Araj GF, et al. Clinical cate-gories of neurobrucellosis. A report of 19 cases. Brain 1987;110(1):213–23.

16. Vajramani GV, Nagmoti MB, Patil CS. Neurobrucellosis presenting as an intramedullary spinal cord abscess. Ann Clin Microbiol Antimicrob 2005;16(4):14–8.

17. Martinez-Chamorro E, Munoz A, Esparza J, et al. Focal cerebral involvement by neurobrucellosis: patholog-ical and MRI findings. Eur J Radiol 2002;43(1):28–30.

18. Povar J, Aguirre JM, Arazo P, et al. Brucelosis con afectacion del sistema nervioso. An Med Interna 1991;8(8):387–90.

19. Guvenc H, Kocabay K, Okten A, et al. Brucellosis in a child complicated with multiple brain abscesses. Scand J Infect Dis 1989;21(3):333–6.

20. Ceran N, Turkoglu R, Erdem I, et al. Neurobrucello-sis: clinical, diagnostic, therapeutic features and outcome. Unusual clinical presentations in an endemic region. Braz J Infect Dis 2011;15(1):52–9.

21. Young JE. Brucella species. In: Mandell GL, Bennett JF, Dolin R, editors. Principles and practice of infectious diseases. 6th edition. Philadelphia (PA): Churchill Livingstone; 2005. p. 2669–74.

22. Lubani MM, Dudin KI, Araj GF, et al. Neurobrucello-sis in children. Pediatr Infect Dis J 1989;8(2):79–82.

23. Karakurum Göksel B, Yerdelen D, Karatas M, et al. Abducens nerve palsy and optic neuritis as initial manifestation in brucellosis. Scand J Infect Dis 2006;38(8):721–5.

24. Seidel G, Pardo CA, Newman-Toker D, et al. Neuro-brucellosis presenting as leukoencephalopathy. Arch Pathol Lab Med 2003;127(9):374–7.

25. Bingol A, Togay Isikay C. Neurobrucellosis as an exceptional cause of transient ischemic attacks. Eur J Neurol 2006;13(5):544–8.

26. Al-Sous MW, Bohlega S, Al-Kawi MZ, et al. Neuro-brucellosis: clinical and neuroimaging correlation. AJNR Am J Neuroradiol 2004;25(3):395–401.

27. Ozkavukcu E, Tuncay Z, Selcuk F, et al. An unusual case of neurobrucellosis presenting with unilateral abducens nerve palsy: clinical and MRI findings. Di-agn Interv Radiol 2009;15(4):236–8.

28. Ozisik HI, Ersoy Y, Refik-Tevfik M, et al. Isolated intracranial hypertension: a rare presentation of neu-robrucellosis. Microbes Infect 2004;6(9):861–3.

29. Namiduru M, Karaoglan I, Yilmaz M. Guillain-Barre syndrome associated with acute neurobrucellosis. Int J Clin Pract 2003;57(10):919–20.

30. Solaroglu I, Kaptanoglu E, Okutan O, et al. Solitary extra-axial posterior fossa abscess due to neurobru-cellosis. J Clin Neurosci 2003;10(6):710–2.

31. Kizilkilic O, Turunc T, Yildirim T, et al. Successful medical treatment of intracranial abscess caused by Brucella spp. J Infect 2005;51(1):77–80.

32. Miyares FR, Deleu D, El Shafie S, et al. Irreversible papillitis and ophtalmoparesis as a presenting mani-festation of neurobrucellosis. Clin Neurol Neurosurg 2007;109(5):439–41.

33. Yilmaz M, Ozaras R, Mert A, et al. Abducent nerve palsy during treatment of brucellosis. Clin Neurol Neurosurg 2003;105(3):218–20.

34. Goktepe AS, Alaca R, Mojur H, et al. Neurobrucello-sis and a demonstration of its involvement in spinal roots via magnetic resonance imaging. Spinal Cord 2003;41(10):574–6.

35. Izadi S. Neurobrucellosis. Shiraz E Medical J 2001; 2:2–6.

36. Ciftci E, Erden I, Akyar S. Brucellosis of the pituitary region: MRI. Neuroradiology 1998;40(6):383–4.

37. Zaidan R, Al Tahan AR. Cerebral venous thrombosis: a new manifestation of neurobrucellosis. Clin Infect Dis 1999;28(2):399–400.

38. Mousa AR, Koshy TS, Araj GF, et al. Brucella meningitis: presentation, diagnosis, and treatment—a prospective study of ten cases. Q J Med 1986; 60(233):873–85.

39. Drevets DA, Leenen PJ, Greenfield RA. Invasion of the central nervous system by intracellular bacteria. Clin Microbiol Rev 2004;17(2):323–47.

40. Kochar DK, Agarwal N, Jain N, et al. Clinical profile of neurobrucellosis—a report on 12 cases from Bika-ner (North-West India). J Assoc Physicians India 2000;48(4):376–80.

41. Baldi PC, Araj GF, Racaro GC, et al. Detection of antibodies to Brucella cytoplasmic proteins in the cerebrospinal fluid of patients with neurobrucellosis. Clin Diagn Lab Immunol 1999;6:756–9.

42. Shaalan MA, Memish ZA, Mahmoud SA, et al. Brucellosis in children: clinical observations in 115 cases. Int J Infect Dis 2002;6(5):182–6.

43. Pappas G, Akritidis N, Bosilkovski M, et al. Brucel-losis. N Engl J Med 2005;352(22):2325–36.

44. Gouider R, Samet S, Triki C, et al. Neurological mani-festations indicative of brucellosis. Rev Neurol (Paris) 1999;155(3):215–8 [in French].

45. Danchaivijitr C, Kennard C. Diplopia and eye move-ment disorders. J Neurol Neurosurg Psychiatry 2004;75(Suppl 4):24–31.

46. Abd Elrazak M. Brucella optic neuritis. Arch Intern Med 1991;151(4):776–8.

47. De Castro CC, Hesselink JR. Tuberculosis. Neuro-imaging Clin N Am 1991;1:119–39.

48. Al- Kawi MZ. Brucellosis. In: Moher JP, Gautier J, editors. Guide to clinical neurology. New York: Churchill Livingstone; 1995. p. 677–80.

49. Bussone G, La Mantia L, Grazzi L, et al. Neurobrucellosis mimicking multiple sclerosis: a case report. Eur Neurol 1989;29(4):238–40.

50. Murrell TG, Matthews BJ. Multiple sclerosis: one manifestation of neurobrucellosis? Med Hypotheses 1990;33(1):43–8.

51. Demaerel P, Wilms G, Casteels K, et al. Childhood neuroborreliosis: clinicoradiological correlation. Neuroradiology 1995;37(7):578–81.

52. Shakir RA. Brucellosis. In: Shakir RA, Neuman PK, Poser CM, editors. Tropical neurology. Cambridge (MA): WB Saunders; 1996. p. 168–79.

53. Hernandez MA, Anciones B, Frank A, et al. Neurobrucellosis and cerebral vasculitis. Neurologia 1988;3(6):241–3.

54. Martin Escudero JC, Gil Gonzalez MI, Aparicio Blanco M. Intra-cranial hypertension and subarachnoid hemorrhage: the forms of presentation of neurobrucellosis. An Med Interna 1990;7(7):358–60 [in Spanish].

55. Guerreiro CA, Scaff M, Callegaro D, et al. Neurobrucellosis: report of three cases. Arq Neuropsiquiatr 1981;39(2):203–13.

56. Milionis H, Christou L, Elisaf M. Cutaneous manifestations in brucellosis: case report and review of the literature. Infection 2000;28(2):124–6.

57. Aguado JM, Barros C, GomezGarces JL, et al. Infective aortitis due to Brucella melitensis. Scand J Infect Dis 1987;19(4):483–4.

58. Jacobs F, Abramowicz D, Vereerstraeten P, et al. Brucella endocarditis: the role of combined medical and surgical treatment. Rev Infect Dis 1990;12(5):740–4.

59. Bahemuka M, Shemena AR, Panayiotopoulos CP, et al. Neurological syndromes of brucellosis. J Neurol Neurosurg Psychiatry 1988;51(8):1017–21.

60. Fincham RW, Sahs AL, Joynt RJ. Protean manifestations of nervous system brucellosis. JAMA 1963;184:269–75.

61. Pascual J, Combarros O, Polo JM, et al. Localized CNS brucellosis: report of 7 cases. Acta Neurol Scand 1988;78(4):282–9.

62. Pfister HW, Borasio GD, Dirnage IU, et al. Cerebrovascular complications of bacterial meningitis in adults. Neurology 1992;42(8):1497–504.

Hirayama Disease

Yen-Lin Huang, MD, Chi-Jen Chen, MD*

KEYWORDS
• Hirayama disease • Cervical myelopathy • Neck flexion
• Adolescent

Hirayama disease is a benign, self-limiting cervical myelopathy first brought to attention by Hirayama[1] in 1959. During the past half century, researches have established this disease as a new entity that differs from motor neuron disease because of spinal cord compression by the posterior dural sac during neck flexion. Primarily affecting male adolescents, it is clinically characterized by a progressive course of distal upper-limb muscular weakness and atrophy, followed by a spontaneous arrest within several years. Early recognition of the disease allows early intervention, which has been shown to stop disease progression. This article reviews the clinical presentation, pathophysiology, image findings, and treatment of Hirayama disease, because a thorough understanding of the disease is essential for early recognition and treatment.

In 1959, Hirayama and colleagues[2] published 12 cases distinguishing a new clinical entity from what was originally thought to be a type of progressive and degenerative motor neuron disease. The term "juvenile muscular atrophy of unilateral upper extremity" was applied. This new clinical entity was further consolidated by following reports of 20 patients in 1963[3] and 38 patients in 1972.[4] The patients are generally in their teens and early twenties, predominantly male, with insidious onset of weakness and muscle wasting involving unilateral distal upper limb, followed by variable period of progression and spontaneous arrest within several years.

Since then, there have been many reports of Hirayama disease, mostly from Japan and other Asian countries, as well as few from other countries.[5–7] However, early reports in the 1960s and 1970s emphasized clinical features and electrophysiological evaluations. It was not until 1982 that the first autopsy case was obtained by Hirayama and colleagues,[8,9] which revealed anterior-posterior flattening of the lower cervical cord associated with ischemic and atrophic changes of the anterior horn cells. Pathologic evidence of focal ischemic cervical poliomyelopathy of the disease prompted neuroradiologic investigation in search of the anatomic pathophysiology of the spinal cord and canal. Earlier studies were conducted using myelography and CT myelograpy.[10,11] Since MR imaging equipment became available and widely accessible in the late 1980s,[11–15] several publications have provided valuable findings in neck-flexion and neutral-position MR imaging of the cervical spine that have assisted the diagnosis of this disease. Imaging findings revealed dynamic changes of the cervical spine, spinal canal, and spinal cord during neck flexion, mainly in the forward displacement of posterior dural sac, causing anterior-posterior flattening and asymmetric atrophy of the lower cervical cord, which corresponded with the pathologic findings.

Several names have been used in publications to describe this disease, including benign juvenile brachial spinal muscular atrophy, juvenile asymmetric segmental spinal muscular atrophy, juvenile muscular atrophy of the distal upper extremity, monomelic amyotrophy, and oblique amyotrophy.[1,5,9,16,17] Hirayama disease is still the most commonly used named throughout publications in neurology and neuroradiology, as well as related fields.

DEMOGRAPHICS

Hirayama disease occurs mainly in people in their teens and early twenties with a significant male predominance. The mean age of onset ranges from 15 to 20 years of age in different

---

The authors report no conflict of interest.
Department of Diagnostic Radiology, Shuang-Ho Hospital, Taipei Medical University, No. 291 Jhong-Jheng Road, 235 Jhonghe District, New Taipei City, Taiwan, Republic of China
* Corresponding author.
E-mail address: ed100975@yahoo.com

Neuroimag Clin N Am 21 (2011) 939–950
doi:10.1016/j.nic.2011.07.009

studies.[5–7,17–21] The degree of male preponderance reported in large series ranged from purely male to a male/female ratio of 2.8:1.[6,22,23] A delay of age of onset after the peak age of normal growth curve was observed in several studies.[5–7] Hirayama[5] observed that the peak of onset age is approximately 2 years later than the peak of longitudinal growth curve of juveniles in Japan. Based on this finding, Hirayama[1,5] speculated that disproportional growth between the vertebral column and the contents of the spinal canal, especially the dural sac, during the juvenile growth spurt underlies this phenomenon. Tashiro and colleagues[24] suggested that the difference in the male and female incidence of the disease could be explained by a more rapid increase in height of males at puberty compared with females.

Hirayama disease is nonfamilial in most patients. There are, however, a few reports of familial cases. Nine familial cases have been reported in the English literature.[25] So far, there are no published reports regarding genetics information that maybe related to familial Hirayama disease. The explanation for the familial occurrence is indeed interesting and needs further studies.

As Hirayama disease became more recognized, several cases and large series have accumulated. There are an exceedingly large number of cases in Japan and more cases reported from other Asian countries in the past 3 decades, particularly in China, Taiwan, Malaysia, India, and Sri Lanka, but relatively fewer cases from Europe and North America.[5–7] Whether there might be an ethnic factor in this disorder is still unclear.

CLINICAL FEATURES OF HIRAYAMA DISEASE

Patients with Hirayama disease present with insidious onset and slow progression of muscle weakness and muscular atrophy of the distal upper limb, including thenar, hypothenar, interossei muscles, and wrist flexors and extensors, with sparing of brachioradialis muscles (**Fig. 1**). The border of muscular atrophy runs obliquely over the volar and dorsal surfaces of the forearm, therefore it is also referred to as oblique amyotrophy.[4] Both extensor and flexor muscles of the fingers and wrists are involved, particularly the finger extensors and wrist flexors. Some investigators reported asymmetric atrophy was more severe on the ulnar than the radial side in the flexor and extensor compartments.[7,16] The phenomenon of cold paresis is widely observed in the patients, characterized by exacerbating of finger weakness on exposure to cold environment.[5,6] Kijima and colleagues[26] proposed that this is caused by conduction block of the muscle fiber membrane

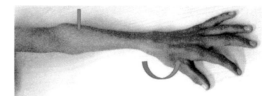

Fig. 1. Photograph of a 19-year-old man, note the wasting of first dorsal interosseous (*curved arrow*) and other small muscles of the hand with preservation of brachioradialis muscles (*straight arrow*) giving an appearance of oblique amyotrophy. (*From* Pradhan S. Bilaterally symmetric form of Hirayama disease. Neurology 2009;72:2083–9; with permission.)

in reinnervated muscles after active denervation. When cold paresis is induced, compound muscle action potentials show delayed latencies and decreased amplitude after high-frequency repetitive nerve stimulation. Resting fasciculation is not observed, but contraction fasciculation is well documented.[7,27,28] It is characterized by fascicular twitching in the extensor side of forearm muscles or tremor-like movement of the fingers during stretching. Fatigue is the most common symptom (33%), followed by cold paresis, atrophy, and tremor.[29] Although most patients reported absence of subjective or objective sensory disturbances, a few patients show slight hypoesthesia in a localized area of the hand.[5,6,30] The muscle stretch reflexes of the arms and legs are within normal range. There are no accompanying neurologic symptoms such as cranial nerve involvement, pyramidal signs, sensory disturbance, and urinary disturbance. Muscle biopsy and needle electromyography show denervation of the atrophied muscles.[5,27] Nerve conduction velocity and analysis of the cerebrospinal fluid are almost normal.

Patients with Hirayama disease commonly show initial unilateral monomelic atrophy, but it is asymmetrically bilateral in some and, occasionally, symmetric.[5] The right upper limb is more frequently involved in Hirayama disease, regardless of the handedness.[3,19,23,30] Huang and colleagues[6] reported more conspicuous manifestation in right upper limb with a right/left ratio of 3:1. Often, the disease progressed to involve the other side in an asymmetric manner.[6,16] A bilateral symmetric form of Hirayama disease has occasionally been reported. The incidence was 3.1% by a National Japan Survey[24] and 10% by Pradhan,[31] who reported 11 cases of bilateral involvement in a series of 106 patients. He proposed that the "bilateral symmetric Hirayama disease" is a more severe variant of Hirayama disease based on more severe and significant clinical and

MR imaging findings. In his series, patients with bilateral involvement showed wider range of involvement, including partial involvement of brachioradialis and biceps brachii. The patients had significant weakness of the forearm and small muscles of the hands; required assistance in daily activities, such as buttoning clothes, holding spoons, and combing hair; had autonomic dysfunction, such as excessive sweating in the hands and cold extremities; and had occasional brisk deep tendon reflexes in the lower limbs.[25] In patients with bilateral involvement, two patterns of progression from one upper limb to the other were observed. The first was that muscle symptoms developed in the other arm during progression of the initial involved arm (with about a 1-year delay in onset). The second was that muscle symptoms developed approximately 2.5 years after cessation of progression in the first arm.[6]

The disease follows a progressive course for a variation of period, with spontaneous arrest within several years. Symptoms generally progress for 2 to 4 years after onset. The duration of progression varies widely, ranging from 16.8 to 73.2 monthes.[17–23] Progression of the disease ceased within 5 years in most patients (around 90%).[6,7] Early arrest of the progression is essential for any possibility of improvement.[5,27]

PATHOPHYSIOLOGY

Pathologic study of this disease was not available until 1982 owing to its benign course. Before neuropathology, there were strenuous debates about whether the disease could be classified as a new disease entity. Some investigators considered the illness to be a variant of degenerative motor neuron disease, traumatic injury of the cervical spinal cord, prolonged survival of acute anterior poliomyelitis, or syringomyelia localized in the anterior horn, in addition to other diseases.[9]

The autopsy case[9] was a 38 year-old patient who experienced left distal upper limb muscular atrophy and weakness associated with cold paresis and fine tremor starting at the age of 15. The symptoms progressed for approximately 1 year before spontaneous arrest. Thereafter, the symptom remained unchanged until the age of 38 when he was diagnosed with lung cancer and died 3 months later. Gross pathology showed evident anterior-posterior flattening of the cervical cord, particularly at C7 and C8. Microscopically, bilateral anterior horns were reduced to less than half of the normal anterior-posterior diameter, most severely at C7 and C8, and predominantly on the left side, corresponding with the patient's clinical symptoms (Fig. 2). The anterior horn

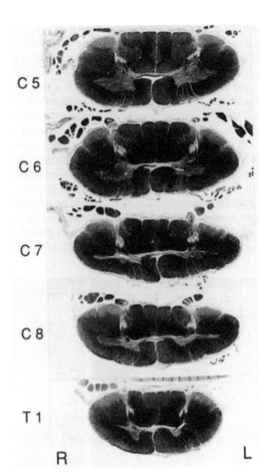

Fig. 2. Transverse sections of cervical spinal cord. Anterior-posterior shrinkage of bilateral anterior horns, most severely at C7 and C8, predominantly on the left. (*From* Hirayama K. Juvenile muscular atrophy of distal upper extremity (Hirayama disease): focal cervical ischemic poliomyelopathy. Neurology 2000;20:S92; with permission.)

lesions were characterized by central necrosis without cavity formation, decrease in the number of large and small nerve cells in the periphery with degenerative changes, and mild astrogliosis without macrophage infiltration. There were no abnormal vascular proliferations or amyloid deposition. The posterior horns, posterior roots, white matter, and the intra medullary and extramedullary vessels were normal. There were no metastatic or spondylolytic changes of the cervical vertebrae and cord. Loss of large and small neurons, a weak gliosis, and central necrosis of the anterior horn were not supportive of degenerative motor neuron disease or other diseases proposed before neuropathology. Hirayama[9] concluded that the changes could be ischemic in origin.

In combination with clinical symptoms, the neuropathological finding of ischemic change of the anterior horn resembles another ischemic neuronal disease, *téphromalacie antérieure* (anterior tephromalacia).[9] Reported by Marie and Foix in 1912,[32] *téphromalacie antérieure* consist of anterior horn infarction of lower cervical cord from occlusion of the spinal arteritis due to syphilitic arteritis or arteriosclerosis. Clinically, *téphromalacie antérieure* also shows muscular wasting restricted to the distal upper limbs, but in middle-aged or elderly people. In 1969, after a study of spinal cord of the aged, Lapresle[33] reported that the anterior horn, particularly the neurons in its central portion, was the most vulnerable to ischemia.[33] Although the mechanisms of cervical cord anterior horn damage may be different, both clinical and pathologic findings suggested a similar pathogenesis between the two diseases owing to circulatory insufficiency of the anterior

horns of lower cervical cord.[9] The name focal ischemic cervical poliomyelopathy was given for diseases with similar pathologic finding of anterior horn ischemia.

After the publication of the first autopsy case of Hirayama disease, the neuropathological findings of ischemic cervical poliomyelopathy encouraged neuroradiologic investigations of the interior changes in the spinal canal. Imaging studies revealed dynamic changes of the spinal cord and dural sac during anterior flexion of the neck in patients with Hirayama disease (**Fig. 3**). These findings include overstretch of the cord, forward displacement of the posterior dural sac, and asymmetric compression and anterior-posterior flattening of the lower cervical cord (see later discussion on

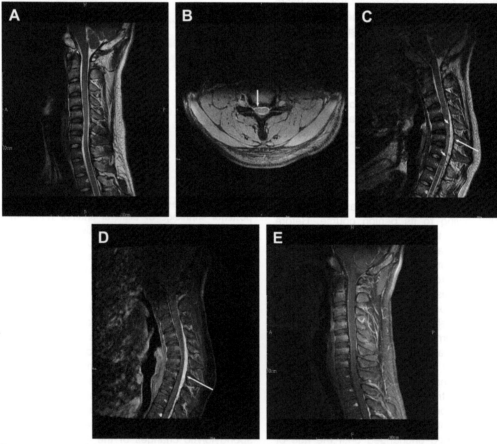

Fig. 3. A 21-year-old man with slowly progressive weakness and atrophy of hands and forearms. (*A*) Nonflexion sagittal T2-weighted MR image (3000/100/2) shows focal cord atrophy at the C5 to C7 levels. The posterior wall of the dural canal is in close contact with the spinal canal. (*B*) Nonflexion axial T2-weighted MR image (542/16/2) reveals atrophy at C7 level, more prominent at right anterior aspect of the cord (*arrow*). (*C*) Flexion sagittal T2-weighted MR image (3000/100/2) shows forward displacement of the posterior wall of the dural canal below C3 (*short arrows*), which causes marked flattening of the lower cervical cord. An epidural mass (*long arrow*) posterior to the shifting dura matter is noted, with small curvilinear flow void signals inside it. (*D*) Contrast-enhanced flexion sagittal T1-weighted MR image (530/12/2) shows strong and homogeneous enhancement of this epidural mass (*arrow*). (*E*) Contrast-enhanced nonflexion sagittal T1-weighted MR image (530/12/2), shows disappearance of the posterior dural mass and recovery of the shifting dura matter to its normal position.

more detailed image findings).[10,16,34,35] The dural displacement decreases gradually with increasing age, which also corresponds well with the duration and clinical course of the disease. These dynamic changes are unequivocal findings confined to early, progressive stage of the disease. The absence of forward displacement of the dural sac and cord compression in elderly patients whose disease had arrested suggested that this dynamic compression has a pathogenetic significance.[5,9]

Although the cause of Hirayama disease is unknown, several mechanisms were proposed. Hirayama[5] suggested that a disproportional growth between the vertebral column and the contents of the spinal canal, especially the dural sac, during the juvenile growth spurt lead to the preponderance for the adolescent population. Although the disproportional growth theory may explain the findings of forward dural sac displacement, asymmetric cord involvement cannot be explained with this theory alone. A "posterior epidural ligament factor" was proposed by Shinomiya and colleagues.[36] Anatomically, there are two kinds of posterior epidural ligaments between the posterior dura matter and the ligamentum flavum. One consists of fine elastic ligaments and the other consists of large ligaments (approximately 1–3 mm in diameter). These ligaments have a tendency to be abundant at C1 through C2, decreased below C2, and sparse at C6 and C7.[37] It has been assumed that these ligaments may contribute to resistance against the separation of the posterior dura matter from the ligamentum flavum. Unequal distribution or lack of these ligaments may be the essential cause of asymmetric cord compression. Tashiro and colleagues[24] proposed that the male prevalence is explained by a more rapid growth spurt during puberty in males. Strenuous exercise of the arms in sports or activities that requires sustained or repeated neck flexions, such as writing at a desk or playing a musical instrument, were frequently noted in patients.[5,22,38] Biondi and colleagues[23] also speculated that repeated subclinical cervical trauma is a cause of chronic microcirculatory disturbances during strenuous physical activities. Elevated serum total immunoglobulin E level (hyperIgEaemia) had also been postulated to be a precipitating factor in Hirayama disease.[39,40]

IMAGING WORK-UP AND FINDINGS

In patients with Hirayama disease, conventional radiographic findings of the cervical spine usually show no specific abnormalities other than straight alignment or scoliosis.[13] Although myelography can confirm the forward movement of the posterior dural wall during neck flexion, this examination is difficult to perform because it is not easy to retain the contrast medium in the cervical subarachnoid space when the neck is flexed, regardless of whether the patient is in a prone, supine, or decubitus position.[34] As MR imaging became more accessible in late 1980s, images in neck flexion and neutral position revealed valuable information and provided a better understanding of the dynamic nature in Hirayama disease.

Neck-flexion MR Imaging

Neck-flexion MR imaging can clearly depict forward displacement of the posterior wall of the lower cervical dural sac (see **Fig. 3**C), which is the hallmark and primary pathogenetic mechanism of Hirayama disease. The shifting dura, then, compresses the lower cervical spinal cord, usually asymmetrically (see **Fig. 3**B). Kikuchi and colleagues[15] explained the mechanism of anteriorly displaced dural canal as a tight dural canal caused by a disproportional length between the vertebrae and the dural canal during flexion. Chen and colleagues[34] explain this phenomenon as follows. The spinal dura matter is a loose sheath that is anchored in the vertebral canal by the nerve roots and by attachment to the periosteum in two places: one at the foramen magnum and the dorsal surfaces of C2 and C3, and another at the coccyx.[41] The remainder of the dura matter is only suspended and cushioned in the spinal canal by the epidural fat, venous plexus, and loose connective tissues.[41] During neck extension, the dura matter of the cervical spine is slack and thrown into accordion-like transverse folds.[42] During neck flexion, the dura tightens as the length of the cervical canal increases while the neck moves from extension to flexion. The difference in length between extension and flexion from T1 to top of the atlas is 1.5 cm at the anterior wall and 5 cm at the posterior wall.[42] Normally, the slack of the dura can compensate for the increased length during flexion. Therefore, although it smoothes out, the dura remains in close contact with the walls of the spinal canal without anterior displacement. In Hirayama disease, the dural canal is no longer slack in extension because of the imbalance in growth of the vertebrae and the dura matter, which cannot compensate for the increased length of the posterior wall during flexion, resulting in a tight dural canal. This causes anterior shifting of the posterior dural wall, and consequently compresses the spinal cord. Chronic compression may cause microcirculatory disturbances in the territory of the anterior spinal artery or in the anterior portion of the spinal cord, which eventually lead to ischemia and necrosis of the anterior horns, as mentioned in the pathophysiology section above.

In association with anterior displacement of posterior dural wall, neck-flexion MR imaging also shows a well-enhanced, crescent-shaped mass in the epidural space of the lower cervical canal with small curvilinear flow-void signals inside it (see **Fig. 3**C, D). This mass vanishes as the neck returns to the neutral position, suggesting that the mass represent congestion of the posterior internal vertebral venous plexus rather than vascular malformation or tumors (see **Fig. 3**E). The flow-void signals inside the crescent-shaped mass indicate the dilated venous plexuses, which was further confirmed by Elsheikh and colleagues[43] using epidural venography. Some pathophysiologic factors are responsible for the engorged venous plexus. First, the negative pressure in the posterior spinal canal resulting from anterior shifting of the dural canal increases the flow to the posterior internal vertebral venous plexus.[44] Second, simultaneously, the anteriorly displaced dural canal compresses the anterior internal vertebral venous plexus and increases the burden of the posterior internal vertebral venous plexus.[34] Third, the posture of neck flexion decreases the venous drainage from internal vertebral venous plexus to the jugular veins.[44] In combination, these factors cause the engorgement of posterior internal vertebral venous plexus,

which also became a striking and characteristic imaging finding of Hirayama disease.

Neutral-position MR Imaging

Despite the characteristic findings on neck-flexion MR imaging, findings on nonflexion neutral-position MR imaging is equally important. The ability to identify abnormalities on routine neutral position MR imaging studies by neuroradiologists can increase the detection rate of Hirayama disease. Chen and colleagues[35] investigated the sensitivity and specificity of these neutral-position MR imaging findings in patients with Hirayama disease (**Table 1**). These include abnormal cervical curvature, loss of attachment (LOA) between the posterior dural sac and subjacent lamina, localized lower cervical cord atrophy, asymmetric cord flattening, and noncompressed intramedullary high-signal intensity on T2-weighted MR images.

Loss of normal cervical lordosis with straight or kyphotic cervical spine alignment is a nonspecific but common finding in patients with Hirayama disease.[13,16,35] According to the principles suggested by Guigui and colleagues[45] and Batzdorf and Batzdorff,[46] cervical curvature can be measured by a line drawn from the dorsocaudal aspect of the C2 vertebral body to the dorsocaudal aspect of the C7 vertebral body and the relationship of the dorsal aspect of the C3 to C6 vertebral body with this line (**Fig. 4**). In normal lordotic cervical curvature, no part of the dorsal aspect of

Table 1
Sensitivity, specificity, accuracy, positive predictive value, and negative predictive value of neutral-position MR imaging findings in diagnosis of Hirayama disease

MR Imaging Finding	Sensitivity (%)	Specificity (%)	Accuracy (%)	Positive Predictive Value (%)	Negative Predictive Value (%)
Localized cord atrophy	58.7 (43.2, 73.0)	100	80.4 (71.1, 87.8)	100	72.9 (60.9, 82.8)
Asymmetric cord flattening	69.6 (54.2, 82.3)	100	85.6 (77.0, 91.9)	100	78.5 (66.5, 87.7)
LOA	93.5 (82.1, 98.6)	98.0 (89.6, 99.9)	95.9 (89.8, 98.9)	97.7 (88.0, 99.9)	94.3 (84.3, 98.8)
Abnormal cervical curvature	82.6 (68.6, 92.2)	47.1 (32.9, 61.5)	63.9 (53.5, 73.4)	58.5 (45.6, 70.6)	75.0 (56.6, 88.5)
Noncompressed intramedullary high-signal intensity on T2-weighted MR images	28.3 (16.0, 43.5)	96.1 (86.5, 99.5)	63.9 (53.5, 73.4)	86.7 (59.5, 98.3)	59.8 (48.3, 70.4)

Data are percentages. Numbers in parentheses are 95% confidence intervals.

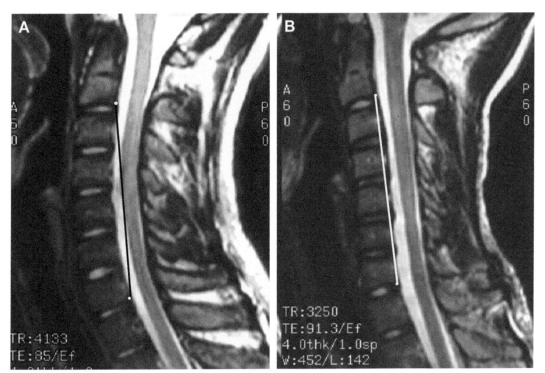

Fig. 4. (A) Sagittal fast-spin-echo T2-weighted MR image (4133/85) in a 17-year-old male control subject. (B) Sagittal fast-spine-echo T2-weighted MR image (3250/9103) in a 17-year-old male patient with slowly progressive weakness and atrophy of the left hand and forearm. Cervical curvature is measured according to the relationship of the dorsal aspect of the vertebral bodies C3 through C6 to a line drawn from the dorsocaudal aspect of the vertebral body C2 to the dorsocaudal aspect of the vertebral body C7 (*black line* in A, *white line* in B). By definition, normal lordotic cervical curvature is curvature in which no part of the dorsal aspect of the vertebral bodies C3 through C6 cross the line from C2 through C7 (A). An abnormal (straight or kyphotic) curvature is curvature in which part or all of the dorsal aspects of the vertebral bodies C3 through C6 meet or cross that line (B). (*From* Chen CJ, Hsu HL, Tseng YC, et al. Hirayama flexion myelopathy: neutral-position MR imaging findings—importance of loss of attachment. Radiology 2004;231:39–44; with permission.)

C3 to C6 vertebral body crosses the line drawn from C2 to C7. In an abnormal straight or kyphotic curvature, all or part of the dorsal aspect of C3 to C6 meet or cross the line drawn from C2 to C7.

The LOA sign is the separation of the posterior dural sac and subjacent lamina in the neutral position possibly related to a tight dural sac (**Fig. 5**). The sign is best evaluated on each side of the lamina at the pedicular level of C4 through C6 on axial T2*-weighted MR images. The degree of separation between the posterior dural sac and its subjacent lamina is evaluated within a range defined medially by the point of junction with the lamina and laterally by a tangential line along the medial aspect of the pedicle. A separation of less than 33.3% at all the observed segments was considered normal, whereas a separation of more than 33.3% at any of the observed segments was considered significant for LOA.[35] The LOA sign, reported by Chen and colleagues,[35] is an

effective finding in the diagnosis of Hirayama disease with sensitivity and specificity of 93.5% and 98%, respectively.

Localized lower cervical cord atrophy and asymmetric cord flattening can be depicted on axial and sagittal MR images, most commonly found at the level of C4 to C7 (**Figs. 6** and **7B**). Localized cord atrophy is defined as a decrease in cord size in comparison with the normal cord above and below the affected level.[35] A note of caution is to verify cord atrophy on sagittal MR images with appropriate contiguous transverse MR images because it is possible to make an erroneous interpretation of cord atrophy on sagittal images if the spinal cord is not truly in the midline. Asymmetric cord flattening can be evaluated most accurately on T2*-weighted MR images, preferably cord flattening without a narrowed or obliterated adjacent subarachnoid space, as the accuracy of this finding is greatly decreased if

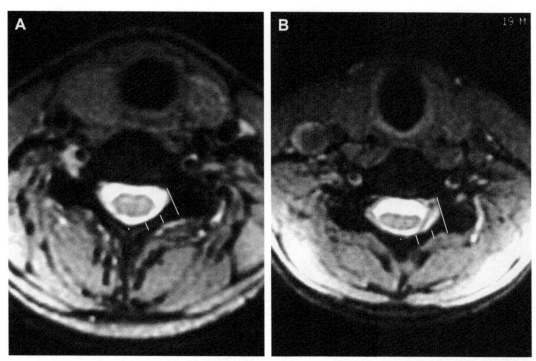

Fig. 5. Transverse neutral-position T2*-weighted MR image (433/17, with 20° flip angle) at the pedicular level. (*A*) Image in 20-year-old male control subject. (*B*) Image in an 18-year-old patient with Hirayama disease. The lamina, defined medially by point of junction of lamina and laterally by tangential line along medial aspect of pedicle (*longest white line* in *A* and *B*), is equally divided into three parts. Images show less than 33.3% LOA between the posterior dural sac and subjacent lamina in *a* and more than 33.3% LOA in *b*. Asymmetrically bilateral cord flattening (more severe on the right side) is also depicted in *b*. (*From* Chen CJ, Hsu HL, Tseng YC, et al. Hirayama flexion myelopathy: neutral-position MR imaging findings—importance of loss of attachment. Radiology 2004;231:39–44; with permission.)

there is presence of adjacent spurs or herniated discs. An elliptic spinal cord is considered normal, a pear-shaped spinal cord is considered asymmetric cord flattening, and a triangular spinal cord is considered symmetric cord flattening.[35]

Noncompressed intramedullary high-signal intensity on T2-weighted MR images in short lengths of 1 to 3 spinal segments is also common at the level of C4 to C7, corresponding with the site of cord atrophy and asymmetric flattening (see **Fig. 7**). Noncompressed intramedullary high-signal intensity is only considered if the surrounding subarachnoid space is patent because intramedullary high-signal intensity associated with cord compression could be due to the force of adjacent spurs or herniated discs.[35] On axial images, these hyperdense signals are mainly localized to bilateral anterior horns or anterior and lateral horns of the gray matter. This abnormality indicates either ischemia or gliosis, which corresponds with the neuropathological finding of ischemic cervical poliomyelopathy.[31,35]

The recognition of these image findings on neutral-position MR imaging should raise suspicion for Hirayama disease. An additional neck-flexion MR imaging study should be arranged to confirm this diagnosis.

TREATMENT

Hirayama disease often occurs with vague initial symptoms, leading to a delay in diagnosis. Though Hirayama disease is self-limiting, early diagnosis is still necessary because it has been shown that early intervention can stop disease progression.[5–7,27] If recognized early, conservative treatment using cervical collar to avoid neck flexion can alleviate muscle weakness, stop progression of the disease in most patients, and even increase of grip strength and improvement of cold paresis in some patients.[5,27] Application of a cervical collar for 3 to 4 years is advised.[27,47] Although some patients could be expected to have a natural, spontaneous arrest, the duration of progression

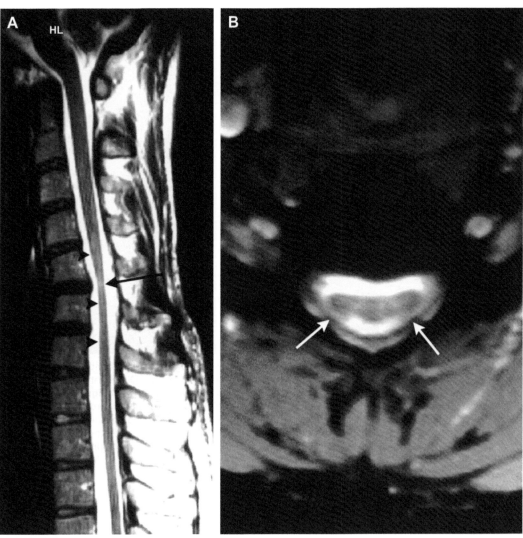

Fig. 6. Neutral-position MR images in a 24-year-old male patient with progressive bilateral weakness and atrophy, which is greater on the right side than on the left, for 3 years. (*A*) Sagittal fast-spin-echo T2-weighted image (4000/85) shows kyphotic cervical curvature, localized cord atrophy at C5 and C6 (*arrowheads*), and faint noncompressed intramedullary high signal intensity at C5-6 disk (*arrow*). (*B*) Transverse T2*-weighted MR image (433/17, with 20° flip angle) at pedicular level of C5 shows symmetric cord flattening and 100% LOA between the posterior dural sac and subjacent lamina (*arrows*). (*From* Chen CJ, Hsu HL, Tseng YC, et al. Hirayama flexion myelopathy: neutral-position MR imaging findings—importance of loss of attachment. Radiology 2004;231: 39–44; with permission.)

was significantly shorter in patients treated (mean 1.8 ± 1.1 years) compared with untreated patients (3.2 ± 2.2 years).[5] Decompressive surgery is indicated only for patients with persistent neurologic deficits and deterioration despite conservative management. Spinal fusion and decompression by surgical procedures are beneficial to the relief of dynamic impairment and static compression. Anterior stabilization of lower cervical vertebrae with corpectomy, discectomy, and supplemented metallic plate fixation, as well as posterior decompression with laminectomy and dural graft augmentation procedures were applied and discussed.[5,27,48,49] However, which route is superior is still debatable. Remarkable arrest of the natural progressive course by early intervention further supported the pathogenetic hypothesis of flexion-induced cervical ischemic poliomyelopathy because this clinical finding is most unlikely in degenerative motor neuron disease.[5,9]

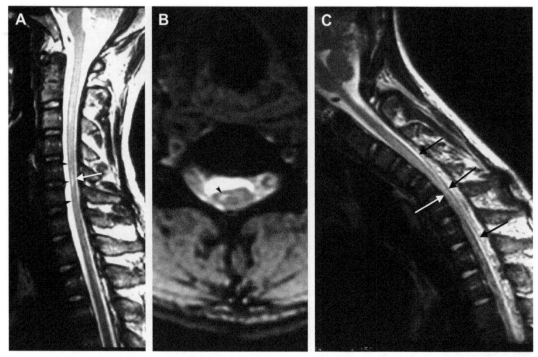

Fig. 7. Neutral-position MR images in 18-year-old male patient with progressive right hand and forearm weakness and atrophy for 2 1/2 years. (*A*) Sagittal fast-spin-echo T2-weighted image (4000/85) shows normal cervical curvature, localized cord atrophy (*arrowheads*), and noncompressed intramedullary high signal intensity (*arrow*). (*B*) Transverse T2*-weighted MR image (433/17, with 20° flip angle) shows asymmetric cord flattening (on right side) and nearly 100% LOA between the posterior dural sac and subjacent lamina. Intramedullary high signal intensity (*arrowhead*) is depicted in right-sided gray matter. (*C*) Sagittal flexion fast-spin-echo T2-weighted image (4000/85) shows anterior displacement of posterior dural sac (*black arrows*) and cord compression (*white arrow*). (*From* Chen CJ, Hsu HL, Tseng YC, et al. Hirayama flexion myelopathy: neutral-position MR imaging findings–Importance of loss of attachment. Radiology 2004;231:39–44; with permission.)

SUMMARY

Hirayama disease is a rare disease presented with slow, progressive asymmetric muscular weakness and atrophy of the distal upper limb predominantly in young male patients, followed by spontaneous arrest within 3 to 5 years. Through the years, this disease has been well established as a new disease entity separated from degenerative motor neuron disease. Neuropathologic findings suggest focal ischemic cervical poliomyelopathy localized to anterior horn of the cervical spinal cord, characterized by necrosis of anterior horn cells, decreased number of large and small nerve cells in the periphery with degenerative changes, and mild astrogliosis without macrophage infiltration. Neuroradiologic investigations revealed compressive flattening of the lower cervical cord due to forward displacement of the cervical dural sac during neck flexion. Although the underlying causative mechanism remains unclear, these findings together suggested flexion-induced cervical myelopathy leading to ischemic changes in the anterior horn of cervical cord. Conservative treatments using a neck collar or spinal fusion and decompression by surgical procedures are targeted to minimize neck flexion and prevent progression of muscular weakness and atrophy.

Hirayama disease is a slow, progressive disease that can have a good prognosis if detected and intervened at an early stage of the disease process. Therefore, early recognition of clinical features, as well as suspicious findings on neutral-position MR imaging, should raise suspicion of the disease; and an additional neck-flexion MR imaging study should be arranged to confirm the diagnosis. Although Hirayama disease is more commonly reported in Japan and other Asian countries, with the increase of Asian population in North America over the past century, clinicians and neuroradiologists in North America should also be aware of and familiarize themselves with the clinical features and image findings of this disease.

REFERENCES

1. Hirayama K. Non-progressive juvenile spinal muscular atrophy of the distal upper limb (Hirayama's disease). In: de Jong JM, editor. Handbook of clinical neurology, vol. 15. Amsterdam: Elsevier Science; 1991. p. 107–20, 59.

2. Hirayama K, Toyokura Y, Tsubaki T. Juvenile muscular atrophy of unilateral upper extremity: a new clinical entity. Psychiatr Neurol Jpn 1959;61:2190–8.

3. Hirayama K, Toyokura Y, Tsubaki T, et al. Juvenile muscular atrophy of unilateral upper extremity. Neurology 1963;13:373–80.

4. Hirayama K. Juvenile non-progressive muscular atrophy localized in the hand and forearm: observations in 38 cases. Rinsho Shinkeigaku 1972;12:313–24 [in Japanese].

5. Hirayama K. Juvenile muscular atrophy of distal upper extremity (Hirayama disease). Intern Med 2000;39:283–90.

6. Huang YC, Ro LS, Chang HS, et al. A clinical study of Hirayama disease in Taiwan. Muscle Nerve 2008; 37:576–82.

7. Zhou B, Chen L, Fan DS, et al. Clinical features of Hirayama disease in mainland China. Amyotroph Lateral Scler 2010;11:133–9.

8. Hirayama K, Tomonaga M, Kitano K, et al. The first autopsy case of "juvenile muscular atrophy of unilateral upper extremity". Shinkei Naika (Neurol Med) 1985;22:85–8.

9. Hirayama K. Juvenile muscular atrophy of distal upper extremity (Hirayama disease): focal cervical ischemic poliomyelopathy. Neuropathology 2000; 20:S91–4.

10. Hirayama K, Tokumaru Y. Cervical dural sac and spinal cord in juvenile muscular atrophy of distal upper extremity. Neurology 2000;54:1922–6.

11. Toma S, Shiozawa Z. Amyotrophic cervical myelopathy in adolescence. J Neurol Neurosurg Psychiatry 1995;58:56–64.

12. Tokumaru Y, Hirayama K. Anterior shift of posterior lower cervical dura mater in patients with juvenile muscular atrophy of unilateral upper extremity. Rinsho Shinkeigaku 1989;29:1237–43 [in Japanese].

13. Mukai E, Sobue I, Muto T, et al. Abnormal radiological findings on juvenile-type distal and segmental muscular atrophy of upper extremities. Rinsho Shinkeigaku 1985;25:620–6 [in Japanese].

14. Mii K, Iida H, Tachibana S, et al. The overstretch syndrome: a new cervical myelopathy caused by the stretch mechanism of the spinal cord. Spinal Surg 1989;3:137–41.

15. Kikuchi S, Tashiro K, Kitagawa M, et al. A mechanism of juvenile muscular atrophy localized in the hand and forearm (Hirayama's disease): flexion myelopathy with tight dural canal in flexion. Rinsho Shinkeigaku 1987;27:412–9 [in Japanese].

16. Pradhan S, Gupta RK. Magnetic resonance imaging in juvenile asymmetric segmental spinal muscular atrophy. J Neurol Sci 1997;146:133–8.

17. Gourie-Devi M, Nalini A. Long-term follow-up of 44 patients with brachial monomelic amyotrophy. Acta Neurol Scand 2003;107:215–20.

18. Misra UK, Kalita J, Mishra VN, et al. A clinical, magnetic resonance imaging, and survival motor neuron gene deletion study of Hirayama disease. Arch Neurol 2005;62:120–3.

19. Peiris JB, Seneviratne KN, Wichremasinghe HR, et al. Non-familial juvenile distal spinal muscular atrophy of upper extremity. J Neurol Neurosurg Psychiatry 1989;52:314–9.

20. Tan CT. Juvenile muscular atrophy of distal upper extremities. J Neurol Neurosurg Psychiatry 1985; 48:285–6.

21. Schroder R, Keller E, Flacke S, et al. MRI findings in Hirayama disease: flexion-induced cervical myelopathy or intrinsic motor neuron disease? J Neurol 1999;246:1069–74.

22. Hashimoto O, Asada M, Ohta M, et al. Clinical observation of juvenile non-progressive muscular atrophy localized in hand and forearm. J Neurol 1976;211: 105–10.

23. Biondi A, Dormont D, Weitzner I Jr, et al. MR imaging of the cervical cord in juvenile amyotrophy of distal upper extremity. AJNR Am J Neuroradiol 1989;10: 263–8.

24. Tashiro K, Kikuchi S, Itoyama Y, et al. Nationwide survey of juvenile muscular atrophy of distal upper extremity (Hirayama disease) in Japan. Amyotroph Lateral Scler Other Motor Neuron Disord 2006;7: 38–45.

25. Atchayaram N, Vasudev MK, Goel G. Familial monomelic amyotrophy (Hirayama disease): two brothers with classical flexion induced dynamic changes of the cervical dural sac. Neurol India 2009;57:810–2.

26. Kijima M, Hirayama K, Nakajima Y. Symptomatic and electrophysiological study on cold paresis in juvenile muscular atrophy of distal upper extremity (Hirayama disease). Rinsho Shinkeigaku 2002;42:841–8 [in Japanese].

27. Lin MS, Kung WM, Chiu WT, et al. Hirayama disease. J Neurosurg Spine 2010;12:629–34.

28. Hosokawa T, Fujieda M, Wakiguchi H, et al. Pediatric Hirayama disease. Pediatr Neurol 2010;43:151–3.

29. Sobue I, Saito N, Ilda M, et al. Juvenile type of distal and segmental muscular atrophy of upper extremities. Ann Neurol 1978;3:429–32.

30. Kao KP, Wu ZA, Chern CM. Juvenile lower cervical spinal muscular atrophy in Taiwan: report of 27 Chinese cases. Neuroepidemiology 1993;12:331–5.

31. Pradhan S. Bilaterally symmetric form of Hirayama disease. Neurology 2009;72:2083–9.

32. Marie P, Foix CH. L'atrophie isolee non-progressive des petits muscles de la main: Téphromalacie

antérieure. Nouv Iconographie Salpêtrière 1912;25: 353–63, 427–53 [in French].

33. Lapresle J. Sur quelques aspects neuropathologiques des troubles de la circulation dans la moelle épinière. Bull Schweiz Akad Med Wiss 1969;24: 512–29 [in French].

34. Chen CJ, Chen CM, Wu CL, et al. Hirayama disease: MR diagnosis. AJNR Am J Neuroradiol 1998;19: 365–8.

35. Chen CJ, Hsu HL, Tseng YC, et al. Hirayama flexion myelopathy: neutral-position MR imaging findings—importance of loss of attachment. Radiology 2004; 231:39–44.

36. Shinomiya K, Dawson J, Spengler DM, et al. An analysis of the posterior epidural ligament role on the cervical spinal cord. Spine 1996;21:2081–8.

37. Shinomiya K, Sato T, Spengler DM, et al. Isolated muscle atrophy of the distal upper extremity in cervical spinal cord compressive disorders. J Spinal Disord 1995;8:311–6.

38. Hirayama K. Juvenile muscular atrophy of distal upper extremity (Hirayama disease). In: Goto F, Takakura K, Kinoshita M, et al, editors. Annual review neurology. Tokyo: Chugai-Igaku; 1996. p. 249–60.

39. Chen TH, Huang CH, Hsieh TJ, et al. Symmetric atrophy of bilateral distal upper extremities and hyperIgEaemia in a male adolescent with Hirayama disease. J Child Neurol 2010;25:371–4.

40. Ito S, Kuwabara S, Fukutake T, et al. HyperIgEaemia in patients with juvenile muscular atrophy of distal extremity (Hirayama disease). J Neurol Neurosurg Psychiatry 2005;76:132–4.

41. Williams PL, Warwick R, Dyson M, et al. Gray's anatomy. 37th edition. London: Churchill Livingstone; 1989. p. 1086–92.

42. Bland JH. Basic anatomy. In: Bland JH, editor. Disorders of the cervical spine: diagnosis and medical management. 2nd editon. Philadelphia: Saunders; 1994. p. 41–70.

43. Elsheikh B, Kissel JT, Christoforidis G, et al. Spinal angiography and epidural venography in juvenile muscular atrophy of the distal arm "Hirayama disease". Muscle Nerve 2009;40:206–12.

44. Mukai E, Matsuo T, Muto T, et al. Magnetic resonance imaging of juvenile-type distal and segmental muscular atrophy of upper extremities. Rinsho Shinkeigaku 1987;27:99–107 [in Japanese].

45. Guigui P, Benoist M, Deburge A. Spinal deformity and instability after multilevel cervical laminectomy for spondylotic myelopathy. Spine 1998;23:440–7.

46. Batzdorf U, Batzdorff A. Analysis of cervical spine curvature in patients with cervical spondylosis. Neurosurgery 1988;22:827–36.

47. Tokumaru Y, Hirayama K. Cervical collar therapy for juvenile muscular atrophy of distal upper extremity (Hirayama disease): results from 38 cases. Rinsho Shinkeigaku 2001;41:173–8 [in Japanese].

48. Imamura H, Matsumoto S, Hayase M, et al. A case of Hirayama's disease successfully treated by anterior cervical decompression and fusion. No To Shinkei 2001;53:1033–8 [in Japanese].

49. Kohno M, Takahashi H, Ide K, et al. Surgical treatment for patients with cervical flexion myelopathy. J Neurosurg 1999;91(Suppl 1):33–42.

Neuroimaging in Acute Transverse Myelitis

Christine Goh, MBBS, FRANZCR[a],*,
Pramit M. Phal, MBBS, FRANZCR[a],
Patricia M. Desmond, MSc, MD, FRANZCR[a,b]

KEYWORDS

- Transverse myelitis • MRI • Spinal cord
- Idiopathic transverse myelitis • Parainfectious myelitis

Transverse myelitis can occur at any age, but is reported to have bimodal peaks in the second and fourth decades.[1] Clinical symptoms of bilateral weakness, sensory disturbance, and autonomic dysfunction typically evolve over hours or days, most progressing to maximal clinical severity within 10 days of onset. A rostral border of sensory loss is usually thoracic, but pediatric cases have a higher rate of cervical cord involvement. At maximal clinical severity, 80% to 94% of patients have numbness, paresthesia, or band-like dysesthesia; half have a paraparesis; and almost all have bladder dysfunction to some degree.[2]

The prognosis is highly variable; postinfectious cases in children typically have good outcomes, while other patients can be left with devastating neurologic deficits. The optimal treatment will depend upon the underlying etiology, but generally immunomodulatory treatments including steroids, immunoglobulins or plasmapheresis play a major role.

Owing to the heterogeneous pathogenesis and prognosis of transverse myelitis, it is vitally important that there be uniformly applied criteria for diagnosis and classification. This is useful, not only to guide individual patient management, but also to assess efficacy of current treatment regimes and allow identification of targets for potential novel therapies.

The diagnostic criteria devised by the Transverse Myelitis Consortium Working Group (**Box 1**) aims to delineate transverse myelitis from the broader spectrum of transverse myelopathies and to divide transverse myelitis into idiopathic and disease-associated groups.

The first requirement of the diagnostic criteria is an appropriate clinical picture, with symptoms referable to the cord and bilateral but not necessarily symmetric involvement. Cases with a history of spinal irradiation and those with a clear arterial distribution to their deficit are excluded. MR imaging is performed urgently to exclude compressive causes and other causes of myelopathy such as spinal arteriovenous malformation.

The second requirement of the diagnostic criteria is that evolution of symptoms to the maximal clinical severity must be between 4 hours and 21 days. The lower limit of 4 hours onset is designed to prevent cases of cord infarction, typically of abrupt onset, from being erroneously diagnosed as transverse myelitis.

The third requirement is confirmation of an active inflammatory process by presence of a cellular infiltrate and/or elevated protein on cerebrospinal fluid (CSF) analysis, or by gadolinium enhancement on MR imaging of the spinal cord.

In patients who meet the criteria for transverse myelitis, idiopathic is separated from disease-associated transverse myelitis by specifying further criteria related to presence of clinical, laboratory, or imaging evidence of connective tissue diseases,

Financial disclosure: None.

[a] Department of Radiology, Royal Melbourne Hospital, Grattan Street, Parkville, Victoria 3050, Australia
[b] University of Melbourne, Royal Melbourne Hospital, Grattan Street, Parkville, Victoria 3050, Australia
* Corresponding author.
E-mail address: christinegoh79@gmail.com

Box 1
Diagnostic criteria for transverse myelitis

Inclusion criteria for diagnosis of transverse myelitis (idiopathic or disease associated)

   Development of sensory, motor, or autonomic dysfunction attributable to the spinal cord

   Bilateral symptoms

   Clearly defined sensory level

   Exclusion of compressive causes by MR imaging or CT myelography

   Spinal cord inflammation demonstrated by cerebrospinal fluid pleocytosis, elevated IgG, or gadolinium enhancement

   Progression to clinical nadir between 4 hours and 21 days from onset of symptoms

Exclusion criteria for diagnosis of transverse myelitis (idiopathic or disease associated)

   History of irradiation to the spine within 10 years

   Clear arterial distribution clinical defect consistent with anterior spinal artery occlusion

   Abnormal flow voids on the surface of the cord consistent with arteriovenous malformation

Exclusion criteria for idiopathic transverse myelitis

   Serologic or clinical evidence of connective tissue disease (sarcoidosis, Behçet disease, Sjögren syndrome, systemic lupus erythematosus, or mixed connective tissue disorder)

   Central nervous system manifestations of syphilis, Lyme disease, HIV, HTLV-1, *Mycoplasma*, or other viral infection.

   Brain abnormalities suggestive of multiple sclerosis

   History of clinically apparent optic neuritis

Data from Transverse Myelitis Consortium Working Group. Proposed diagnostic criteria and nosology of acute transverse myelitis. Neurology 2002;59:499–505.

---

infective conditions, multiple sclerosis, and optic neuritis.

Thus, the diagnostic work-up of transverse myelitis begins with contrast-enhanced MR imaging of the spinal cord and brain, CSF analysis including cell count and protein, an autoimmune screen, and specialized tests such as serum and CSF culture, serology, and polymerase chain reaction (PCR).

A study evaluating the diagnostic criteria found that patients presenting with transverse myelopathy could be grouped as 15.6% idiopathic, 20.5% systemic disease, 17.3% infectious or parainfectious, 10.8% multiple sclerosis, and 17% neuromyelitis optica, with a further 18.8% found to have spinal cord infarct instead of transverse myelitis.[3]

IDIOPATHIC TRANSVERSE MYELITIS

Idiopathic transverse myelitis made up 16.5% of acute myelopathy presentations in one large series.[3] Heterogeneity in patient demographics, response to therapy, and outcome suggest that this group remains diverse in its pathogenesis. It is expected that better understanding of the various known causes of transverse myelitis and the development of more sensitive and specific microbial assays and autoimmune markers will cause this percent to shrink. It is yet to be determined whether there is a unified pathogenetic entity of idiopathic transverse myelitis.

Prognosis

Outcomes have been heterogeneous in this group of patients—nearly equally divided between little-to-no residual disability, moderate residual disability, and severe disability.[4] However, the reported rates of good outcomes have ranged between 20% and 64% in different studies.[3,5,6]

Studies have found that elevated CSF interleukin (IL)-6 levels in transverse myelitis patients correlate with and are strongly predictive of disability,[7] suggesting that IL-6 may be the central mediator of tissue injury in transverse myelitis. Protein 14-3-3, thought to be a marker of axonal damage and a sensitive marker of Creutzfeldt-Jakob disease, has also been found in the CSF of transverse myelitis patients. Some, but not all, studies have found that this may correlate with worse outcome or progression to multiple sclerosis.[8–10]

Imaging Features

MR imaging of the spinal cord

MR imaging demonstrates T2-hyperintense spinal cord lesions in almost all reported cases of idiopathic transverse myelitis. The classic lesion is predominantly central, extends over more than two segments, and involves more than two-thirds the cross-sectional area of the cord (**Fig. 1**).[4,6,11,12] The typical description includes a preference for the thoracic cord[12]; however, two studies[3,6] have found cervical lesions are more common than thoracic (44% cervical vs 37% thoracic, and 60% cervical vs 33% thoracic, respectively).

Cord expansion is described in approximately half of cases. Enhancement is present in 37% to 74% and has been reported to be more frequent in the subacute stage than at initial acute presentation.[3,4,6] The pattern of enhancement is variable, and has been described as moderate diffuse enhancement, poorly defined heterogeneous enhancement, nodular enhancement or peripheral enhancement.

Diffusion tensor imaging

Although not currently a routine part of imaging assessment of transverse myelitis, MR diffusion tensor imaging has recently been described in transverse myelitis and, in the future, may assist in characterization of the lesion and in assessment of prognosis. A small study by Renoux and colleagues[13] compared healthy subjects to 15 patients who had a diverse range of inflammatory

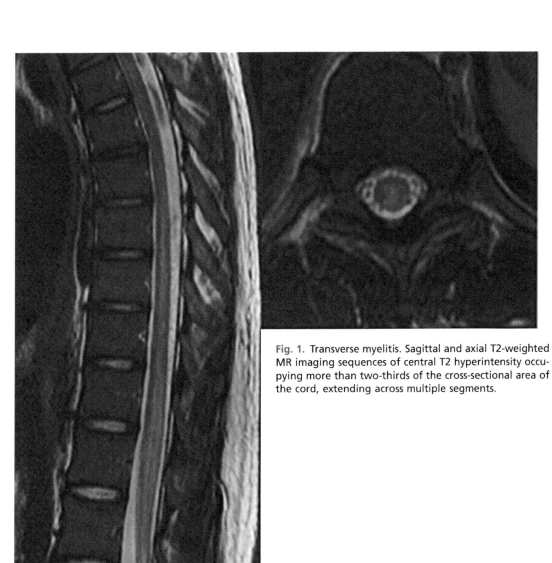

Fig. 1. Transverse myelitis. Sagittal and axial T2-weighted MR imaging sequences of central T2 hyperintensity occupying more than two-thirds of the cross-sectional area of the cord, extending across multiple segments.

myelopathies, confirming that fractional anisotropy (FA) is reduced within the cord lesion of myelitis patients. They also found that diffusion tensor imaging was more sensitive than T2-weighted imaging in identifying lesions. In 80% of patients, additional FA lesions were identified and, in 41.6% of these, the T2-occult lesion better correlated with the level of clinical manifestation than the T2-apparent lesion. A more recent study compared 10 patients with idiopathic transverse myelitis to healthy subjects.[14] The degree of FA reduction within the lesion and presence of reduced FA in distal normal-appearing cord both correlated with worse outcomes.

Longitudinally extensive versus acute partial transverse myelitis

The length of the cord lesion, not currently specified in the diagnostic criteria, may be turn out to be an important discriminator in terms of pathogenesis and prognosis. Some researchers have differentiated between the so-called longitudinally extensive transverse myelitis (LETM), which extends over more than three segments and is centrally located involving all or most of the cross section of the cord, and acute partial myelitis, which has fewer than two segments of cord involvement and is eccentrically located or asymmetric, suggesting the prognosis may be worse in the patients with a centrally located long-segment lesion.[15,16]

The morphology of the cord lesion and presence of abnormalities on the MR imaging of the brain have also been found to correlate with the risk of relapsing disease that eventually satisfies criteria for multiple sclerosis. When the cord lesion is long-segment and central in location, the risk of progression to clinically definite multiple sclerosis is low, at less than 2%. An asymmetric cord lesion less than two segments in length in combination with a normal initial MR imagining of the brain has 10% risk of progression to clinically definite multiple sclerosis over 61 months follow-up[17]; this increases to 21% risk of progression at 20 years follow-up according to another study of clinically isolated syndromes such as transverse myelitis and optic neuritis.[18] When the initial MR imaging of the brain shows the presence of nonspecific white matter lesions, the risk of progression to multiple sclerosis is substantially increased, with rates of up to 88% reported.[18]

MULTIPLE SCLEROSIS AND NEUROMYELITIS OPTICA
Multiple Sclerosis

Rarely, transverse myelitis may be the initial presentation of multiple sclerosis, a multiphasic, inflammatory, demyelinating disorder affecting brain, cord, and optic nerves, with the highest incidence seen in young-adult females. Diagnosis requires clinical and MR imaging evidence of characteristic lesions demonstrating dissemination in time and space. The diagnosis is supported by the presence of oligoclonal bands in CSF, which are found in more than 80% of patients.[19] Visually evoked response testing may reveal subclinical optic nerve involvement.

In contrast to transverse myelitis, the classic spinal cord lesions in multiple sclerosis are small, involve less than two segments, and predominantly affect the peripheral cord in a dorsal and lateral location (**Fig. 2**).[20] Active lesions are T2 hyperintense, with gadolinium enhancement. In the subacute to chronic phase, enhancement and swelling resolves. Old lesions may become T1 hypointense or be associated with focal atrophy. This dissemination in time is a key concept in differentiating multiple sclerosis from transverse myelitis. In the rare instances where multiple sclerosis presents as transverse myelitis, follow-up imaging will demonstrate new lesions occurring in cord and brain.

Neuromyelitis Optica

This severe relapsing demyelinating condition, previously referred to as Devic disease, affects the cord and optic nerves with relative sparing of the brain. The disease is demographically and clinically distinct from multiple sclerosis, affecting an older age group (39 years compared with 29 years), with more pronounced female predominance, and with disproportionate representation from the nonwhite population.[21,22] Attacks are frequently more severe than in multiple sclerosis and lead to greater residual disability, with more than 50% of patients visually impaired and requiring ambulatory assistance at 5 years from diagnosis. CSF analysis reveals pleocytosis with high proportion of neutrophils, and oligoclonal bands are present in only 15% to 30% of neuromyelitis optica (NMO) cases compared with 85% of multiple sclerosis cases.[21]

The concept of NMO as a condition discrete from other forms of demyelination has been strengthened by the discovery of an NMO-specific autoantibody that binds to aquaporin 4, the water channel protein most abundant in the CNS, which is highly specific (91%) and sensitive (73%) to NMO.[23] Further refinements to the immunoassay have achieved sensitivity and specificity of 91% and 100%, and higher titers of the antibody have been demonstrated to correlate with disease severity and clinical relapse.[24] The 2006

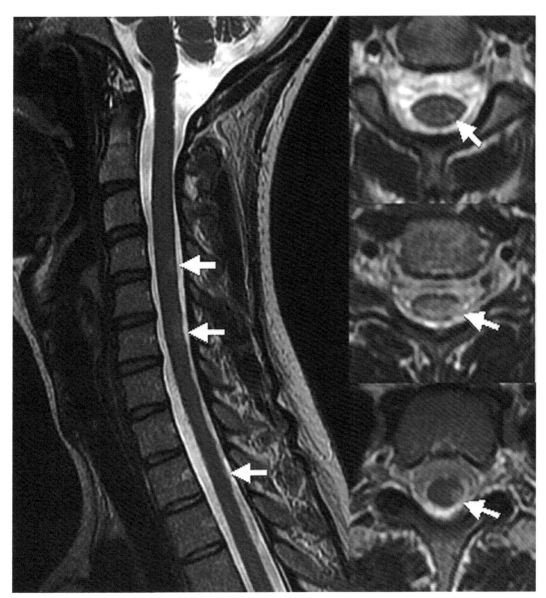

Fig. 2. Multiple sclerosis. Sagittal and axial T2-weighted sequences through the cervical spine of multiple, short-segment T2 hyperintense lesions that are peripheral in location (*arrows*).

revised diagnostic criteria for NMO reflects these developments. The diagnostic combination of two out of three criteria provides 99% sensitivity and 90% specificity for the NMO.[25] These include NMO IgG positivity, longitudinally extensive cord lesion, or onset MR imaging of the brain which is nondiagnostic for multiple sclerosis.

On MR imaging, the T2-hyperintense cord lesions are typically centrally located and span more than three segments. Enhancement is variable, but patchy central enhancement and expansion is common in the acute phase.[22] The myelitis can extend cranially to involve brainstem with resultant hiccups, nausea, and respiratory failure.

MR imaging evidence of brain involvement is uncommon at presentation, but the most patients will develop nonspecific and clinically silent white matter lesions later in the course. In 10% of patients, multiple sclerosis-like cerebral lesions have been described, but were reported to have a subtly differing appearance on postgadolinium T1 sequences, described as "cloud-like" with patchy enhancement and indistinct margins.[26] In another 10%, involvement of the hypothalamus and periaqueductal gray matter has been described. This is thought to be typical of NMO and is explained with reference to the high expression of aquaporin 4 at these sites.[27]

Of NMO patients, 10% to 40% have a coexistent autoimmune disorder such as SLE, Sjögren syndrome or myasthenia gravis, presumably reflecting susceptibility to autoimmune conditions.[28,29]

NMO IgG has become a very useful tool in the work-up of transverse myelitis. The combination of NMO-IgG positivity and LETM implies that NMO is the underlying cause. Patients can receive the optimal treatment for their myelopathy and are excluded from the idiopathic transverse myelitis cohort in research projects.

SYSTEMIC AUTOIMMUNE CONDITIONS

Transverse myelitis in autoimmune conditions has most frequently been described in SLE, with and without antiphospholipid syndrome, but well-documented cases have implicated Sjögren syndrome, mixed connective tissue disease, antiphospholipid syndrome, sarcoidosis, Behçet disease, rheumatoid arthritis, and ankylosing spondylitis. Although transverse myelitis is an uncommon complication of connective tissue diseases, sufferers bear a 1000-fold greater risk than the general population. It is also important to note that transverse myelitis may be the initial presentation; in one study of transverse myelitis presentations, almost half of those eventually attributed to a systemic autoimmune disease were not aware of the diagnosis at presentation.[5]

The pathogenesis of transverse myelitis in this population is not well understood. Scarce autopsy studies in SLE patients have described ischemic necrosis, infarction, or myelomalacia of the cord, and perivascular inflammatory cells and occasionally thrombi in small vessels. Historically, the favored hypothesis has been that vasculitis and arterial thrombi related to autoimmunologic phenomena result in ischemic necrosis within the cord.[30]

Advances in the understanding of the pathogenesis of NMO have given rise to an alternative hypothesis. Pointing to the well-documented high incidence of optic neuritis and the more recent evidence of NMO-IgG positivity in many cases, it has been suggested that, in most cases, myelitis in patients with a connective tissue disorder may represent coexistent NMO instead of a direct complication of the autoimmune disorder.[28,31]

However, more recent work on a cohort of SLE patients described two clinical pictures of myelopathy.[32] One was a profound acute onset weakness with poor prognosis that occurred in the setting of active SLE. The other had a more subacute course of progressive weakness associated with optic neuritis and NMO positivity. A review of Sjögren-associated myelopathy cases[33]

postulated a similar division. This suggests that although coexistent NMO is an important cause of myelopathy in the setting of systemic autoimmune diseases, there is a separate entity of transverse myelitis related to the underlying vasculitic process.

SLE

CNS manifestations in SLE are common, occurring in more than half of patients and including aseptic meningitis, cerebrovascular disease, seizures, cranial and peripheral neuropathy, cognitive and psychological disorders, and headache. Myelopathy is an uncommon manifestation, with 1% to 3% incidence but, importantly, is the initial presentation in almost half of cases.[30,34,35]

The clinical presentation of acute SLE-associated myelitis has been described as acute in onset, accompanied by a short prodrome of fever, headache, and malaise. Coexistent optic neuritis is present in 21% to 48%, and CSF protein levels are elevated without oligoclonal bands.[30,34] Correlation with markers of lupus activity and autoantibodies such as antiphospholipid antibodies is variable in the reported literature.

Prognosis is variable, with complete recovery in 50%, partial recovery in 29%, and no improvement or deterioration in 21%.[34] Worse outcomes have been described in patients with rapid onset of profound weakness at presentation, and in those with initial MR imaging findings of extensive diffuse spinal cord involvement. Conversely, rapid resolution of MR imaging of the lesions following the institution of immunosuppressive therapy suggests a favorable outcome.[30]

MR imaging findings also vary in the reported literature. MR imaging of the spinal cord is normal at presentation in 16% to 30% of patients with clinical myelitis.[34,36] Of the remainder, most of the reported cases identify long-segment central T2 hyperintensity and expansion, with enhancement common but variable; whereas isolated cases demonstrate small multifocal T2-hyperintense lesions.[5,30,32,34]

Birnbaum and colleagues[32] described two distinct subtypes of myelitis within a cohort of 22 patients with SLE and myelitis, the largest such cohort yet studied. One group had a rapid onset (<6 hours in 72.7%) of flaccid paralysis, hyporeflexia, and urinary retention, leading to a poor outcome with persistent paraplegia. The second group had a more subacute onset of spasticity, hyperreflexia, and mild-to-moderate weakness for 1 to 30 days, followed by a relapsing course.

Group 1 was differentiated by a febrile prodrome, evidence of active SLE based on clinical grounds and erythrocyte sedimentation rate (ESR), and CSF profile of neutrophilic pleocytosis and elevated protein. Incidence of optic neuritis (0% in group 1 and 54.5% in group 2) and NMO-IgG positivity (12.5% in group 1 and 57.1% in group 2) was also strikingly different between the two groups. These findings suggest both NMO and disease-associated transverse myelitis exist in SLE.

Sjögren Syndrome

The sicca complex of keratoconjunctivitis sicca, xerostomia, and salivary gland inflammation is the hallmark of this chronic progressive autoimmune-mediated inflammatory exocrinopathy, but systemic disease can affect all organ systems. The syndrome is divided into primary and secondary Sjögren syndrome, with the latter most commonly associated with rheumatoid arthritis, although other autoimmune disorders such as SLE are also associated. Women are affected more frequently than men (ratio 9:1), with onset commonly at 40 to 50 years of age.[37]

CNS involvement has been described in 25% to 30% of patients, and includes demyelination, autonomic dysfunction, stroke, peripheral neuropathy, and myelopathy.[35] Transverse myelitis is rare, occurring in up to 1% of patients with Sjögren syndrome, and the experience within medical literature is limited to case reports.[37]

Williams and Butler[33] reviewed the 17 previously reported cases and divided cases into two clinical patterns. The first is a rapid onset of severe sensory and motor deficit accompanied by neck and interscapular pain, with poor outcome and high mortality. The second is a subacute progression from gait, sensory, and urinary disturbance to eventual paraplegia, associated with optic neuritis in four out of five cases. As in SLE, NMO and disease-associated transverse myelitis both seem to be represented in this population.

Most of the cases that have undergone MR imaging demonstrate a long-segment central cord lesion with cord expansion and variable enhancement, but multifocal lesions have also been described.[5,33,38,39]

Behçet Disease

The clinical triad of uveitis with recurrent oral and genital ulcers is the hallmark of Behçet disease, an episodic systemic inflammatory disease that can involve almost all tissues. The disease is most prevalent in the eastern Mediterranean, Middle East, and eastern Asia, with the highest prevalence in Turkey (80–370 cases per 100,000 population). The disease is rare in the western world (0.12–0.33 cases per 100,000 population in the United States).[40] Age at onset is typically between 20 to 40 years, and the disease is twice as common in men as in women.[41,42]

CNS manifestations arise in around 10% of patients and are usually divided into parenchymal, including meningoencephalitis (in 75%) or myelitis (in 10%), and nonparenchymal, including venous thrombosis (in 18%), idiopathic intracranial hypertension, and, rarely, intracranial aneurysm formation. CNS manifestations are reportedly twice as common in male as in female patients.[42]

Myelitis makes up approximately 10% of cases of neuro-Behçet disease. The diagnosis in an acute transverse myelitis presentation may be suspected based on known history or presence of uveitis and ulcers, but is occasionally the presenting condition. Typically, patients have a CSF pleocytosis with normal CSF glucose. ESR correlates with active disease and is usually elevated.[41]

MR imaging of the spinal cord shows T2-hyperintense lesions, predominantly of the posterolateral cord, which usually extend over more than two segments.[41–43] Myelitis in neuro-Behçet disease has been an isolated CNS manifestation in most reports and so MR imaging of the brain is generally normal. However, some cases of spinal involvement have been identified as part of a severe case of meningoencephalitis, with the typical MR imaging findings of unilateral T2 hyperintensity, edema, and enhancement within the brainstem, thalamus, and basal ganglia. In these cases, brainstem involvement will tend to dominate the clinical picture.[42]

Sarcoidosis

Sarcoidosis is a noncaseating granulomatous disease of uncertain cause. The African American population has a higher incidence (35–80 per 100,000) and younger onset (30–50 years) compared with white Americans (3–10 per 100 000 and onset of 40–60 years). Incidence also increases in the lower latitudes (15–20 per 100,000 in northern Europe compared with 1–5 per 100,000 in southern Europe). Women have an approximately 30% greater risk.[44]

CNS involvement in sarcoidosis occurs in 5% to 10% of patients and, in half of these, it will be part of the presenting illness. Spinal involvement is considered relatively uncommon, estimated to occur in 6% to 8% of patients with neurosarcoidosis. However, this may be an underestimation because cases are increasingly reported in newer studies using MR imaging criteria.[45] Indeed, Spencer and colleagues[46] found that spinal involvement was the most common manifestation in their cohort of 21 patients with neurosarcoidosis, occurring in 43%.

The most common clinically apparent abnormalities described on MR imaging are intramedullary lesions with patchy enhancement extending more than three levels with a preference for cervical segments, although nonenhancing lesions and multifocal short-segment lesions have also been described. Associated leptomeningeal enhancement is a common finding, whereas extradural mass lesions and multiple cauda equine lesions have less commonly been described.[46–52]

PARAINFECTIOUS TRANSVERSE MYELITIS

Parainfectious myelitis is the term used for transverse myelitis that is temporally related to and presumed caused by a systemic infection, although in many cases the infective agent cannot be identified. Up to 40% of cases of pediatric transverse myelitis are preceded by clinical signs or serologic evidence of a systemic infection, with viral infections most commonly implicated.[11,53] In the adult population, parainfectious causes have been implicated in 6% to 45% of presentations of acute transverse myelitis.[5,12,54]

In practice, cases of transverse myelitis related to direct infection are difficult to delineate from those occurring in the convalescent phase; therefore the term covers those cases due to direct microbial infection with neuronal injury resulting from either the infection itself or from the systemic immune process against the agent, as well as those cases occurring in the convalescent phase due to an immune-mediated response to a recent infection. The diagnosis can be made in clinical presentations of transverse myelitis with a history of an infectious syndrome within 4 weeks preceding clinical onset, accompanied by culture, serologic, or PCR evidence of infection.

MR imaging features are often nonspecific, mirroring those in idiopathic transverse myelitis. Table 1 lists some of the more commonly implicated viral, bacterial, and fungal pathogens, with a description of common imaging findings. The most common and least specific finding is of long-segment T2 hyperintensity within the cord, usually with some degree of edema. Enhancement may be diffuse, patchy, peripheral, or absent. Associated leptomeningeal and/or nerve root enhancement has been described in infection with some pathogens, including herpes simplex virus (HSV), Epstein-Barr virus, varicella-zoster virus (VZV), mycobacterium tuberculosis, Lyme disease, and parasitic agents (Figs. 3 and 4).

In recent years, outbreaks of Western Nile virus and enterovirus 71 in North America[55–58] have focused increasing attention on microbial diseases that cause a poliomyelitis-like syndrome,

characterized by an acute flaccid paralysis with MR imaging and nerve-conduction studies implicating involvement of the anterior horn cells. Autopsy studies have confirmed the presence of inflammation and necrosis localized to the anterior horn cells. The archetypical infective agent is, of course, poliovirus; however, recognized causes include other picornaviruses, including enterovirus 71, coxsackie virus A and B, and echovirus, as well as flaviviruses, such as Western Nile virus, tick-borne encephalitis virus, and Japanese encephalitis virus.[59] Many studies have been able to demonstrate characteristic MR imaging findings of T2 hyperintensity localized to the anterior horn (Fig. 5) in these patients.[60–66]

Another reason for increased attention on infectious myelitis is the rise in HIV/AIDS. In addition to HIV-associated myelopathy, opportunistic infections with cytomegalovirus, VZV, HSV, toxoplasmosis, and tuberculosis may involve the cord.[67,68] Occurring in 5% of AIDS patients, HIV myelitis is due to direct infection of the cord and is often associated with HIV encephalitis. MR imaging findings are central T2 hyperintensity that predominates in the thoracic cord and may have patchy enhancement.[69]

Vacuolar myelopathy is a painless spastic paraparesis with sensory ataxia, slowly progressive for weeks to months. Pathogenesis remains unclear, but it is usually temporally associated with the AID dementia complex, and is more likely to be due to secondary metabolic disturbance than direct infection.[70,71] Although present at autopsy in half of AIDS patients, it is symptomatic in 5% to 10%. MR imaging reveals nonenhancing symmetric dorsolateral T2-signal hyperintensity of the midthoracic to distal thoracic cord, correlating with the distribution of vacuolar degeneration at histologic analysis.[72,73] The subacute time course and lack of definite inflammatory component make vacuolar myelopathy a differential for transverse myelitis instead of a cause.

Pathogenesis

In some cases, direct microbial infection of the CNS has been suggested by CSF-PCR positivity or by histopathological evidence at biopsy or autopsy. These limited cases include incidents of cytomegalovirus, VZV, herpes simplex virus 1 and 2, human herpesvirus 6, Epstein-Barr virus, human T-cell lymphotropic virus 1, HIV 1, *Borrelia burgdorferi*, and *Treponema pallidum*.[53,74]

Immune-mediated mechanisms such as molecular mimicry, microbial superantigen-mediated infection, and derangements in humoral immunity are likely to play a significant role in many cases

Table 1
Infective organisms implicated in transverse myelitis

	Clinical Features	Imaging Features on MR Imaging Spinal Cord
Herpes Viruses[98–104]		
Herpes Simplex Virus 1	Most common cause of viral encephalitis. Myelitis is rare and may occur as part of meningoencephalomyelitis	Long-segment ↑T2 signal with variable enhancement Case reports of intramedullary hemorrhage
Herpes Simplex Virus 2	Ascending myelitis is more common than in Herpes simplex virus 1 infection	Long-segment ↑T2 signal with variable enhancement
Human Herpesvirus 6 and 7	Encephalitis and meningoencephalitis are rare. Myelitis is extremely rare	Isolated case reports have showed normal MR imaging or long-segment ↑T2 signal
Varicella-Zoster Virus	*Primary disease:* cerebellar ataxia, meningoencephalitis, transverse myelitis, and aseptic meningitis occur in <1% *Reactivation:* radiculomyelitis is accompanied by dermatomal rash in only half of cases *HIV/AIDS:* disseminated disease with rash and extensive cord involvement	Long-segment ↑T2 signal centered at level of dermatome Enhancement is common Changes are most severe at dorsal root entry zone and posterior horn of the involved dermatome
Cytomegalovirus	CNS disease is rare in the immunocompetent Manifestations include radiculitis/radiculomyelitis (most common), myelitis, encephalomyelitis, and ventriculoencephalitis	Thickening, clumping, and enhancement of nerve roots and leptomeninges, often with associated long-segment cord ↑T2 signal, favoring conus Case reports of isolated long-segment cord ↑T2 signal and expansion
Epstein Barr Virus	Symptomatic CNS involvement occurs in 5%, including meningitis, encephalitis, myelitis, cranial neuritis, ADEM, and GBS	↑T2 signal and enhancement is usually long-segment and may be multifocal Nerve root and/or leptomeningeal enhancement may be present
Orthomyxoviruses[105]		
Influenza A	Encephalitis is rare, and myelitis very rare	Isolated case reports of ↑T2 signal and enhancement
Paramyxoviruses[106–108]		
Measles Virus	Encephalitis and encephalomyelitis are rare manifestations	Isolated case reports describe long-segment ↑T2 signal and expansion with variable enhancement
Mumps Virus	Meningoencephalitis is a rare manifestation and myelitis is very rare	Long-segment ↑T2 signal and expansion
Picornaviruses[56,59–61,63,65,109–113]		
Poliovirus	Symptomatic CNS involvement in 1%–2%, manifesting as spinal poliomyelitis (in 75%), bulbar poliomyelitis, meningitis, or polioencephalitis	Few MR imaging studies, showing ↑T2 signal of the anterior horns

(continued on next page)

Table 1
(continued)

	Clinical Features	Imaging Features on MR Imaging Spinal Cord
Enterovirus 71	CNS involvement in up to 30%, manifested by meningitis, encephalitis, and poliomyelitis-like syndrome. Rarely transverse myelitis and GBS	Poliomyelitis-like syndrome Unilateral or bilateral ↑T2 signal of the anterior horns Occasional ventral nerve root enhancement
Coxsackie Virus A and B	Rare cases of poliomyelitis-like syndrome and transverse myelitis.	Case reports of transverse myelitis. Long-segment ↑T2 signal. There
Echovirus	Rare cases of poliomyelitis-like syndrome and transverse myelitis	may be patchy or peripheral enhancement
Flaviviruses[64,66,114–119]		
West Nile virus	CNS complications are common and may manifest as rhombencephalitis (50%), aseptic meningitis (20%), or poliomyelitis-like syndrome (5%–10%)	Poliomyelitis-like syndrome: Unilateral or bilateral ↑T2 signal of the anterior horns across multiple segments. Enhancement is uncommon
Tick-Borne Encephalitis Virus	Meningitis (49%), meningoencephalitis (41%), meningoencephalomyelitis (10%), poliomyelitis-like syndrome	Encephalitis: Initial MR imaging is normal in up to half of cases, with yield increasing on MR imaging later in the clinical course
Japanese Encephalitis Virus	Encephalitis is the most common CNS manifestation, with poliomyelitis-like syndrome occurring less commonly than in West Nile virus	Bilateral thalamic ↑T2 lesions are the classic finding. Brainstem and basal ganglia are also frequently involved
Murray Valley Encephalitis Virus St Louis Encephalitis Virus		
Dengue Virus	CNS involvement is uncommon, but may manifest as encephalitis, myelitis, ADEM, or GBS	Patchy parenchymal enhancement and leptomeningeal or periventricular enhancement may be present
Retroviruses[67,120–123]		
HTLV 1	<5% of carriers develop symptomatic neurologic involvement	Long-segment ↑T2 signal of lateral columns, less commonly extending to dorsal columns, occasionally with enhancement. Progresses to atrophy of lateral columns with no signal change or enhancement
HIV	*HIV myelitis:* isolated or with cerebral involvement *Vacuolar myelopathy:* present in up to 50% AIDS patients, but symptomatic in 5%–10%. Likely a metabolic complication rather than due to direct infection	*HIV myelitis:* Long-segment ↑T2 signal with multifocal enhancement *Vacuolar myelopathy:* MR imaging normal or dorsolateral ↑T2 signal over multiple segments
Bacterial[124–137]		
Borrelia burgdorferi	CNS involvement in 20% of untreated cases. Meningitis, meningoencephalitis, meningoencephalomyelitis, cranial nerve palsies, and painful radiculopathy. Meningitis and meningoencephalitis are more common in European than North American strains	Nerve root enhancement plus cord ↑T2 signal of adjacent segments. Leptomeningeal or nerve root enhancement may be present Rarely transverse myelitis picture with long-segment diffuse ↑T2 signal with patchy enhancement

(continued on next page)

Table 1
(continued)

	Clinical Features	Imaging Features on MR Imaging Spinal Cord
Treponema pallidum	Neurosyphilis in 5%–10% of untreated cases. Meningitis, meningovascular disease (endarteritis), myelitis, meningomyelitis, tabes dorsalis	Short-segment peripheral and long-segment ↑T2 signal with enhancement have both been described. Leptomeningeal enhancement may be seen
Mycoplasma pneumoniae	Encephalomyelitis is common in children. Myelitis is a rare complication	Long-segment ↑T2 signal
Mycobacterium tuberculosis	CNS involvement may include meningitis, tuberculoma or, less commonly, myelitis	80% involve thoracic cord, majority with ↑T2 signal, but may have ↓T2 signal lesions Diffuse, nodular, or ring-like enhancement Cavitation may occur Leptomeningeal and dural enhancement may be present
Parasites[138–146]		
Neurocysticercosis	Intracranial involvement is most common, with spinal involvement occurring in 1%–5% Intramedullary lesions are far less common than extramedullary intradural lesions	*Intramedullary:* cystic lesion that may develop irregular peripheral enhancement and edema as it degenerates *Extramedullary:* clusters of cystic lesions, or thick irregular leptomeningeal enhancement
Schistosomiasis	Spinal involvement is uncommon	↑T2 signal and mild-to-moderate expansion of the distal cord and conus. Enhancement patterns may include nodular intramedullary foci, leptomeningeal enhancement, and enhancing thickening of nerve roots
Gnathostomiasis	Organism endemic in Southeast Asia Eosinophilic meningitis, myelitis, and painful radiculitis May present with subarachnoid hemorrhage	↑T2 signal long-segment expanded lesions of the central cord. Enhancement and hemorrhage are common. Scattered intracranial lesions may coexist

Abbreviations: ADEM, acute disseminated encephalomyelitis; GBS, Guillain-Barre syndrome; HTLV, human T-lymphotropic virus.

of parainfectious transverse myelitis.[2,53,75] Molecular mimicry refers to cross-reactivity, which can occur between microbial antigens and cell-wall components of human neuronal tissue. Microbial superantigen-mediated antigens differ from the behavior of classic agents in two ways. First, they bind with a different site on the T cell receptor, which is better conserved. Second, they are able to activate T cells in the absence of costimulatory molecules, resulting in activation of 200-fold greater numbers of circulating T cells. This can result in activation of autoreactive T cells with resultant autoimmune-mediated tissue damage.

Humoral derangements also play a role in many cases. High levels of circulating antibodies may form immune complexes that cause damage due to deposition within the cord. Infectious agents may also induce autoimmunity by polyclonal activation of B lymphocytes or via bystander activation increasing cytokine production and the activation of autoreactive T cells.

POSTVACCINATION TRANSVERSE MYELITIS

Up to 30% of children with transverse myelitis have a history of recent vaccination. In most

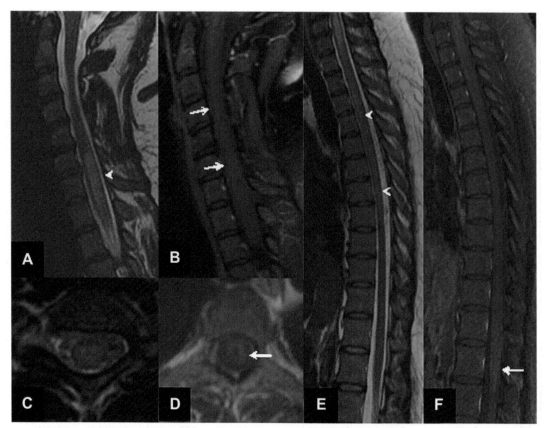

Fig. 3. Viral myelitis. Although the pathogen was not isolated, the diagnosis was made based upon the clinical picture of concurrent febrile illness with CSF lymphocytosis and elevated protein. T2-weighted (*A, C, E*) and gadolinium-enhanced T1-weighted (*B, D, F*) MR imaging sequences demonstrate central T2 hyperintensity extending from C6 to T1 and T2 to T8 (*arrowheads*) with leptomeningeal enhancement (*arrows*). Follow-up MR imaging at 1 month showed complete resolution of signal abnormality and enhancement.

cases, this reflects the high rates of immunization in this age group instead of a direct causation, with vaccines having an excellent safety profile. Postvaccination transverse myelitis seems to be a rare complication of vaccination. A literature review of English-language articles published between 1970 and 2009 found only 43 cases, most presenting within 1 month of vaccination.[75] The vaccines implicated were, in order of frequency, anti-HBV, measles-mumps-rubella or rubella, diphtheria-tetanus-pertussis or tetanus, rabies, oral poliovirus, influenza, typhoid, and Japanese B encephalitis.

The pathogenesis is likely similar to the proposed mechanisms of immune-mediated neural damage described in parainfectious transverse myelitis. In the case of vaccine-related myelitis, adjuvant agents included in the vaccine with the aim of augmenting the immune response to the vaccine antigens may also play a role.[75]

OTHER ENTITIES TO CONSIDER IN THE DIFFERENTIAL DIAGNOSIS OF TRANSVERSE MYELITIS
Vascular Conditions

Cord ischemia
The typical clinical picture of cord infarction is of sudden onset motor, sensory, and autonomic disturbance with an identifiable level. The abrupt onset and presence of associated features, such as temporally related systemic hypotension, severe atherosclerotic disease, aortic dissection, thoracoabdominal aortic aneurysm, vasculitis, prothrombotic diseases, and endocarditis will prompt

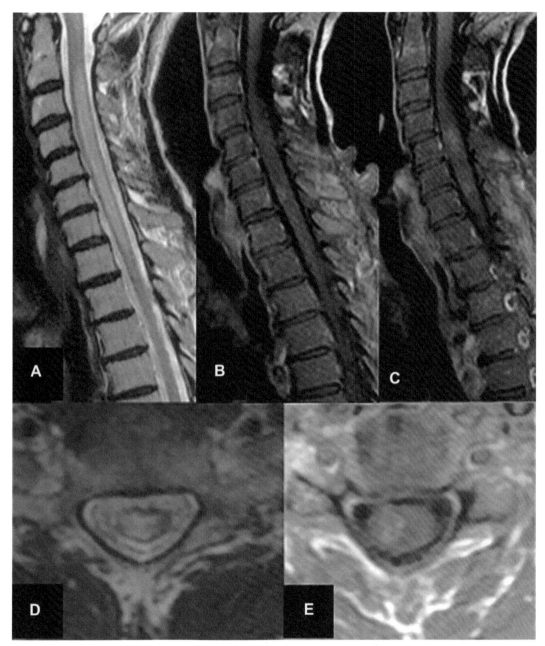

Fig. 4. Zoster myelitis. T2-weighted (A, D) and gadolinium-enhanced T1-weighted (B, C, E) MR imaging sequences through the cervical spine demonstrate cord expansion and T2 hyperintensity extending from C2 to T1, with patchy and ring-like areas of enhancement. The most pronounced T2-signal change and enhancement (E) was in the posterior horn region at the level of dermatomal rash.

clinical suspicion of the diagnosis. Embolism of a fibrocartilaginous disc fragment is a rare cause.

The anterior spinal artery supplies the corticospinal tracts and all gray matter apart from the posterior horn and is almost invariably the site of occlusion. The central gray matter of the cord is also more prone to ischemia than the peripheral white matter due to the greater metabolic demand of cell bodies. This is reflected in the usual distribution of abnormal T2 hyperintensity in cord ischemia that, in order of increasing severity, involves the anterior columns ("snake-eyes" appearance), central gray matter, or central cord with rim of spared peripheral white matter.[76] Initial MR

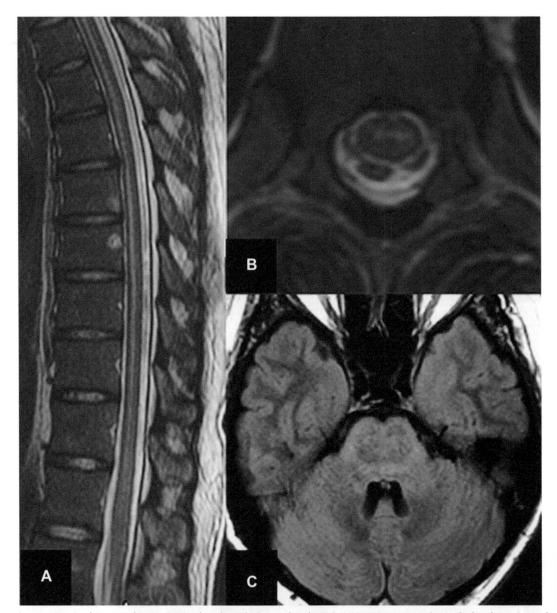

Fig. 5. Anterior horn syndrome. Sagittal and axial T2-weighted MR imaging sequences through the thoracic cord (*A, B*) in a patient with acute flaccid paralysis demonstrate T2 hyperintensity without expansion, centered on the anterior horns bilaterally. There was no enhancement on postgadolinium sequences. The neurologic impairment and cord signal change had completely resolved at 3 months follow-up. Axial fluid-attenuated inversion recovery (FLAIR) sequence at the level of the pons (*C*) shows high signal peripherally and within pontine nuclei and the dentate nuclei bilaterally. At 3 month follow-up, appearances had improved with residual, mild, patchy central pontine signal abnormality. Brainstem involvement is a typical finding in flavivirus encephalitis and may coexist with myelitis.

imaging may be normal, with T2 hyperintensity and expansion evolving in hours and enhancement developing in the subacute setting.[77,78] The midthoracic to lower thoracic cord is most vulnerable to occlusion of the artery of Adamkiewicz,[79,80] whereas watershed ischemia typically involves the midthoracic to upper thoracic cord.[78]

The diagnosis of cord ischemia is often difficult on imaging grounds alone because the more specific snake-eyes appearance is not common

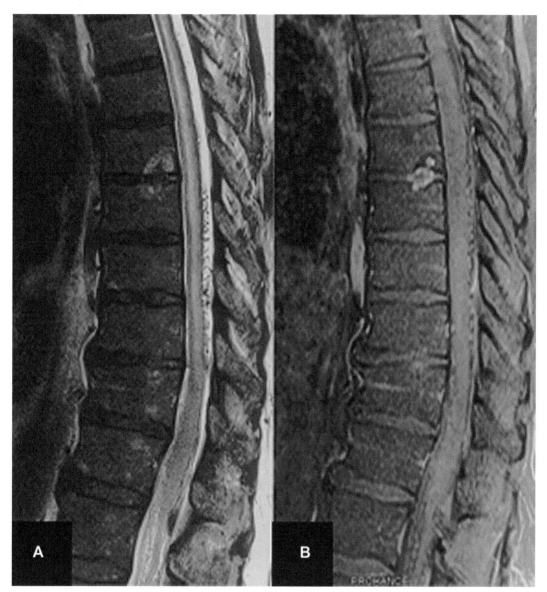

Fig. 6. Spinal dural arteriovenous fistula: Sagittal T2 weighted (*A*) and gadolinium enhanced T1 weighted (*B*) sequences through the thoracic spine demonstrate long-segment central T2 hyperintensity with expansion. Numerous abnormal flow voids and vascular enhancement are identified within the spinal canal. Linear low T2 signal applied to the surface of the cord suggests hemosiderin deposition related to previous subarachnoid hemorrhage.

and MR imaging findings of normal cord signal or long-segment central T2 hyperintensity are not helpful in narrowing the differential diagnosis. Diffusion-weighted imaging (DWI) of the spine has the potential to allow earlier and more confident diagnosis of infarction. Spinal cord DWI has been slow to be accepted into clinical practice, presumably because greater technical difficulties are involved than in cerebral DWI, requiring optimization of specialized pulse sequences. The

reported literature on spinal DWI for ischemia includes few small case series demonstrating feasibility of the technique. These suggest it is a highly sensitive tool that is able to identify infarction before the evolution of T2-signal change.[81,82] Most study protocols have utilized single-shot echo planar imaging at 1.5 T, but two researchers have suggested that multishot, interleaved echo planar imaging may have advantages over single-shot echo planar imaging and fast-spin

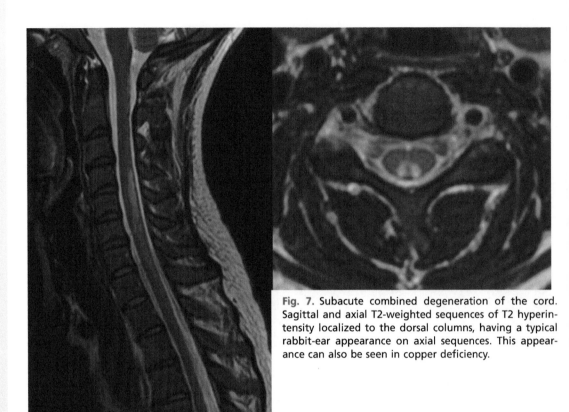

Fig. 7. Subacute combined degeneration of the cord. Sagittal and axial T2-weighted sequences of T2 hyperintensity localized to the dorsal columns, having a typical rabbit-ear appearance on axial sequences. This appearance can also be seen in copper deficiency.

echo techniques, with better signal-to-noise ratio and reduced artifact.[81,83]

Vascular malformations

Spinal vascular malformations may cause intramedullary or subarachnoid hemorrhage, with abrupt onset of symptoms, or cause progressive myelopathy related to venous congestion or arterial steal syndrome. Spinal dural arteriovenous fistula is the most common subtype, making up 70% of spinal vascular malformations, and tends to occur in men between the ages of 40 and 60 years with a progressive subacute clinical course.[84]

MR imaging findings of prominent vascular flow voids and numerous enhancing vessels suggest the diagnosis of arteriovenous malformation (Fig. 6), which is confirmed by spinal angiography. Cord expansion and T2 hyperintensity related to venous congestion and ischemia are common and may be associated with diffuse enhancement. Additional findings may be siderosis or intramedullary foci of T2-hypointense hemosiderin related to previous hemorrhage.[85–87] Contrast-enhanced MR angiography is useful in identifying the level of the lesion and may facilitate spinal digital

subtraction angiography, which remains the gold standard.[88]

Radiation Myelopathy

Delayed radiation myelopathy has been reported beyond 10 years after radiotherapy[5] and is characterized by focal swelling and diffuse, high T2 signal on MR imaging corresponding to the irradiation port, often containing patchy or ring-like areas of enhancement.[89–91] Follow-up demonstrates normalization of cord signal intensity with severe atrophy.[90] A useful clue for the radiologist given an incomplete clinical history is fatty marrow signal within adjacent vertebral bodies, with a sharp border correlating with the radiation port.

Cobalamin and Copper Deficiency

Vitamin B12 (cobalamin) deficiency causes impairment of normal DNA and fatty acid synthesis with results including megaloblastic anemia and subacute combined-degeneration of the cord.[92] Deficiency may occur in pernicious anemia, ileal or gastric fundal resection, or because of severely restricted diet. Nitrous oxide administration can provoke symptomatic B12 deficiency in patients

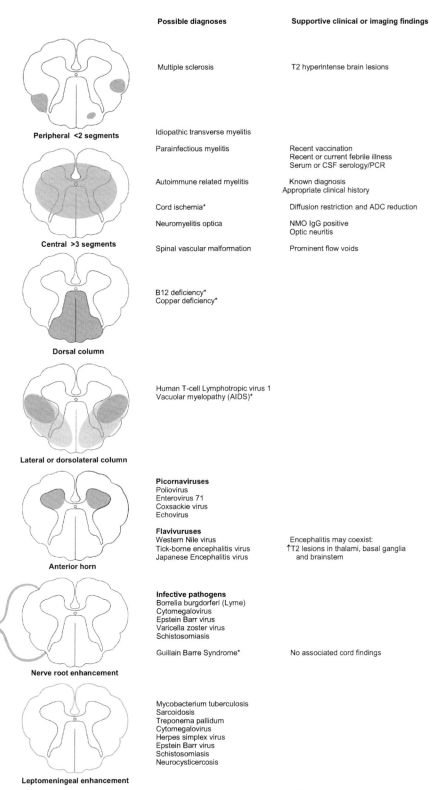

Possible diagnoses

Supportive clinical or imaging findings

Peripheral <2 segments

Multiple sclerosis — T2 hyperintense brain lesions

Central >3 segments

Idiopathic transverse myelitis

Parainfectious myelitis — Recent vaccination / Recent or current febrile illness / Serum or CSF serology/PCR

Autoimmune related myelitis — Known diagnosis / Appropriate clinical history

Cord ischemia* — Diffusion restriction and ADC reduction

Neuromyelitis optica — NMO IgG positive / Optic neuritis

Spinal vascular malformation — Prominent flow voids

Dorsal column

B12 deficiency* / Copper deficiency*

Lateral or dorsolateral column

Human T-cell Lymphotropic virus 1 / Vacuolar myelopathy (AIDS)*

Anterior horn

Picornaviruses
Poliovirus
Enterovirus 71
Coxsackie virus
Echovirus

Flavivuruses
Western Nile virus — Encephalitis may coexist:
Tick-borne encephalitis virus — ↑↑T2 lesions in thalami, basal ganglia
Japanese Encephalitis virus — and brainstem

Nerve root enhancement

Infective pathogens
Borrelia burgdorferi (Lyme)
Cytomegalovirus
Epstein Barr virus
Varicella zoster virus
Schistosomiasis

Guillain Barre Syndrome* — No associated cord findings

Leptomeningeal enhancement

Mycobacterium tuberculosis
Sarcoidosis
Treponema pallidum
Cytomegalovirus
Herpes simplex virus
Epstein Barr virus
Schistosomiasis
Neurocysticercosis

Fig. 8. Morphologic patterns of signal abnormality and enhancement within the spinal cord which may provide clues to etiology. Asterisks indicate that these entities lie outside the diagnosis of transverse myelitis, but may be important in the differential diagnosis.

with previously subclinical deficiency due to its action in oxidizing active cobalamin into its inactive form.[93] Copper deficiency, most commonly related to reduced absorption after gastric surgery, can cause an indistinguishable clinical and radiological appearance.[94]

The demyelination usually predates the appearance of anemia and preferentially involves the dorsal columns of the cord, causing loss of proprioception and vibration sense with sensory disturbance. The MR imaging appearance is of long-segment, bilateral T2 hyperintensity of the dorsal columns described as an "inverted V" or "rabbit-ear" appearance (**Fig. 7**),[92,95,96] with case reports of extension into the lateral columns, brainstem, pyramidal tracts, and cerebellum.[97] Treatment results in improvement of the areas of signal abnormality, preceding clinical improvement.

THE ROLE OF NEUROIMAGING IN TRANSVERSE MYELITIS

The often nonspecific imaging features of transverse myelitis belie the vital importance of MR imaging in its assessment and treatment. Imaging findings are an essential component of the current diagnostic criteria, which explicitly require exclusion of cord compression and absence of characteristic brain lesions of multiple sclerosis, and will accept gadolinium enhancement as evidence of active inflammation. Beyond this basic role, imaging assessment may lead to clues regarding the underlying cause, which prompts directed clinical questioning and the use of specialized tests to confirm the diagnosis. One of the rare wild-type poliomyelitis cases in the Western world after eradication was diagnosed by a radiologist in a patient being treated for Guillain-Barre syndrome.[65]

The role of the radiologist in transverse myelopathy is to:

1. Urgently exclude cord compression
2. Search for other causes of acute myelopathy
3. Look for imaging features that may point to a disease-associated cause that will benefit from specific therapy
4. Provide follow-up imaging to assess temporal evolution and response to treatment.

Exclude Cord Compression

Cord compression is a surgical emergency, with a brief window of time in which decompressive surgery will allow clinical improvement or halt progression of neurologic impairment. Common causes of compression include disc herniation and extramedullary mass lesions arising from the spine or dura, such as metastasis, myeloma, and meningioma. MR imaging of the cord should be performed urgently in all cases of acute myelopathy. If MR imaging is not available or if there are MR imaging contraindications, CT myelography is an acceptable alternative in the emergent setting.

Characterize the Pattern of Spinal Cord Involvement and Any Associated Intracranial Disease

If no cord compressive lesion is identified, contrast-enhanced MR imaging of the cord and MR imaging of the brain can then be performed in a less urgent manner, but will still be required to complete the assessment. Imaging characteristics of idiopathic and subtypes of disease-associated transverse myelitis have been described in detail above. A pattern-based approach to the differential diagnosis based on the location of the T2-hyperintense lesion within the cord and the associated enhancement characteristics, outlined in **Fig. 8**, may assist in narrowing the differential diagnosis.

In the future, advanced techniques such as diffusion-weighted and diffusion tensor imaging of the spinal cord may add to the capability of neuroimaging to define the cause in an acute presentation of transverse myelitis or transverse myelopathy. In the meantime, a good clinical history remains an invaluable tool in the formulation of a useful differential diagnosis.

Importance of Follow-Up Neuroimaging

Interval follow-up is of use in assessing response to treatment, but is also an important diagnostic tool in difficult or equivocal cases. A suspected diagnosis can be confirmed by rapid response to a specific treatment, such as antimicrobial therapy or vitamin B12 replacement. Resolution of expansion and enhancement over time is very helpful in excluding cord neoplasm in those cases of ischemia, radiation myelopathy, and inflammatory myelitis with a unicentric lesion and a concerning enhancement pattern on initial MR imaging. Follow-up brain and spinal cord MR imaging may also demonstrate the appearance of new lesions, which will confirm progression of an isolated cord syndrome to clinically definite multiple sclerosis.

SUMMARY

Transverse myelitis is an acute inflammatory condition characterized by rapid onset of bilateral motor, sensory, and autonomic dysfunction. Although a relatively rare condition, having a reported incidence of 1 to 8 cases per million, the diversity of its underlying causes makes it an important diagnostic challenge. Historically, transverse myelitis has been a complex and sometimes convoluted topic, with interchangeable use of terms such as acute transverse myelitis and transverse myelopathy. An approach to the classification and workup of transverse myelitis outlined by the Transverse Myelitis Consortium Working Group in 2002[1] aims to standardize the diagnostic criteria and terminology to facilitate the design and analysis of clinical research, and forms a useful tool in the clinical workup patients at presentation. The pathogenesis of transverse myelitis can be grouped into four broad categories: multiple sclerosis and NMO; systemic autoimmune syndromes such as SLE and Sjögren; infectious causes; and idiopathic. Radiation myelopathy and vascular conditions, such as cord ischemia and spinal vascular malformation, are other conditions that often fall within the differential diagnosis, but are classified separately to transverse myelitis. Imaging appearances in transverse myelitis can be relatively nonspecific; however, the morphology of cord involvement, enhancement pattern, and presence of coexistent abnormalities on MR images of the brain can provide clues as to the underlying cause. Together with the clinical background and specialized tests, neuroimaging is extremely important in identifying subgroups who may benefit from specific treatment.

REFERENCES

1. Transverse Myelitis Consortium Working Group. Proposed diagnostic criteria and nosology of acute transverse myelitis. Neurology 2002;59:499–505.
2. Kerr DA, Ayetey H. Immunopathogenesis of acute transverse myelitis. Curr Opin Neurol 2002;15: 339–47.
3. de Seze J, Lanctin C, Lebrun C, et al. Idiopathic acute transverse myelitis: application of the recent diagnostic criteria. Neurology 2005;65:1950–3.
4. Choi K, Lee K, Chung S. Idiopathic transverse myelitis: MR characteristics. AJNR Am J Neuroradiol 1996;17:1151–60.
5. de Seze J, Stojkovic T, Breteau G, et al. Acute myelopathies: clinical, laboratory and outcome profiles in 79 cases. Brain 2001;124:1509–21.
6. Krishnan C, Kaplin A, Deshpande D, et al. Transverse myelitis: pathogenesis, diagnosis and treatment. Front Biosci 2004;9:1483–99.
7. Kaplin AI. IL-6 induces regionally selective spinal cord injury in patients with the neuroinflammatory disorder transverse myelitis. J Clin Invest 2005; 115:2731–41.
8. Dujmovic I. Cerebrospinal fluid and blood biomarkers of neuroaxonal damage in multiple sclerosis. Multiple Sclerosis International 2011;2011: 1–18. DOI:10.1155/2011/767083.
9. de Seze J, Peoc'h K, Ferriby D, et al. 14-3-3 protein in the cerebrospinal fluid of patients with acute transverse myelitis and multiple sclerosis. J Neurol 2002;249:626–7.
10. Irani DN, Kerr DA. 14-3-3 protein in the cerebrospinal fluid of patients with acute transverse myelitis. Lancet 2000;355:901.
11. Alper G, Petropoulou KA, Fitz CR, et al. Idiopathic acute transverse myelitis in children: an analysis and discussion of MRI findings. Mult Scler 2011;17:74–80.
12. Harzheim M. Discriminatory features of acute transverse myelitis: a retrospective analysis of 45 patients. J Neurol Sci 2004;217:217–23.
13. Renoux J, Facon D, Fillard P, et al. MR diffusion tensor imaging and fiber tracking in inflammatory diseases of the spinal cord. AJNR Am J Neuroradiol 2006;27:1947–51.
14. Lee JW, Park KS, Kim JH, et al. Diffusion tensor imaging in idiopathic acute transverse myelitis. AJR Am J Roentgenol 2008;191:W52–7.
15. Pittock SJ, Lucchinetti CF. Inflammatory transverse myelitis: evolving concepts. Curr Opin Neurol 2006;19:362–8.
16. Scott TF. Nosology of idiopathic transverse myelitis syndromes. Acta Neurol Scand 2007;115:371–6.
17. Scott TF, Kassab SL, Singh S. Acute partial transverse myelitis with normal cerebral magnetic resonance imaging: transition rate to clinically definite multiple sclerosis. Mult Scler 2005;11:373–7.
18. Fisniku LK, Brex PA, Altmann DR, et al. Disability and T2 MRI lesions: a 20-year follow-up of patients with relapse onset of multiple sclerosis. Brain 2008; 131:808–17.
19. Bergamaschi R, Tonietti S, Franciotta D, et al. Oligoclonal bands in Devic's neuromyelitis optica and multiple sclerosis: differences in repeated cerebrospinal fluid examinations. Mult Scler 2004;10:2–4.
20. Tartaglino LM, Friedman DP, Flanders AE, et al. Multiple sclerosis in the spinal cord: MR appearance and correlation with clinical parameters. Radiology 1995;195:725–32.
21. Wingerchuk DM, Lennon VA, Lucchinetti CF, et al. The spectrum of neuromyelitis optica. Lancet Neurol 2007;6:805–15.
22. Collongues N, Marignier R, Zephir H, et al. Neuromyelitis optica in France: a multicenter study of 125 patients. Neurology 2010;74:736–42.
23. Lennon VA, Wingerchuk DM, Kryzer TJ, et al. A serum autoantibody marker of neuromyelitis optica: distinction from multiple sclerosis. Lancet 2004; 364:2106–12.
24. Takahashi T, Fujihara K, Nakashima I, et al. Anti-aquaporin-4 antibody is involved in the

pathogenesis of NMO: a study on antibody titre. Brain 2007;130:1235–43.

25. Wingerchuk DM, Lennon VA, Pittock SJ, et al. Revised diagnostic criteria for neuromyelitis optica. Neurology 2006;66:1485–9.

26. Ito S, Mori M, Makino T, et al. "Cloud-like enhancement" is a magnetic resonance imaging abnormality specific to neuromyelitis optica. Ann Neurol 2009;66:425–8.

27. Pittock SJ, Weinshenker BG, Lucchinetti CF, et al. Neuromyelitis optica brain lesions localized at sites of high aquaporin 4 expression. Arch Neurol 2006; 63:964–8.

28. Pittock SJ, Lennon VA, de Seze J, et al. Neuromyelitis optica and non organ-specific autoimmunity. Arch Neurol 2008;65:78–83.

29. Matà S, Lolli F. Neuromyelitis optica: an update. J Neurol Sci 2011;303:13–21.

30. Łukjanowicz M, Brzosko M. Myelitis in the course of systemic lupus erythematosus: review. Pol Arch Med Wewn 2009;119:67–72.

31. Kim S, Waters P, Vincent A, et al. Sjogren's syndrome myelopathy: spinal cord involvement in Sjogren's syndrome might be a manifestation of neuromyelitis optica. Mult Scler 2009;15:1062–8.

32. Birnbaum J, Petri M, Thompson R, et al. Distinct subtypes of myelitis in systemic lupus erythematosus. Arthritis Rheum 2009;60:3378–87.

33. Williams C, Butler E. Treatment of myelopathy in Sjögren syndrome with a combination of prednisone and cyclophosphamide. Arch Neurol 2001; 58:815–9.

34. Kovacs B, Lafferty TL, Brent LH, et al. Transverse myelopathy in systemic lupus erythematosus: an analysis of 14 cases and review of the literature. Ann Rheum Dis 2000;59:120–4.

35. Cikes N, Bosnic D, Sentic M. Non-MS autoimmune demyelination. Clin Neurol Neurosurg 2008;110: 905–12.

36. Lu X, Gu Y, Wang Y, et al. Prognostic factors of lupus myelopathy. Lupus 2008;17:323–8.

37. Rogers SJ, Williams CS, Román GC. Myelopathy in Sjögren syndrome: role of nonsteroidal immunosuppressants. Drugs 2004;64:123–32.

38. Hermisson M, Klein R, Schmidt F, et al. Myelopathy in primary Sjögren syndrome: diagnostic and therapeutic aspects. Acta Neurol Scand 2002;105:450–3.

39. Anantharaju A, Baluch M, Van Thiel DH. Transverse myelitis occurring in association with primary biliary cirrhosis and Sjogren's syndrome. Dig Dis Sci 2003;48:830–3.

40. Sakane T, Takeno M, Suzuki N. Behçet's disease. N Engl J Med 1999;341:1284–91.

41. Riera-Mestre A, Martínez-Yelamos S, Martínez-Yelamos A, et al. Clinicopathologic features and outcomes of neuro-Behçet disease in Spain: a study of 20 patients. Eur J Intern Med 2010;21:536–41.

42. Al-Araji A, Kidd DP. Neuro-Behçet disease: epidemiology, clinical characteristics, and management. Lancet Neurol 2009;8:192–204.

43. Calguneri M, Onat AM, Ozturk MA, et al. Transverse myelitis in a patient with Behcet's disease: favorable outcome with a combination of interferon-α. Clin Rheumatol 2004;24:64–6.

44. Rybicki B, Iannuzzi M. Epidemiology of sarcoidosis: recent advances and future prospects. Semin Respir Crit Care Med 2007;28:022–35.

45. Lower EE, Weiss KL. Neurosarcoidosis. Clin Chest Med 2008;29:475–92.

46. Spencer TS, Campellone JV, Maldonado I, et al. Clinical and magnetic resonance imaging manifestations of neurosarcoidosis. Semin Arthritis Rheum 2005;34:649–61.

47. Hashmi M, Kyritsis AP. Diagnosis and treatment of intramedullary spinal cord sarcoidosis. J Neurol 1998;245:178–80.

48. Christoforidis G, Spickler E. MR of CNS sarcoidosis: correlation of imaging features to clinical symptoms and response to treatment. AJNR Am J Neuroradiol 1999;20:655–69.

49. Kumar N, Frohman EM. Spinal neurosarcoidosis mimicking an idiopathic inflammatory demyelinating syndrome. Arch Neurol 2004;61:586–9.

50. Rieger J. Spinal cord sarcoidosis. Neuroradiology 1994;36:627–8.

51. Saleh S, Saw C, Marzouk K, et al. Sarcoidosis of the spinal cord: literature review and report of eight cases. J Natl Med Assoc 2006;98:965–76.

52. Yamamoto T, Ito S, Hattori T. Acute longitudinal myelitis as the initial manifestation of Sjögren's syndrome. J Neurol Neurosurg Psychiatry 2006; 77:780.

53. Trecker CC, Kozubal DE, Kaplin AI, et al. Transverse myelitis: pathogenesis, diagnosis, and management. In: Lucchinetti CF, Hohlfeld R, editors. Multiple Sclerosis 3, vol. 35. Butterworth-Heinemann; 2010. p. 237–57.

54. Jeffery DR, Mandler RN, Davis LE. Transverse myelitis: retrospective analysis of 33 cases, with differentiation of cases associated with multiple sclerosis and parainfectious events. Arch Neurol 1993;50:532–5.

55. Tyler KL. Emerging viral infections of the central nervous system: part 1. Arch Neurol 2009;66:939–48.

56. McMinn PC. An overview of the evolution of enterovirus 71 and its clinical and public health significance. FEMS Microbiol Rev 2002;26:91–107.

57. Gordon SM, Isada CM. West nile fever: lessons from the 2002 season. Cleve Clin J Med 2003;70: 449–54.

58. Borchardt SM, Feist MA, Miller T, et al. Epidemiology of West Nile virus in the highly epidemic state of North Dakota, 2002–2007. Public Health Rep 2010;125:246–9.

59. Solomon T, Willison H. Infectious causes of acute flaccid paralysis. Curr Opin Infect Dis 2003;16: 375–81.

60. Chen C, Chang Y, Huang C. Acute flaccid paralysis in infants and young children with enterovirus 71 infection: MR imaging findings and clinical correlates. AJNR Am J Neuroradiol 2001;22:200–5.

61. McMinn P, Stratov I, Nagarajan L. Neurological manifestations of enterovirus 71 infection in children during an outbreak of hand, foot, and mouth disease in Western Australia. Clin Infect Dis 2001; 32:236–42.

62. Mullins JA, Khetsuriani N, Nix WA, et al. Emergence of echovirus type 13 as a prominent enterovirus. Clin Infect Dis 2004;38:70–7.

63. Shen WC, Tsai C, Chiu H, et al. MRI of Enterovirus 71 myelitis with monoplegia. Neuroradiology 2000; 42:124–7.

64. Sejvar JJ, Bode AV, Marfin AA, et al. West Nile Virus-associated flaccid paralysis. Emerg Infect Dis 2005;11:1021–7.

65. Stewardson AJ. Imported case of poliomyelitis, Melbourne, Australia, 2007. Emerg Infect Dis 2009;15:63–5.

66. Roos KL. West Nile encephalitis and myelitis. Curr Opin Neurol 2004;17:343–6.

67. Thurnher MM, Post MJ, Jinkins JR. MRI of infections and neoplasms of the spine and spinal cord in 55 patients with AIDS. Neuroradiology 2000;42: 551–63.

68. McCutchan J. Cytomegalovirus infections of the nervous system in patients with AIDS. Clin Infect Dis 1995;20:747–54.

69. DeSanto J, Ross JS. Spine infection/inflammation. Radiol Clin North Am 2011;49:105–27.

70. Brew B. The pathogenesis of the neurological complications of HIV-1 infection. Genitourin Med 1993;69:333–40.

71. McArthur JC, Brew BJ, Nath A. Neurological complications of HIV infection. Lancet Neurol 2005;4:543–55.

72. Santosh CG, Bell JE, Best JJK. Spinal tract pathology in AIDS: postmortem MRI correlation with neuropathology. Neuroradiology 1995;37:134–8.

73. Sartoretti-Schefer S, Blättler T, Wichmann W. Spinal MRI in vacuolar myelopathy, and correlation with histopathological findings. Neuroradiology 1997; 39:865–9.

74. Andersen O. Myelitis. Curr Opin Neurol 2000;13: 311–6.

75. Agmon-Levin N, Kivity S, Szyper-Kravitz M, et al. Transverse myelitis and vaccines: a multi-analysis. Lupus 2009;18:1198–204.

76. Mawad ME, Rivera V, Crawford S, et al. Spinal cord ischemia after resection of thoracoabdominal aortic aneurysms: MR findings in 24 patients. AJR Am J Roentgenol 1990;155:1303–7.

77. Hirono H, Yamadori A, Komiyama M, et al. MRI of spontaneous spinal cord infarction: serial changes in gadolinium-DTPA enhancement. Neuroradiology 1992;34:95–7.

78. Friedman DP, Tartaglino LM, Fisher AR, et al. MR imaging in the diagnosis of intramedullary spinal cord diseases that involve specific neural pathways or vascular territories. AJR Am J Roentgenol 1995;165:515–23.

79. Fujikawa A, Tsuchiya K, Takeuchi S, et al. Diffusion-weighted MR imaging in acute spinal cord ischemia. Eur Radiol 2004;14:2076–8.

80. Stepper F, Lövblad K. Anterior spinal artery stroke demonstrated by echo-planar DWI. Eur Radiol 2001;11:2607–10.

81. Thurnher MM, Bammer R. Diffusion-weighted MR imaging (DWI) in spinal cord ischemia. Neuroradiology 2006;48:795–801.

82. Loher TJ, Bassetti CL, Lövblad KO, et al. Diffusion-weighted MRI in acute spinal cord ischaemia. Neuroradiology 2003;45:557–61.

83. Bammer R, Augustin M, Prokesch RW, et al. Diffusion-weighted imaging of the spinal cord: interleaved echo-planar imaging is superior to fast spin-echo. J Magn Reson Imaging 2002;15:364–73.

84. Krings T, Thron AK, Geibprasert S, et al. Endovascular management of spinal vascular malformations. Neurosurg Rev 2009;33:1–9.

85. Hasuo K, Mizushima A, Mihara F, et al. Contrast-enhanced MRI in spinal arteriovenous malformations and fistulae before and after embolisation therapy. Neuroradiology 1996;38:609–14.

86. Isu T, Iwasaki Y, Akino M, et al. Magnetic resonance imaging in cases of spinal dural arteriovenous malformation. Neurosurgery 1989;24:919–23.

87. Sener RN, Larsson EM, Backer R, et al. MRI of intradural spinal arteriovenous fistula associated with ischemia and infarction of the cord. Clin Imaging 1993;17:73–6.

88. Saraf-Lavi E, Bowen BC, Quencer RM, et al. Detection of spinal dural arteriovenous fistulae with MR imaging and contrast-enhanced MR angiography: sensitivity, specificity, and prediction of vertebral level. AJNR Am J Neuroradiol 2002;23:858–67.

89. Wang PY, Shen WC, Jan JS. Serial MRI changes in radiation myelopathy. Neuroradiology 1995;37: 374–7.

90. Koehler PJ, Verbiest H, Jager J, et al. Delayed radiation myelopathy: serial MR-imaging and pathology. Clin Neurol Neurosurg 1996;98:197–201.

91. Michikawa M, Wada Y, Sano M, et al. Radiation myelopathy: significance of gadolinium-DTPA enhancement in the diagnosis. Neuroradiology 1991;33:286–9.

92. Hemmer B, Glocker FX, Schumacher M, et al. Subacute combined degeneration: clinical, electrophysiological, and magnetic resonance imaging

findings. J Neurol Neurosurg Psychiatry 1998;65: 822–7.

93. Renard D, Dutray A, Remy A, et al. Subacute combined degeneration of the spinal cord caused by nitrous oxide anaesthesia. Neurol Sci 2009;30: 75–6.

94. Jaiser S. Copper deficiency masquerading as subacute combined degeneration of the cord and myelodysplastic syndrome. Adv Clin Neurosci Rehabil 2007;7:20–1.

95. Rabhi S, Maaroufi M, Khibri H, et al. Magnetic resonance imaging findings within the posterior and lateral columns of the spinal cord extended from the medulla oblongata to the thoracic spine in a woman with subacute combined degeneration without hematologic disorders: a case report and review of the literature. J Med Case Reports 2011;5:166.

96. Tan L, Ho K, Fong G. Subacute combined degeneration of the spinal cord. Hong Kong J Emerg Med 2010;17:79–81.

97. Katsaros VK, Glocker FX, Hemmer B, et al. MRI of spinal cord and brain lesions in subacute combined degeneration. Neuroradiology 1998;40:716–9.

98. Bulakbasi N, Kocaoglu M. Central nervous system infections of herpesvirus family. Neuroimaging Clin N Am 2008;18:53–84, viii.

99. Nakajima H, Furutama D, Kimura F, et al. Herpes simplex virus type 2 infections presenting as brainstem encephalitis and recurrent myelitis. Intern Med 1995;34:839–42.

100. Portolani M, Pecorari M, Gennari W, et al. Case report: primary infection by human herpesvirus 6 variant a with the onset of myelitis. Herpes 2006; 13:72–4.

101. Ward KN, White RP, Mackinnon S, et al. Human herpesvirus-7 infection of the CNS with acute myelitis in an adult bone marrow recipient. Bone Marrow Transplant 2002;30:983–5.

102. Fux CA, Pfister S, Nohl F, et al. Cytomegalovirus-associated acute transverse myelitis in immunocompetent adults. Clin Microbiol Infect 2003;9: 1187–90.

103. Karacostas D, Christodoulou C, Drevelengas A, et al. Cytomegalovirus-associated transverse myelitis in a non-immunocompromised patient. Spinal Cord 2002;40:145–9.

104. Phowthongkum P, Phantumchinda K, Jutivorakool K, et al. Basal ganglia and brainstem encephalitis, optic neuritis, and radiculomyelitis in Epstein-Barr virus infection. J Infect 2007;54:e141–4.

105. Salonen O, Koshkiniemi M, Saari A, et al. Myelitis associated with influenza A virus infection. J Neurovirol 1997;3(1):83–5.

106. Endo A, Fuchigami T, Imai Y, et al. A case of acute transverse myelitis due to measles virus. J Pediatr Infect Dis 2009;4:405–8.

107. Bansal R, Kalita J, Misra UK, et al. Myelitis: a rare presentation of mumps. Pediatr Neurosurg 1998; 28:204–6.

108. Venketasubramanian N. Transverse myelitis following mumps in an adult—a case report with MRI correlation. Acta Neurol Scand 1997;96:328–31.

109. Alexander JP, Baden L, Pallansch MA, et al. Enterovirus 71 infections and neurologic disease–United States, 1977-1991. J Infect Dis 1994;169: 905–8.

110. Ku B, Lee K. Acute transverse myelitis caused by Coxsackie virus B4 infection: a case report. J Korean Med Sci 1998;13:449–53.

111. Minami K, Tsuda Y, Maeda H, et al. Acute transverse myelitis caused by Coxsackie virus B5 infection. J Paediatr Child Health 2004;40:66–8.

112. Starakis I, Marangos M, Giali S, et al. Acute transverse myelitis due to Coxsackie virus. J Clin Neurosci 2005;12:296–8.

113. Takahashi S, Miyamoto A, Oki J, et al. Acute transverse myelitis caused by ECHO virus type 18 infection. Eur J Pediatr 1995;154:378–80.

114. Leis AA, van Gerpen JA, Sejvar JJ. The aetiology of flaccid paralysis in West Nile virus infection. J Neurol Neurosurg Psychiatry 2004;75:940 [author reply: 940–1].

115. Bender A. Severe tick borne encephalitis with simultaneous brain stem, bithalamic, and spinal cord involvement documented by MRI. J Neurol Neurosurg Psychiatry 2005;76:135–7.

116. Solomon T, Dung NM, Kneen R, et al. Japanese encephalitis. J Neurol Neurosurg Psychiatry 2000; 68:405–15.

117. Misra UK, Kalita J, Syam UK, et al. Neurological manifestations of dengue virus infection. J Neurol Sci 2006;244:117–22.

118. Wasay M, Channa R, Jumani M, et al. Encephalitis and myelitis associated with dengue viral infection clinical and neuroimaging features. Clin Neurol Neurosurg 2008;110:635–40.

119. Einsiedel L, Kat E, Ravindran J, et al. MR findings in Murray Valley encephalitis. AJNR Am J Neuroradiol 2003;24:1379–82.

120. Umehara F, Nose H, Saito M, et al. Abnormalities of spinal magnetic resonance images implicate clinical variability in human T-cell lymphotropic virus type I-associated myelopathy. J Neurovirol 2007; 13:260–7.

121. Watanabe M, Yamashita T, Hara A, et al. High signal in the spinal cord on T2-weighted images in rapidly progressive tropical spastic paraparesis. Neuroradiology 2001;43:231–3.

122. Quencer RM. AIDS-associated myelopathy: clinical severity, MR findings, and underlying etiologies. AJNR Am J Neuroradiol 1999;20:1387–8.

123. Bakshi R. Neuroimaging of HIV and AIDS related illnesses: a review. Front Biosci 2004;9:632–46.

124. Tullman MJ, Delman BN, Lublin FD, et al. Magnetic resonance imaging of meningoradiculomyelitis in early disseminated Lyme disease. J Neuroimaging 2003;13:264–8.

125. Piesman J, Gern L. Lyme borreliosis in Europe and North America. Parasitology 1999;129:S191–220.

126. Makhani N, Morris SK, Page AV, et al. A twist on Lyme: the challenge of diagnosing European Lyme neuroborreliosis. J Clin Microbiol 2010;49:455–7.

127. Mantienne C, Albucher JF, Catalaa I, et al. MRI in Lyme disease of the spinal cord. Neuroradiology 2001;43:485–8.

128. Bigi S, Aebi C, Nauer C, et al. Acute transverse myelitis in Lyme neuroborreliosis. Infection 2010;38:413–6.

129. Lesca G, Deschamps R, Lubetzki C, et al. Acute myelitis in early Borrelia burgdorferi infection. J Neurol 2002;249:1472–4.

130. Lowenstein D, Mills C. Acute syphilitic transverse myelitis: unusual presentation of meningovascular syphilis. Genitourin Med 1987;63:333–8.

131. Tsui E, Ng S, Chow L, et al. Syphilitic myelitis with diffuse spinal cord abnormality on MR imaging. Eur Radiol 2002;12:2973–6.

132. Tsiodras S, Kelesidis T, Kelesidis I. Mycoplasma pneumoniae-associated myelitis: a comprehensive review. Eur J Neurol 2006;13:112–24.

133. Weng WC, Peng SS, Wang SB, et al. Mycoplasma pneumoniae-associated transverse myelitis and rhabdomyolysis. Pediatr Neurol 2009;40:128–30.

134. Goebels N, Helmchen C, Abele-Horn M, et al. Extensive myelitis associated with Mycoplasma pneumoniae infection: magnetic resonance imaging and clinical long-term follow-up. J Neurol 2001;248:204–8.

135. Suda S, Ueda M, Komaba Y, et al. Tuberculous myelitis diagnosed by elevated adenosine deaminase activity in cerebrospinal fluid. J Clin Neurosci 2008;15:1068–9.

136. Wasay M, Arif H, Khealani B, et al. Neuroimaging of tuberculous myelitis: analysis of ten cases and review of literature. J Neuroimaging 2006;16:197–205.

137. Sawanyawisuth K, Tiamkao S, Kanpittaya J, et al. MR imaging findings in cerebrospinal gnathostomiasis. AJNR Am J Neuroradiol 2004;25:446–9.

138. Leite C, Jinkins J, Escobar B. MR imaging of intramedullary and intradural-extramedullary spinal cysticercosis. AJR Am J Roentgenol 1997;169:1713–7.

139. Singhi P. Neurocysticercosis in children. Indian J Pediatr 2009;76:537–45.

140. Singh P, Sahai K. Intramedullary cysticercosis. Neurol India 2004;52:264–5.

141. Wallin MT, Kurtzke JF. Neurocysticercosis in the United States: review of an important emerging infection. Neurology 2004;63:1559–64.

142. Saleem S, Belal AI, el-Ghandour NM. Spinal cord schistosomiasis: MR imaging appearance with surgical and pathologic correlation. AJNR Am J Neuroradiol 2005;26:1646–54.

143. Bennett G, Provenzale JM. Schistosomal myelitis: findings at MR imaging. Eur J Radiol 1998;27:268–70.

144. Bunyaratavej K, Pongpunlert W, Jongwutiwes S, et al. Spinal gnathostomiasis resembling an intrinsic cord tumor/myelitis in a 4-year-old boy. Southeast Asian J Trop Med Public Health 2008;39:800–3.

145. Sawanyawisuth K, Tiamkao S, Nitinavakarn B, et al. MR imaging findings in cauda equina gnathostomiasis. AJNR Am J Neuroradiol 2005;26:39–42.

146. Schmutzhard E, Boongird P. Eosinophilic meningitis and radiculomyelitis in Thailand, caused by CNS invasion of Gnathostoma spinigerum and Angiostrongylus cantonensis. J Neurol Neurosurg Psychiatry 1988;51:80–7.

Pyomyositis

Vikas Agarwal, MD, DM[a],*, Sandeep Chauhan, MD, FICP[b],
Rakesh K. Gupta, MD[c]

KEYWORDS

- Tropical pyomyositis • Myositis • Muscle abscess
- Muscle infections • Diffusion-weighted imaging
- *Staphylococcus aureus*

Key Points: Pyomyositis

- Pyomyositis is the primary infection of the skeletal muscle/s.
- It is more common in tropical countries, but is increasingly being reported worldwide.
- It can affect immunocompromised and immunocompetent individuals.
- *Staphylococcus aureus* is the most common causative organism.
- Ultrasound is a simple, readily available, good technique for diagnosis, but it may miss early lesions.
- MR imaging is the preferred imaging technique for detection.
- MR imaging is highly sensitive, can image large areas of the body, and detect subclinical involvement. It has the added advantage of detecting adjacent bone and joint involvement and excluding other soft tissue disorders, such as tumors and lymphedema.

Pyomyositis (also known as *tropical myositis, temperate myositis, pyogenic myositis, suppurative myositis, myositis purulenta tropica,* and *epidemic abscess*) is a primary infection of skeletal muscle and often associated with abscess formation. Intermuscular abscesses, abscesses extending into muscles from adjoining tissues such as bone or subcutaneous tissues, and those secondary to previous septicemia are not classified as pyomyositis.

In the 1800s, both Virchow and Osler reported cases of "diffuse purulent infiltration of the muscles"; however, the first detailed description of pyomyositis is attributed to Scriba[1,2] in 1885. Pyomyositis was entirely thought to be confined to tropical areas predominantly affecting young and healthy populations. Levin and colleagues[3] described a case in the United States for the first time in 1971. Since then increasingly more cases are being described from temperate areas where the incidence seems to mirror the increase in the number of immunocompromised persons, particularly those with HIV infection, diabetes, organ transplantation, malignancies, chemotherapy, and rheumatologic diseases (temperate pyomyositis).[4–19] These immunosuppressed states account for three-fourths of cases in temperate areas, with HIV being responsible for nearly a quarter of all these cases. Because of these differences, tropical and temperate pyomyositis were considered separate entities, but this distinction is more or less superficial, and

---

Conflict of interest: The authors have nothing to disclose.
[a] Department of Clinical Immunology, Sanjay Gandhi Postgraduate Institute of Medical Sciences, Raebareli Road, Lucknow 226014, Uttar Pradesh, India
[b] Department of Rheumatology, Nobles Hospital, The Strang IM4 4RJ, Isle of Man 01624 650000, UK
[c] Department of Radiodiagnosis, Sanjay Gandhi Postgraduate Institute of Medical Sciences, Rae Bareli Road, Lucknow 226014, Uttar Pradesh, India
* Corresponding author.
E-mail address: vikasagr@sgpgi.ac.in

therefore suggestions were made to rename this entity more appropriately as *pyomyositis* (which we will be used in this article), *infectious myositis*, or *spontaneous bacterial myositis*.

PREVALENCE

Exact prevalence and incidence rates are not known because of the lack of epidemiologic studies. Information in the literature is restricted to case reports and case series from individual hospitals or Medline searches. Studies from Africa estimate that pyomyositis is responsible for 1% to 4% of all hospital admissions in tropical countries.[9,20] A Medline database search in the United States from 1981 to 2002 revealed 84 cases of pyomyositis in people infected with HIV, 119 in those who had non-HIV underlying immunosuppressive states, and 127 in normal healthy individuals.[9] Unnikrishnan and colleagues[21] reported 13 cases of pyomyositis in children younger than 16 years from a large tertiary orthopedic center in the United Kingdom between 1998 and 2007. A study from Australia estimates annual incidence of 0.5 cases per 100 000 person-years.[22] In a retrospective analysis conducted by Tanir and colleagues,[23] among 242 patients who were hospitalized with a soft tissue diagnosis, pyomyositis accounted for 6 (2.5%) cases.

ETIOLOGY

Staphylococcus aureus is the causative organism in up to 90% of cases from tropical areas and 75% from temperate areas, detected in either blood cultures or surgical specimens.[3,6,9,24] A recent spurt has occurred in community-acquired, methicillin-resistant *Staphylococcus aureus* (MRSA) causing pyomyositis.[11,18,19,25–27] The second most common type of bacteria implicated in causing pyomyositis is group A streptococci.[6] Streptococci (groups B, C, and G), *Pneumococcus, Neisseria, Haemophilus, Aeromonas, Pseudomonas, Klebsiella,* and *Escherichia* have also been implicated, albeit uncommonly.[6,16,28–30] Mycobacteria (*M avium* complex, *M Tuberculosis,* and *M haemophilium*), fungi (*Blastomycosis, Cryptococcus neoformans, Aspergillus, Candida, Fusarium, Pneumocystis Jiroveci*), and anaerobes (*Salmonella, Vibrio, Enterococci, Capnocytophaga sputigena, Stenotrophomonas maltophilia,* and *Burkholderia cenocepacia*) remain subjects of anecdotal case reports.[12,14,31–45] Chiu and colleagues[46] reported a higher incidence of gram-negative bacterial pyomyositis in patients with underlying diseases. Crum[9] had similar findings in a retrospective analysis from the United

States. However, *Staphylococcus, Bartonella,* and *Salmonella* species were the causative agents most commonly isolated with the diagnosis in patients with HIV.

PATHOGENESIS

The exact pathogenesis is currently poorly understood, causing tropical pyomyositis to be difficult to differentiate from temperate pyomyositis. Factors such as preceding viral and protozoal infections and nutritional deficiencies have been proposed, but evidence in this regard is sketchy.[47] The pathogenesis involves the presence of transient bacteremia in a setting of muscle injury.

Skeletal muscles are intrinsically very resistant to infections. In 1904, investigators showed that pyomyositis could only occur in *S aureus*–inoculated animal muscles that had been initially traumatized by electric shock, pinching, or ischemia.[48] Even direct inoculation of staphylococcus in skeletal muscles failed to produce an abscess.[49] More evidence comes from the fact that pyomyositis was seen is fewer than 1% cases of fatal Staphylococcal septicemia.[50]

In addition to blunt trauma, muscular injuries from overuse may be a risk factor for the development of pyomyositis. Cases of pyomyositis have been documented in young healthy individuals after vigorous exercises concurrent with asymptomatic episodes of bacteremia possibly from skin abrasions.[51–53] In 20% to 50% of cases, patients had a history of blunt trauma or rigorous exercise.[54,55] The most plausible explanation seems to be that sequestered iron is released from myoglobin in traumatized muscles. This released iron provides a nutrient that is essential for rapid growth and proliferation of organisms in an appropriate circumstance (transient bacteremia), hence leading to the development of pyomyositis. In addition, formation of small hematomas around the site may provide a favorable site for the binding of staphylococci and other bacteria, and the surrounding damaged and devitalized tissue might also impede the host immune response.

Conflicting studies by Bickels and colleagues[56] and Scharschmidt and colleagues[57] have added more to the already prevalent confusion. In their review of 676 patients, Bickels and colleagues[56] reported trauma in fewer than 5% of cases, thereby ruling out muscle trauma as a prerequisite for myositis. This observation was also supported by Scharschmidt and colleagues.[57] Furthermore, in 11 cases of pyomyositis from Australia, none had history of antecedent muscle trauma.[22] Therefore, given the infrequency of pyomyositis compared with the number of athletic events, muscle injury may have some role, but evidence is still inconclusive.

Other mechanisms postulated, though not fully substantiated, include lack of immunity against staphylococcus, as evidenced by defective T-lymphocyte responses.[58] Patients with HIV have an increased incidence of pyomyositis compared with the general population. The reasons could be multifactorial (higher colonization rates with *S aureus*, neutropenia, defective immune responses, use of intravenous lines, direct damage to the muscle [HIV myopathy],or reactions to anti-retroviral medications, such as mitochondrial myopathy associated with zidovudine).[59]

HISTOPATHOLOGY

Microscopically, patchy myocytolysis with inflammatory infiltrate is seen, with areas of complete disintegration and edematous separation of muscle fibers with interfiber infiltration. The process is not diffuse, and is followed by either a reparative process or complete degeneration with suppuration. The pathologic hallmark of pyomyositis is myositis without abscess in biopsied muscle specimens.[60]

CLINICAL FEATURES

Pyomyositis is seen more commonly in young men, with a male-to-female ratio of 1.5:1.[9,61] No age group is immune, and increasingly more cases are being reported in pediatric age groups.[21,62] Falesi and colleagues[63] reported pyomyositis in a neonate. Commonly, a single muscle is affected, but involvement of multiple muscles is not unusual (12%–40% of cases).[24] Although the most common site of pyomyositis is the thigh, it commonly affects other bulky muscles, such as the gastrocnemius, glutei, pectorals, and biceps, with a propensity for lower limbs.[64] Involvement of the muscles of forearm, abdominal wall, sternocleidomastoid, intercostals muscles, paraspinal, and pelvic muscles, and even extraocular muscles, has been anecdotally reported.[65–70]

The evolution of myositis can be clinically divided into three discrete stages.[24]

Invasive Stage

The invasive stage is subacute, occurring over 1 to 3 weeks, and characterized by local painful swelling with a wooden consistency with or without erythema (because infection is deep-seated). Fever and leukocytosis are invariably present. Aspiration at this stage will not yield pus because the bacterial seeding has just begun and purulent collection has not developed. This stage may resolve, remaining undiagnosed in most patients, or can progress to the next stage. It is often overlooked, and differentials vary from hematoma to thrombosis to osteomyelitis.

Suppurative Stage

The suppurative stage is the one at which the diagnosis of pyomyositis is usually established. High spiky swinging temperatures herald the onset, which usually occurs between the second and third weeks. The area is extremely painful and tender. An abscess is seen on imaging studies. Aspiration, if attempted at this stage, will yield pus. However, because the infection is deep-seated, classical characteristics of abscess, such as erythema and fluctuation, are generally absent. The presence of regional lymphadenopathy suggests an alternative diagnosis.

Late Stage

If the suppurative stage remains undiagnosed and untreated, the infection disseminates, leading to multiple abscesses, septicemia, septic shock, and multiorgan system failure, marking the late stage.

Differential Diagnosis

Pyomyositis may have myriad presentations besides the typical one (only local symptoms, only fever and leukocytosis, acute fever with chills, pyrexia of unknown origin [in absence of local symptoms], compartment and compression syndromes, and septic shock). A review of the literature showed that the diagnosis of pyomyositis has been missed; for instance, pyomyositis of iliopsoas muscle presented like appendicitis.[71] Likewise, septic arthritis of the hip, epidural abscess or sciatica, osteomyelitis, and inflammatory myositis have been erroneously diagnosed in the presence of pyomyositis.[72–76]

Therefore, lest the diagnosis be missed, resulting in adverse outcomes for a potential treatable entity, physicians in all spheres must maintain a high degree of vigil for this entity.[77–79] Other conditions, such as deep vein thrombosis, cellulitis, muscle contusion, muscle hematoma, muscle or tendon rupture, septic arthritis, osteomyelitis, osteosarcoma, polymyositis, spontaneous gangrenous myositis trichinosis, cysticercus cellulose, and leptospirosis, may often have similar presentations to pyomyositis, especially in the invasive stage, often leading to a diagnostic dilemma.

DIAGNOSIS

Early diagnosis is the key to success but is commonly missed. The reasons include lack of awareness, nonspecific features in the invasive stage, atypical manifestations, and a wide range of differential diagnoses.

Leukocytosis is variable, especially in the invasive stage, but a shift to left occurs with suppurative stage leukocytosis. Half of the HIV-positive patients will not have leukocytosis.[9] Keeping up with inflammation, inflammatory markers such as erythrocyte sedimentation rate and C-reactive protein are also elevated but are nonspecific. Some clues can be obtained from blood tests; for instance, the presence of eosinophilia suggests parasitic infection, and deranged liver and renal functions favor the diagnosis of leptospirosis. Muscle enzymes such as creatinine kinase and aldolase are not raised despite evidence of muscle inflammation and destruction.[56,80,81]

Blood cultures are sterile in approximately 90% of patients from tropical areas and up to 70% patients from temperate regions.[82,83] Even if positive, blood cultures support the diagnosis in an appropriate clinical setting but are not diagnostic for pyomyositis. Poor yield in blood cultures may occur because bacteremia is usually transient in pyomyositis. Better yields are from temperate countries, probably because of better microbiological techniques. Despite the poor yield, blood cultures should be taken to test for aerobic and anaerobic bacteria, mycobacteria, and fungi, especially in immunocompromised patients.

Aspiration and culture of the pus remains the standard diagnostic method, but in the early stages minimal or no suppuration occurs, and therefore pus may not be aspirated. Pus cultures may not yield any organism in up to 30% of cases.[60]

Muscle biopsy with culture of tissue remains the gold standard.[60] In addition to confirming the diagnosis of pyomyositis, other diagnosis such as polymyositis, osteosarcoma, and intermuscular abscesses can be confidently excluded.

Imaging

Noninvasive radiologic methods, such as ultrasound, CT, or MR imaging, are useful in confirming the diagnosis and monitoring patients during follow-up. Plain radiographs are not sensitive, but in a few cases may suggest muscle enlargement, loss of muscle definition, obliteration of deep fat planes, gas in soft tissues, and reactive changes in adjacent bone. Plain radiographs are more useful in excluding other processes, such as osteomyelitis or bone tumor.

Ultrasound remains the preferred initial screening tool because it is easily available and cost-effective. It shows hypoechoic areas with increased muscle bulk, but the early invasive stage may be missed.[84] CT can visualize pyomyositis as areas of low attenuation with loss of muscle plain surrounded by a rim of contrast enhancement, but it cannot differentiate abscess from swollen muscles.[25]

MR imaging is more specific and sensitive compared with CT. It usually presents as ill-defined muscle enlargement with hyperintensity on T2-weighted images, which may be associated with swelling of fascial planes, abnormal signal intensity of the nearby bone, or fluid in the joint. Reactive bone edema is difficult to differentiate from osteomyelitis even after contrast study. Occasionally, fluid collection within the muscle may be visible as hyperintense on T2-weighted images and isointense to hypointense on T1-weighted images (Figs. 1 and 2). Postcontrast T1-weighted imaging study shows rim enhancement, suggesting an abscess along with uniform enhancement of the involved muscles.[84–86] Diffusion-weighted imaging (DWI) has been reported to help in differentiating abscess from tumor in various body locations; however, its role in pyomyositis is unknown. DWI shows a hyperintense signal from the involved muscles, which shows a hypointense signal on an apparent diffusion coefficient trace and is referred to as *restriction of diffusion* (see Figs. 1 and 2), similar to the description of the abscess anywhere else in the remainder of the organs. The authors routinely use DWI as part of their imaging protocol in suspected cases of pyomyositis, and have found it to be extremely useful. Moreover, because the disease process may be patchy and widespread at times, MR imaging may have an additional advantage of showing the exact extent of the disease noninvasively, and is useful in monitoring the response to therapy. MR imaging is also useful in detecting pyomyositis in the pelvic region and ruling out other pathologies effectively.[87] Gallium scintigraphy may also help to localize inflammation, but it is nonspecific and expensive.[88]

Once the diagnosis is made, common immunosuppressive states (diabetes, HIV, rheumatologic conditions, and malignancies) must be ruled out along with serum immunoglobulin levels.

TREATMENT

As with any serious infection, antibiotic therapy cannot be delayed and should be instituted immediately once the diagnosis is confirmed (Fig. 3). Although pyomyositis is rarely diagnosed during the invasive stage, antibiotics alone will suffice at this stage. Once the abscess has formed, ultrasound-guided or CT-guided percutaneous

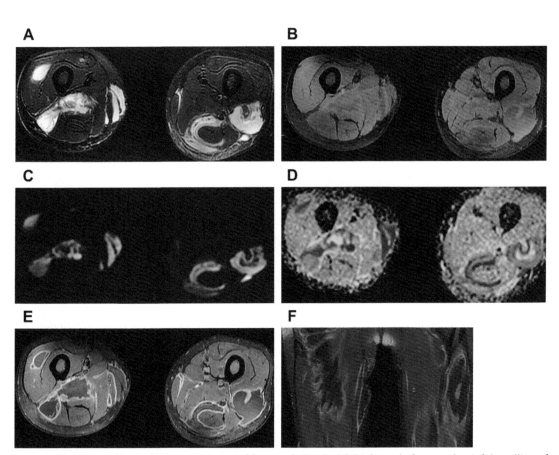

Fig. 1. MR imaging of both thighs in a 20-year-old man admitted with high-grade fever and painful swelling of thighs. Axial fat-saturated T2-weighted image (*A*) at mid-thigh level shows bright signal in anterior and posterior compartment of both thighs, mainly in the vastus group of muscles. Axial T1-weighted image (*B*) shows hypointense signal intensity in these involved areas. Diffusion-weighted image (*C*) shows restricted diffusion with corresponding low apparent diffusion coefficient (ADC) value on ADC map (*D*). Axial postcontrast fat-saturated T1-weighted image (*E*) shows peripheral rim enhancement in vastus medialis, lateralis, and intermedius muscles, with central areas of liquefaction suggestive of fluid collections. Coronal postcontrast fat-saturated T1-weighted image (*F*) shows craniocaudal extent of the lesion.

drainage should be performed emergently to ensure complete drainage. Traditional methods such as surgical incision and drainage are rarely used, for instance, in the presence of significant necrosis with large areas of involvement.

Choice of antibiotics must be guided by the treating physician's judgment. While awaiting culture and sensitivity reports, cloxacillin is recommended as first-line therapy, with first-generation cephalosporins such as cefazolin as an alternative for penicillin-sensitive individuals. Coverage for MRSA using vancomycin or teicoplanin should be considered in severely ill patients who are at a high risk for MRSA or whose culture sensitivity report shows MRSA.[89] Furthermore, considering the increased incidence of community-acquired MRSA causing pyomyositis, vancomycin or teicoplanin may be used as first-line therapy. Linezolid,

dalfopristin-quinupristin, daptomycin, and tigecycline should be reserved for vancomycin intermediate-sensitive *Staphylococcus*.[89] Adding a second drug against *Staphylococcus* does not confer any benefit.

Penicillin remains the first-line antimicrobial agent for streptococcus. Gram-negative organisms require two drugs, usually consisting of a combination of a third-generation cephalosporin with aminoglycosides. For anaerobes, either metronidazole or clindamycin is the preferred agent. If the patient is immunosuppressed or very toxic, empirical treatment is started with broad-spectrum antibiotics covering staphylococcus, streptococcus, gram-negative bacteria, and anaerobes. In these situations, vancomycin with an antipseudomonal carbapenem or β-lactam combination is the most appropriate therapy.

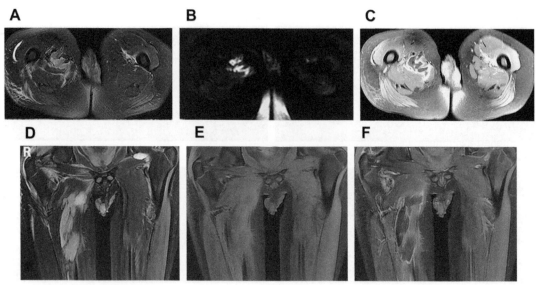

Fig. 2. MR imaging of both upper thighs in a 20-year-old man admitted with high-grade fever and painful swelling of thighs. Axial (*A*) and coronal (*D*) fat-suppressed T2W MR images show ill-defined hyperintensity in the vastus medialis muscles of both upper thighs, predominantly involving the right thigh. Hyperintensity is also noted in the skin and subcutaneous tissue of lateral aspect of right thigh. Diffusion-weighted image (*B*) shows restricted diffusion in right medial thigh. Axial postcontrast fat-saturated T1-weighted images (*C*) show peripheral rim enhancement with central areas of liquefaction, suggestive of fluid collections in right vastus medialis muscle. Ill-defined enhancement is also noted in the subcutaneous tissue of right thigh, suggestive of cellulites. No significant enhancement is noted on left side. Coronal pre (*E*) and postcontrast fat-saturated T1-weighted images (*F*) show craniocaudal extent of the lesion.

Other antimicrobials, such as aztreonam fluoroquinolone, aminoglycoside, cephalosporin, or clindamycin, alone or in combination, have been used successfully.

Failure of fever to normalize indicates metastatic infection, drug resistance, or drug fever. Imaging may be used to assess the course of the disease and to determine metastatic infection. Using

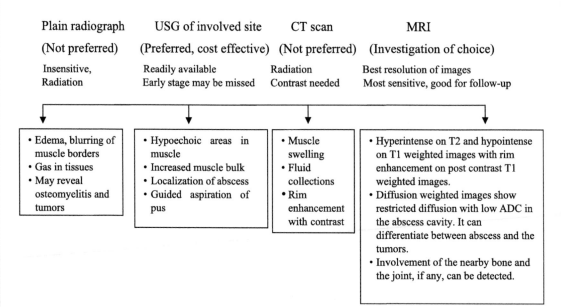

Plain radiograph	USG of involved site	CT scan	MRI
(Not preferred)	(Preferred, cost effective)	(Not preferred)	(Investigation of choice)
Insensitive, Radiation	Readily available Early stage may be missed	Radiation Contrast needed	Best resolution of images Most sensitive, good for follow-up
• Edema, blurring of muscle borders • Gas in tissues • May reveal osteomyelitis and tumors	• Hypoechoic areas in muscle • Increased muscle bulk • Localization of abscess • Guided aspiration of pus	• Muscle swelling • Fluid collections • Rim enhancement with contrast	• Hyperintense on T2 and hypointense on T1 weighted images with rim enhancement on post contrast T1 weighted images. • Diffusion weighted images show restricted diffusion with low ADC in the abscess cavity. It can differentiate between abscess and the tumors. • Involvement of the nearby bone and the joint, if any, can be detected.

Fig. 3. Approach to a patient with suspected pyomyositis.

topical mupirocin or systemic rifampicin to eliminate the nasal carriage of staphylococcus in patients with past episodes of pyomyositis or staphylococcus septicemia and in immunocompromised persons can prevent further episodes.[90]

PROGNOSIS

Heightened awareness, newer diagnostic modalities, and effective chemotherapeutic agents have considerably reduced the mortality associated with pyomyositis. The fatality rate still varies from as low as 0.5% to as high as 10%. Patients who recover even from severe disease have surprisingly little or no dysfunction in the affected part.

REFERENCES

1. Scriba J. Beitrang zur, Aetiologie der myositis acuta. Deutsche Zeit Chir 1885;22:497–502 [in German].
2. Traquair RN. Pyomyositis. J Trop Med Hyg 1947;50: 81–9.
3. Levin MJ, Gardner P, Waldvogel FA. An unusual infection due to staphylococcus aureus. N Engl J Med 1971;284:196–8.
4. Garcia-Mata S, Hidalgo A, Esparza J. Primary pyomyositis of the psoas muscles in a temperate climate. Review of two cases in children followed up over the long term. An Sist Sanit Navar 2006; 29:419–31.
5. Bonafede P, Butler J, Kimbrough R, et al. Temperate zone pyomyositis. West J Med 1992;156:419–23.
6. Christin L, Sarosi GA. Pyomyositis in North America: case reports and review. Clin Infect Dis 1992;15:668–77.
7. Ansaloni L, Acaye GL, Re MC. High HIV seroprevalence among patients with pyomyositis in northern Uganda. Trop Med Int Health 1996;1:210–2.
8. Smith PG, Pike MC, Taylor E, et al. The epidemiology of tropical pyomyositis in Mengo districts of Uganda. Trans R Soc Trop Med Hyg 1978;72:46–53.
9. Crum NF. Bacterial pyomyositis in the United States. Am J Med 2004;117:420–8.
10. Marath H, Yates M, Lee M, et al. Pyomyositis. J Diabetes Complications. PMID: 21106397. [Epub ahead of print].
11. Zalavras CG, Rigopoulos N, Poultsides L, et al. Increased oxacillin resistance in thigh pyomyositis in diabetic patients. Clin Orthop Relat Res 2008; 466:1405–9.
12. Jang EY, Lee SO, Choi SH, et al. Case of pyomyositis due to Mycobacterium haemophilum in a renal transplant recipient. J Clin Microbiol 2007;45:3847–9.
13. McRae M, Sharma S. Forearm pyomyositis in a breast cancer patient on chemotherapy. J Plast Reconstr Aesthet Surg 2010;63:e737–9.
14. Khosla P, Aroaa N, Jain S. Tubercular pyomyositis in a case of rheumatoid arthritis being treated with infliximab. Int J Rheum Dis 2010;13:82–5.
15. Ravindran V, Duke O. Non-tropical pyomyositis in a patient with systemic lupus erythematosus. Lupus 2009;18:379–80.
16. Yassin M, Yadavalli GK, Alvarado N, et al. Streptococcus anginosus (Streptococcus milleri Group) Pyomyositis in a 50-year-old man with acquired immunodeficiency syndrome: case report and review of literature. Infection 2010;38:65–8.
17. Traina ED, Crider MF, Berman D, et al. Pyomyositis as the presenting feature of acute lymphocytic leukemia. Clin Pediatr (Phila) 2008;47:167–70.
18. Fukushima T, Iwao H, Nakazima A, et al. MRSA-pyomyositis in a patient with acute myelogenous leukemia after intensive chemotherapy. Anticancer Res 2009;29:3361–4.
19. Kalambokis G, Theodorou A, Kosta P, et al. Multiple myeloma presenting with pyomyositis caused by community-acquired methicillin-resistant Staphylococcus aureus: report of a case and literature review. Int J Hematol 2008;87:516–9.
20. Horn CV, Master S. Pyomyositis tropicans in Uganda. East Afr Med J 1968;45:463–71.
21. Unnikrishnan PN, Perry DC, George H, et al. Tropical primary pyomyositis in children of the UK: an emerging medical challenge. Int Orthop 2010;34: 109–13.
22. Block AA, Marshall C, Ratcliffe A, et al. Staphylococcal pyomyositis in a temperate region: epidemiology and modern management. Med J Aust 2008; 189:323–5.
23. Tanir G, Tonbul A, Tuygun N, et al. Soft tissue infections in children: a retrospective analysis of 242 hospitalized patients. Jpn J Infect Dis 2006;59: 258–60.
24. Cheidozi LC. Pyomyositis: review of 205 cases in 112 patients. Am J Surg 1979;137:255–9.
25. Pannaraj PS, Hulten KG, Gonzalez BE, et al. Infective pyomyositis and myositis in children in the era of community-acquired, methicillin-resistant Staphylococcus aureus infection. Clin Infect Dis 2006;43: 953–60.
26. Kulkarni GB, Pal PK, Veena Kumari HB, et al. Community-acquired methicillin-resistant Staphylococcus aureus pyomyositis with myelitis: a rare occurrence with diverse presentation. Neurol India 2009;57:653–6.
27. Woodward JF, Sengupta DJ, Cookson BT, et al. Disseminated community-acquired USA300 methicillin-resistant Staphylococcus aureus pyomyositis and septic pulmonary emboli in an immunocompetent adult. Surg Infect (Larchmt) 2010;11:59–63.
28. Yahalom G, Guranda L, Meltzer E. Internal obturator muscle abscess caused by Klebsiella pneumoniae. J Infect 2007;54:157–60.

29. Sarubbi FA, Gafford GD, Bishop DR. Gram negative bacterial pyomyositis: unique case and review. Rev Infect Dis 1989;11:789–92.

30. Wong SL, Anthony EY, Shetty AK. Pyomyositis due to Streptococcus pneumonia. Am J Emerg Med 2009;27:633.e1–3.

31. Couzigou C, Lacombe K, Girard PM, et al. Non-O:1 and non-O:139 Vibrio cholerae septicemia and pyomyositis in an immunodeficient traveler returning from Tunisia. Travel Med Infect Dis 2007;5:44–6.

32. Mootsikapun P, Mahakkanukrauh A, Suwannaroj S, et al. Tuberculous pyomyositis. J Med Assoc Thai 2003;86:477–81.

33. Minami K, Sakiyama M, Suzuki H, et al. Pyomyositis of the vastus medialis muscle associated with Salmonella enteritidis in a child. Pediatr Radiol 2003;33:492–4.

34. Pearl GS, Sieger B. Granulomatous *Pneumocystis carinii* myositis presenting as an intramuscular mass. Clin Infect Dis 1996;22:577–8.

35. Macher AM, Neafie R, Angritt P, et al. Microsporidial myositis and the acquired immunodeficiency syndrome (AIDS): a four-year follow-up. Ann Intern Med 1988;109:343.

36. Vandenbos F, Roger PM, Mondail-Miton V, et al. *Aspergillus fumigatus* muscle abscess revealing invasive aspergillus in a patient expectant of AIDS. Presse Med 1998;27:1844.

37. O'Neill KM, Ormsby AH, Prayson RA. Cryptococcal myositis: a case report and review of the literature. Pathology 1998;30:316–7.

38. Pérez-Rodríguez MT, Sopeña B, Longueira R, et al. Calf pyomyositis caused by Enterococcus faecalis. QJM 2011;104(6):527–9.

39. Chan JF, Wong SS, Leung SS, et al. Capnocytophaga sputigena primary iliopsoas abscess. J Med Microbiol 2010;59:1368–70.

40. Wong VK, Lissack ME, Turmezei TD, et al. Salmonella pyomyositis complicating sickle cell anemia: a case report. J Med Case Reports 2010;4:198.

41. Sen RK, Tripathy SK, Dhatt S, et al. Primary tuberculous pyomyositis of forearm muscles. Indian J Tuberc 2010;57:34–40.

42. Thomas J, Prabhu VN, Varaprasad IR, et al. Stenotrophomonas maltophilia: a very rare cause of tropical pyomyositis. Int J Rheum Dis 2010;13:89–90.

43. Lin MY, Chihara S, Smith KY, et al. Classic pyomyositis of the extremities as an unusual manifestation of Blastomyces dermatitidis: a report of two cases. Mycoses 2010;53:356–9.

44. El-Laboudi AH, Etherington C, Whitaker P, et al. Acute Burkholderia cenocepacia pyomyositis in a patient with cystic fibrosis. J Cyst Fibros 2009;8:273–5.

45. Tsai SH, Peng YJ, Wang NC. Pyomyositis with hepatic and perinephric abscesses caused by Candida albicans in a diabetic nephropathy patient. Am J Med Sci 2006;331:292–4.

46. Chiu SK, Lin JC, Wang NC, et al. Impact of underlying diseases on the clinical characteristics and outcome of primary pyomyositis. J Microbiol Immunol Infect 2008;41:286–93.

47. Dunkerley GR, Older J, Onwochei B, et al. Pyomyositis. Am Fam Physician 1996;54:565–9.

48. Miyake H. Beitrage zur Kenntnis der sogenannten Myositis infectiosa. Mitt Grenzgeb Med Chir 1904;13:155–98 [in German].

49. Halsted WS. Surgical papers. Baltimore (MD): John Hopkins University Press; 1924.

50. Smith MI, Vickers AB. Natural history of treated and untreated patients with septicaemia. Lancet 1960;1:1318–22.

51. Burkhart BG, Hamson KR. Pyomyositis in a 69-year-old tennis player. Am J Orthop 2003;32:562–3.

52. Jayoussi R, Bialik V, Eyal A, et al. Pyomyositis caused by vigorous exercise in a boy. Acta Paediatr 1995;84:226–7.

53. Koutures CG, Savoia M, Pedowitz RA. Staphylococcus aureus thigh pyomyositis in a collegiate swimmer. Clin J Sport Med 2000;10:297–9.

54. Gibson RK, Rosenthal SJ, Lukert BP. Pyomyositis. Increasing recognition in temperate climates. Am J Med 1984;77:768–72.

55. Hall RL, Callaghan JJ, Moloney E, et al. Pyomyositis in a temperate climate, presentation, diagnosis and treatment. J Bone Joint Surg Am 1990;72:1240–4.

56. Bickels J, Ben–Sira L, Kessler A, et al. Primary pyomyositis. J Bone Joint Surg Am 2002;84-A:2277–86.

57. Scharschmidt TJ, Weiner SD, Myers JP. Bacterial Pyomyositis. Curr Infect Dis Rep 2004;6:393–6.

58. Idoko JA, Oyeyinka GO, Giassuddin AS, et al. Neutrophil cell function and migration inhibition study in Nigerian patients with tropical pyomyositis. J Infect 1987;15:33–7.

59. Schwartzman WA, Lambertus MW, Kennedy CA, et al. Staphylococcal pyomyositis in patients infected by the human immunodeficiency virus. Am J Med 1991;90:595–600.

60. Shepherd JJ. Tropical myositis, is it an entity and what is its causes? Lancet 1983;2:1240–2.

61. Sharma A, Kumar S, Wanchu A, et al. Clinical characteristics and predictors of mortality in 67 patients with primary pyomyositis: a study from North India. Clin Rheumatol 2010;29:45–51.

62. Chiu NC, Hsieh MC, Chi H, et al. Clinical characteristics of pyomyositis in children: 20-year experience in a medical center in Taiwan. J Microbiol Immunol Infect 2009;42:494–9.

63. Falesi M, Regazzoni BM, Wyttenbach M, et al. Primary pelvic pyomyositis in a neonate. J Perinatol 2009;29:830–1.

64. Ovadia D, Ezra E, Ben-Sira L, et al. Primary pyomyositis in children: a retrospective analysis of 11 cases. J Pediatr Orthop B 2007;16:153–9.

65. Collier S, Vig N, Collier J. Two cases of tropical pyomyositis of the sternocleidomastoid muscle occurring in the UK. Br J Oral Maxillofac Surg 2010;48:216–7.

66. Acharya IG, Jethani J. Pyomyositis of extraocular muscle: case series and review of the literature. Indian J Ophthalmol 2010;58:532–5.

67. Ntusi NB, Khaki A. Primary multifocal pyomyositis due to Staphylococcus aureus. QJM 2011;104:163–5.

68. Prasad R, Verma N, Mishra OP. Pyomositis: a report of three cases. Ann Trop Paediatr 2009;29:313–6.

69. Phoon ES, Sebastin SJ, Tay SC. Primary pyomyositis (bacterial myositis) of the pronator quadratus. J Hand Surg Eur Vol 2009;34:549–51.

70. Hassan FO, Shannak A. Primary pyomyositis of the paraspinal muscles: a case report and literature review. Eur Spine J 2008;17:S239–42.

71. Wysoki MG, Angeid-Backman E, Izes BA. Iliopsoas myositis mimicking appendicitis: MRI diagnosis. Skeletal Radiol 1997;26:316–8.

72. Bansal M, Bhaliak V, Bruce CE. Obturator internus muscle abscess in a child: a case report. J Pediatr Orthop B 2008;17:223–4.

73. Chen WS, Wan YL. Iliacus pyomyositis mimicking septic arthritis of the hip joint. Arch Orthop Trauma Surg 1996;115:233–5.

74. Casetta I, Cesnik E, Fainardi E, et al. An unusual cause of a common symptom: pyomyositis presenting with sciatica. Joint Bone Spine 2009;76:427–8.

75. Abdullah ZS, Khan MU, Kodali SK, et al. Pyomyositis mimicking osteomyelitis detected by SPET/CT. Nucl Med 2010;13:277–9.

76. Walji S, Rubenstein J, Shannon P, et al. Disseminated pyomyositis mimicking idiopathic inflammatory myopathy. J Rheumatol 2005;32:184–7.

77. Park S, Shatsky JB, Pawel BR, et al. A traumatic compartment syndrome: a manifestation of toxic shock and infectious pyomyositis in a child. A case report. J Bone Joint Surg Am 2007;89:1337–42.

78. Colmegna I, Justiniano M, Espinoza LR, et al. Piriformis pyomyositis with sciatica: an unrecognized complication of "unsafe" abortions. J Clin Rheumatol 2007;13:87–8.

79. Immerman RP, Greenman RL. Toxic shock syndrome associated with pyomyositis caused by a strain of Staph aureus that does not produce toxic shock syndrome toxin. J Infect Dis 1987;156:505–7.

80. Gupta B, Khanna SK, Sharma BK. Pyomyositis. J Assoc Physicians India 1980;28:91–4.

81. Meena AK, Rajashekhar S, Reddy JJ, et al. Pyomyositis-clinical and MRI characteristics report of three cases. Neurol India 1999;47:324–6.

82. Gambhir IS, Singh DS, Gupta SS, et al. Tropical pyomyositis in India, a clinico-histopathological study. J Trop Med Hyg 1992;95:42–6.

83. Brown JD, Wheeler B. Pyomyositis: report of 18 cases in Hawaii. Arch Intern Med 1984;144:1749–51.

84. Trusen A, Beissert M, Schultz G, et al. Ultrasound and MRI features of pyomyositis in children. Eur Radiol 2003;13:1050–5.

85. Gordon BA, Martinez S, Collins AJ. Pyomyositis: characteristics at CT and MR imaging. Radiology 1995;197:279–86.

86. Theodorou SJ, Theodorou DJ, Resnick D. MR imaging findings of pyogenic bacterial myositis (pyomyositis) in patients with local muscle trauma: illustrative cases. Emerg Radiol 2007;14:89–96.

87. Karmazyn B, Loder RT, Kleiman MB, et al. The role of pelvic magnetic resonance in evaluating nonhip sources of infection in children with acute nontraumatic hip pain. J Pediatr Orthop 2007;27:158–64.

88. Schiff RG, Silver L. Tropical pyomyositis: demonstration of extent and distribution of disease by gallium scintigraphy. Clin Nucl Med 1990;15:542–4.

89. Robert L, Reresiewiscz, Parosenet J. Staphylococcal infections. In: Fauci AS, Braunwald E, Martin JB, et al, editors. 15th edition, Harrison's principles of internal medicine. New York: McGraw-Hill; 2001. p. 889–900.

90. Hudson IR. The efficacy of intranasal mupirocin in the prevention of staphylococcal infections: a review of recent experience. J Hosp Infect 1994;27:81–98.

Index

Note: Page numbers of article titles are in **boldface** type.

Neuroimag Clin N Am 21 (2011) 985–987
doi:10.1016/S1052-5149(11)00147-X
1052-5149/11/$ – see front matter © 2011 Elsevier Inc. All rights reserved.

United States Postal Service

Statement of Ownership, Management, and Circulation
(All Periodicals Publications Except Requestor Publications)

1. Publication Title	2. Publication Number	3. Filing Date
Neuroimaging Clinics of North America	0 1 0 - 5 4 8	9/16/11

4. Issue Frequency	5. Number of Issues Published Annually	6. Annual Subscription Price
Feb, May, Aug, Nov	4	$314.00

7. Complete Mailing Address of Known Office of Publication (*Not printer*) (*Street, city, county, state, and ZIP+4®*)

Elsevier Inc.
360 Park Avenue South
New York, NY 10010-1710

Contact Person
Amy S. Beacham

Telephone (Include area code)
215-239-3687

8. Complete Mailing Address of Headquarters or General Business Office of Publisher (*Not printer*)

Elsevier Inc. 360 Park Avenue South, New York, NY 10010-1710

9. Full Names and Complete Mailing Addresses of Publisher, Editor, and Managing Editor (*Do not leave blank*)

Publisher (*Name and complete mailing address*)

Kim Murphy, Elsevier, Inc., 1600 John F. Kennedy Blvd. Suite 1800, Philadelphia, PA 19103-2899

Editor (*Name and complete mailing address*)

Joanne Husovski, Elsevier, Inc., 1600 John F. Kennedy Blvd. Suite 1800, Philadelphia, PA 19103-2899

Managing Editor (*Name and complete mailing address*)

Barton Dudlick, Elsevier, Inc., 1600 John F. Kennedy Blvd. Suite 1800, Philadelphia, PA 19103-2899

10. Owner (*Do not leave blank. If the publication is owned by a corporation, give the name and address of the corporation immediately followed by the names and addresses of all stockholders owning or holding 1 percent or more of the total amount of stock. If not owned by a corporation, give the names and addresses of the individual owners. If owned by a partnership or other unincorporated firm, give its name and address as well as those of each individual owner. If the publication is published by a nonprofit organization, give its name and address.*)

Full Name	Complete Mailing Address
Wholly owned subsidiary of	4520 East-West Highway
Reed/Elsevier, US holdings	Bethesda, MD 20814

11. Known Bondholders, Mortgagees, and Other Security Holders Owning or Holding 1 Percent or More of Total Amount of Bonds, Mortgages, or Other Securities. If none, check box ☐ None

Full Name	Complete Mailing Address
N/A	

12. Tax Status (*For completion by nonprofit organizations authorized to mail at nonprofit rates*) (*Check one*)
The purpose, function, and nonprofit status of this organization and the exempt status for federal income tax purposes:
☐ Has Not Changed During Preceding 12 Months
☐ Has Changed During Preceding 12 Months (*Publisher must submit explanation of change with this statement*)

PS Form 3526, September 2007 (Page 1 of 3 (Instructions Page 3)) PSN 7530-01-000-9931 PRIVACY NOTICE: See our Privacy policy in www.usps.com

---

13. Publication Title	14. Issue Date for Circulation Data Below
Neuroimaging Clinics of North America	August 2011

15. Extent and Nature of Circulation		Average No. Copies Each Issue During Preceding 12 Months	No. Copies of Single Issue Published Nearest to Filing Date
a. Total Number of Copies (*Net press run*)		1958	1519
b. Paid Circulation (By Mail and Outside the Mail)	(1) Mailed Outside-County Paid Subscriptions Stated on PS Form 3541. (*Include paid distribution above nominal rate, advertiser's proof copies, and exchange copies*)	998	920
	(2) Mailed In-County Paid Subscriptions Stated on PS Form 3541 (*Include paid distribution above nominal rate, advertiser's proof copies, and exchange copies*)		
	(3) Paid Distribution Outside the Mails Including Sales Through Dealers and Carriers, Street Vendors, Counter Sales, and Other Paid Distribution Outside USPS®	284	252
	(4) Paid Distribution by Other Classes Mailed Through the USPS (e.g. First-Class Mail®)		
c. Total Paid Distribution (*Sum of 15b (1), (2), (3), and (4)*)	▶	1282	1172
d. Free or Nominal Rate Distribution (By Mail and Outside the Mail)	(1) Free or Nominal Rate Outside-County Copies Included on PS Form 3541	64	60
	(2) Free or Nominal Rate In-County Copies Included on PS Form 3541		
	(3) Free or Nominal Rate Copies Mailed at Other Classes Through the USPS (e.g. First-Class Mail)		
	(4) Free or Nominal Rate Distribution Outside the Mail (Carriers or other means)		
e. Total Free or Nominal Rate Distribution (Sum of 15d (1), (2), (3) and (4))	▶	64	60
f. Total Distribution (Sum of 15c and 15e)	▶	1346	1232
g. Copies not Distributed (See instructions to publishers #4 (page #3))	▶	612	287
h. Total (Sum of 15f and g)	▶	1958	1519
i. Percent Paid (15c divided by 15f times 100)		95.25%	95.13%

16. Publication of Statement of Ownership
☐ If the publication is a general publication, publication of this statement is required. Will be printed ☐ Publication not required
in the November 2011 issue of this publication.

17. Signature and Title of Editor, Publisher, Business Manager, or Owner

[signature]

Amy S. Beacham – Senior Inventory Distribution Coordinator

Date: September 16, 2011

I certify that all information furnished on this form is true and complete. I understand that anyone who furnishes false or misleading information on this form or who omits material or information requested on the form may be subject to criminal sanctions (including fines and imprisonment) and/or civil sanctions (including civil penalties).

PS Form 3526, September 2007 (Page 2 of 3)

Moving?

Make sure your subscription moves with you!

To notify us of your new address, find your **Clinics Account Number** (located on your mailing label above your name), and contact customer service at:

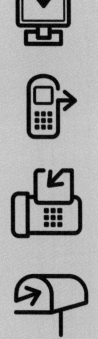

Email: journalscustomerservice-usa@elsevier.com

800-654-2452 (subscribers in the U.S. & Canada)
314-447-8871 (subscribers outside of the U.S. & Canada)

Fax number: 314-447-8029

Elsevier Health Sciences Division
Subscription Customer Service
3251 Riverport Lane
Maryland Heights, MO 63043

ELSEVIER

Printed and bound by CPI Group (UK) Ltd, Croydon, CR0 4YY

03/10/2024

01040356-0002